Multislice
Computed Tomography

A Practical Approach
To Clinical Protocols

Multislice Computed Tomography

A Practical Approach To Clinical Protocols

Editor

Paul M. Silverman, M.D.
Professor of Radiology
Chief, Section of Body Imaging
Gerald D. Dodd, Jr., Distinguished Chair in Diagnostic Imaging
Department of Radiology
University of Texas M.D. Anderson Cancer Center
Houston, Texas

Contributing Authors

Sanjeev Bhalla	Donna M. Moxley
James A. Brink	David P. Naidich
Dianna D. Cody	Rendon C. Nelson
William Davros	Geoffrey D. Rubin
Elliot K. Fishman	Ilona M. Schmalfuss
Anthony A. Mancuso	Marilyn J. Siegel
Georgeann McGuinness	Paul M. Silverman

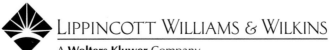

LIPPINCOTT WILLIAMS & WILKINS
A **Wolters Kluwer** Company
Philadelphia • Baltimore • New York • London
Buenos Aires • Hong Kong • Sydney • Tokyo

Acquisitions Editor: Beth Barry
Developmental Editor: Lisa Consoli
Production Editor: Penny Bice
Manufacturing Manager: Colin Warnock
Cover Designer: Diana Andrews
Compositor: Maryland Composition Co., Inc.
Printer: Maple Press

Library of Congress Cataloging-in-Publication Data

Multislice computed tomography : a practical approach to clinical protocols/[edited by] Paul M. Silverman,
     p. cm.
   Includes bibliographical references and index.
   ISBN 0-7817-3312-X (alk. paper)
     1. Tomography. I. Silverman, Paul M.

   RC78.7.T6 M85 2002b
   616.07′57—dc21   2002066078

---

10 9 8 7 6 5 4 3 2 1

To my family for their love and support
so that we might be able to pursue all our dreams together.
Special love to my wife Amy,
and to my children Zachary and Rebecca.

"Life is not a dress rehearsal"
Rose Tremain

Thoughts. . . .From Fly Fishing Through the Midlife Crisis

—Howell Raines

The art of fly-fishing is a distinct separation from the work that most of us do on a day-to-day basis. It is within this time of solitude that we can embrace nature and measure our accomplishments. . .

Of course, I am not the first person to discover in fly-fishing a framework for thinking about life. On its surface the analogy is obvious if we can discipline ourselves to cast a line with perfection, perhaps we can oppose order on–or perceive some inherit order within–the chaos of daily existence. What do we seek when we fish with the most fragile of rods in the most difficult water we can find?

–Hoover fly fishing while the country goes to hell, casting frantically, not understanding the frustration that churned within him and produced his lust for deeper pools, more fish, bigger fish. The President of the United States transformed himself into a follower of Redneck Way. I often wondered if he ever learned how deeply he erred with his stalking of these big, innocent hatchery trout. For he was already in the presence of a perfect thing, the Eastern Brook trout living as it lived while the centuries rolled over the earth living as it lived in those very waters before Christ, before Caesar, before the Pharaohs.

To embrace this knowledge in one's inmost heart is to depart from the Redneck Way and to know, that one's "fishing is not about food." It is a way of interrupting the invisibility of these shining creatures and existing for a moment with them in their wildness and transience, their indifference to our approval and their dependence on our restraint if they are to add another hour to their thousandth year.

Contents

Contributing Authors

Sanjeev Bhalla, M.D. *Instructor of Radiology, Co-Director Emergency Radiology, Assistant Residency Program Director (CT, MR, Emergency and Thoracic Imaging) Mallinckrodt Institute of Radiology, Washington University School of Medicine, 510 South Kingshighway, St. Louis, MO 63110*

James A. Brink, M.D. *Professor of Radiology, Vice Chairman, Clinical Affairs, Chief, Abdominal Imaging, Department of Radiology, Yale University School of Medicine, 333 Cedar Street, New Haven, Connecticut 06510*

Dianna D. Cody, Ph.D. *Associate Professor, Diagnostic Imaging Physics, University of Texas M.D. Anderson Cancer Center, Division of Diagnostic Imaging, 1515 Holcombe, Box 57, Houston, Texas 77030*

William Davros, Ph.D., ABMP(D) *Section Head, Diagnostic Clinical Medical Physics, Division of Radiology (L-10), The Cleveland Clinic Foundation, 9500 Euclid Avenue, Cleveland, Ohio 44195*

Elliot K. Fishman, M.D., *Department of Radiology, Johns Hopkins Hospital, 600 North Wolfe Street, Baltimore, Maryland 21287*

Anthony A. Mancuso, M.D. *Professor and Chairman, Department of Radiology, Professor of Otolaryngology, Staff Neuroradiologist, University of Florida, College of Medicine, P.O. Box 100327, JHMHC, Gainesville, Florida 32610*

Georgeann McGuinness, M.D. *Associate Professor of Radiology, Co-Director, Section of Thoracic Imaging, New York University Medical Center, Department of Radiology, 560 First Avenue, New York, NY 10016*

Donna M. Moxley, M.S., DABR, *Medical Physicist, University of Texas M.D. Anderson Cancer Center, Division of Diagnostic Imaging, 1515 Holcombe Blvd., Box 57, Houston, Texas 77030*

David P. Naidich, M.D. *Professor of Radiology, Director, Computed Tomography, Department of Radiology, Bellevue Hospital, 462 1st Avenue, New York, New York 10016*

Rendon C. Nelson, M.D. *Professor of Radiology, Director, Division of Abdominal Imaging, Duke University Medical Center, Box 3808, Durham, North Carolina 27710*

Geoffrey D. Rubin, M.D. *Assistant Professor of Radiology, Department of Radiology, Stanford University School of Medicine, 300 Pasteur Drive, Room S072B, Stanford, California 94305*

Ilona M. Schmalfuss, M.D. *Assistant Professor of Radiology, Division of Neuroradiology, Department of Radiology, University of Florida, College of Medicine, 1600 SW Archer Road, Gainesville, Florida 32610*

Marilyn J. Siegel, M.D. *Professor of Radiology and Pediatrics, Department of Radiology, Mallinckrodt Institute of Radiology, Washington University School of Medicine, 510 South Kingshighway Boulevard, St. Louis, Missouri 63110*

Paul M. Silverman, M.D. *Professor of Radiology, Chief, Section of Body Imaging, Gerald D. Dodd, Jr., Distinguished Chair in Diagnostic Imaging, Department of Radiology, University of Texas M.D. Anderson Cancer Center, 1515 Holcombe, Box 57, Houston, Texas 77030*

Preface

The recent introduction of multislice CT in the 1990s has had a profound impact on the utilization of CT scanning to solve diagnostic problems. The earlier introduction of helical (spiral) CT had a similar impact over conventional step and shoot CT when introduced in the 1980's by virtue of its ability to dramatically increase the speed of CT examinations. Multislice CT (MSCT), sometimes referred to as multi-detector or multi-detector–row CT, has had a similar, if not more pronounced clinical impact. With the wide dissemination of 4-slice helical units, the increase in speed over conventional helical CT is in the range of 4- to 6-fold. More recently, 8-, 16-, and even 32-slice units have further increased CT speed. The result is that patients are better able to tolerate examinations and the quality and flexibility of examinations is significantly broadened.

Multislice CT now provides for the ability to scan an organ in a single breath-hold. In the case of patients who are ill or have difficulty in holding their breath, as well as the pediatric and trauma population, these patients now are able to receive accurate examinations because of the faster scan times and the ability to perform the overall examination of the entire body in just minutes. This technology also allows new flexibility in scanning in multiple phases of contrast enhancement. In the liver this improves one's ability to detect hypervascular metastases that previously might have gone undetected or required more invasive techniques. In the area of pulmonary embolism, the ability to perform thinner section scans in the same or less time than conventional thicker slices has improved the detection of pulmonary emboli to the point of detection of not only segmental but also smaller branches. The increased speed also has provided the flexibility to allow one to scan the pelvis and legs to identify the presence of deep venous thrombosis.

Although three-dimensional (3-D) imaging had been performed with helical units, the use of MSCT scanners has now made 3-D imaging a routine application for enhancing the visibility of certain lesions and, most importantly, disseminating this information in a convincing fashion to our clinical colleagues. The clinical impact is most pronounced to surgeons, assisting them in making the best possible operative decisions. Three-dimensional vascular examinations now can be used in the staging of various tumors to determine resectability, as well as to evaluate vascular abnormalities such as aortic dissection. Three-dimensional exams can even be used in performing peripheral vascular "run-offs" because of the ability to stack numerous thin images without misregistration artifacts into a 3-D representation. The world of three-dimensional imaging now includes CT colonography, virtual endoscopy, and angioscopy. MSCT has also opened up the area of cardiac imaging as a reality.

Further technical improvements have already shown the ability for the major manufacturers to produce even faster scanners, which will lead to truly volumetric scanning acquisitions, likely within this decade.

This textbook contains seven distinct chapters. The seven areas covered include: *Principles of Multislice Computed Tomographic Technology, Multislice Computed Tomography of the Head and Neck, Multislice Computed Tomography of the Chest, Multislice Computed*

Tomography of the Abdomen and Pelvis, Multislice Computed Tomography in Pediatrics, Multislice Imaging of the Musculoskeletal System, and Multislice Imaging for Three-Dimensional Examinations. Each chapter has a text component followed by numerous references. The chapters related to specific organ systems have separate sections with generically constructed protocols that can be used by radiologists regardless of the type of multislice scanner purchased. The organization of the protocols is such that they lend themselves to ready application in the clinical environment. The book follows the format of its successful predecessor *Helical (Spiral) Computed Tomography: A Practical Approach to Clinical Protocols*, but now brings the reader into the new world of multislice technology.

The organization of protocols includes information all the major parameters needed to perform high quality multislice examinations including: *Indications, Scanner settings, oral contrast, phase of respiration, rotation time, acquisition slice thickness, pitch, reconstruction slice thickness/interval for filming, superior and inferior extent of anatomic coverage, IV contrast protocols (concentration, rate, scan delays, total volume)* and a *comments section including "pearls"* related to multislice imaging. For purposes of making this book user-friendly and generic in nature certain formats have been adopted. Example, a pitch of 0.75 is listed as 0.75 (HQ=3:1) and a pitch of 1.5 as 1.5 (HS=6:1). A thorough discussion of this is found in the introductory chapter on ***Principles of Multislice Computed Tomographic Technology***. In the case where there are vendor specific differences, General Electric CT scanner nomenclature is provided within parenthesis (i.e. HQ=3:1). We have elected to use the terminology in parentheses that corresponds to a 4-slice scanner. Generic pitch can be arrived at with any slice GE scanner (4-slice, 8-slice, etc.) by dividing the GE pitch by 4, 8, etc. In the chapter ***Multislice Computed Tomography in Pediatrics***, additional information is given regarding: *sedation, contrast administration rates, catheter size,* and *dose of oral contrast.* In the chapter, ***Multislice Computed Tomography of the Chest*** additional information provided for *reconstruction algorithms*, and in the chapter ***Multislice Imaging for Three-Dimensional Examinations*** detailed information is provided to allow the reader to generate the highest quality 3-D images.

It is my hope and firm belief that this book will serve as a foundation for radiologists to use as a practical guide for clinical protocols when employing multislice CT (MSCT). Readers should feel free to apply these protocols and refine them for their own distinct clinical practices.

Paul M. Silverman, M.D.

Acknowledgments

I would like to take this opportunity to personally thank all of my colleagues at the University of Texas, M.D. Anderson Cancer Center for their support during the preparation of this textbook. Their commitment and dedication to patient care is unsurpassed in my clinical career in radiology. The Body Imaging Section, now numbering 23 faculty, with their unique dedication to the field of oncologic radiology, and our clinical colleagues, continue to challenge each one of us to be better each and every day providing the highest level of care to our patients.

I also wish to thank my colleagues in the Society of Computed Body Tomography and Magnetic Resonance (SCBT/MR) whose dedication to advancing this field is foremost in the mission statement of this society. I acknowledge the major vendors of CT equipment for the information provided regarding the technical aspects of scanning, particularly General Electric Medical Systems, Siemens Medical Systems, Philips Medical Systems, Elscint Medical Systems, and Toshiba Medical Systems. Despite the underlying competitive aspects of their business, my experience with the directors of CT operations from each of these companies has always been one of full commitment to the advancement of the radiology, providing the best diagnostic tools to radiologists. I applaud them for their diligence. I would also like to thank Ryan Hennan from Vital Images (Plymouth, Minnesota) for his assistance with material for the cover. Special recognition to my Administrative Assistants, Charlotte A. Burrell and Brenda J. Sommerville, for their invaluable assistance in editing and compiling the materials necessary to make this textbook a success. Finally, I would like to thank all my co-authors.

1

Principles Of Multislice Computed Tomographic Technology

Dianna D. Cody*, Donna M. Moxley*, William Davros**,
and Paul M. Silverman***

*Division of Diagnostic Imaging, University of Texas M. D. Anderson Cancer Center,
Houston, Texas 77030
**Diagnostic Clinical Medical Physics Division of Radiology, The Cleveland Clinic
Foundation, Cleveland, Ohio 44195
***Department of Radiology, Section of Body Imaging, Gerald D. Dodd, Jr.
Distinguished Chair Diagnostic Imaging, and the Department of Radiology,
University of Texas M. D. Anderson Cancer Center, Houston, Texas 77030

Since the introduction of multislice helical computed tomographic (MSCT) scanners in 1998, this technology has achieved widespread clinical acceptance across the country and around the world. The ability to acquire four or more images with each rotation of the computed tomography (CT) gantry has made a significant impact in patient throughput, particularly when combined with high-heat-capacity x-ray tubes. The frequently heard marketing promise of nonstop CT scanning with no more delays for x-ray tubes to cool has finally arrived in busy clinical radiology departments.

Clinical applications that have experienced the most improvement with this technology are those in which the data-acquisition time factor is critical. This new technology is also referred to as multidetector or multirow or multidetector-multirow CT; we will use the term multislice CT (MSCT) to reflect the outcome, rather than the scanner design. This new technology can decrease examination times by as much as eightfold. Fields such as trauma, pediatrics, and chest imaging have enjoyed particular success with the use of this technology. Vascular studies have also benefited from the fast image-acquisition rates (1). Triple-phase protocols are now routinely available to more thoroughly evaluate liver lesions with the advent of MSCT scanners (2). Coronal imaging, important for head and neck exams, can now be achieved with routine reformatting using MSCT systems (3).

The most striking difference between the single-slice helical technology and the MSCT system design is the configuration of the radiation detectors. In the past, these detectors were long and narrow, with the length of a single detector element aligned in the z-axis direction (Tables 1 and 2; Fig. 1). This geometry allowed the collimation of the x-ray beam to create images of varying slice thickness, all using the same set of detectors. MSCT technology has incorporated a detector array that is segmented in the z-axis direction, forming a mosaic of elements in the detector assembly. This physical separation of detector elements allows for simultaneous acquisition of multiple images in the scan plane with one rotation of the x-ray tube about the patient (Fig. 2).

MSCT systems also offer flexible image-reconstruction options. Single-slice helical CT (SSCT) has the ability to reconstruct images of the same thickness but with different image

TABLE 1. *Reconstruction options for General Electric lightspeed platform and Siemens*

Detector configuration	Image thickness choices (mm)	Table speed per rotation (mm/rotation)
A. General Electric Lightspeed		
4 × 1.25 mm	1.25, 2.5	3.75 or 7.5
4 × 2.5 mm	2.5, 3.75, 5.0	7.5 or 15
4 × 3.75 mm	3.75, 5.0, 7.5	11.25
4 × 3.75 mm	5.0, 7.5	22.5
4 × 5 mm	5.0, 7.5, 10.0	15 or 30
B. Siemens		
2 × 0.5 mm	0.5, 0.75, 1.0, 1.25, 2	Variable from 0 to 2
4 × 1.0 mm	1.0, 1.25, 1.5, 2, 3, 4, 5	Variable from 0 to 8
4 × 2.5 mm	3, 4, 5, 6, 7, 8, 10	Variable from 0 to 20
4 × 5.0 mm	6, 7, 8, 10	Variable from 0 to 40

indexing (table-increment intervals). MSCT scanners by their nature acquire three-dimensional (3D) raw projection data that are contiguous in space. It is therefore possible to use these projection data to reconstruct images at various image thicknesses and at different intervals along the z-axis. For example, four images per gantry rotation can be acquired with the total z-axis detector dimension being 20 mm (four rows by 5 mm). These data can then

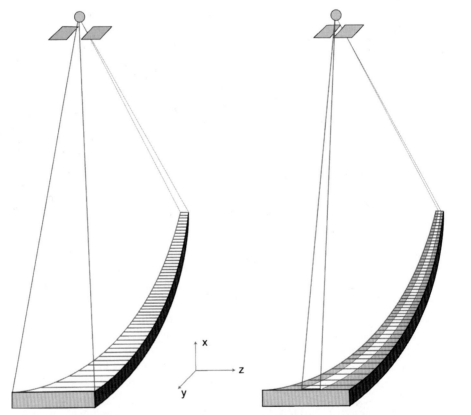

FIG. 1. These illustrations depict the detector configuration in conventional single-slice computed tomographic systems. The slice width is controlled by the pre–patient collimation assembly, which is open to the full slice width **(left)** and pinched to a narrower image thickness **(right)**.

TABLE 2. *Examples of General Electric collimator settings, image width, and images per rotation, as well as table travel with 0.75 (HQ = 3.0) and 1.5 (HS = 6.0) pitches*

Collimator (mm)	Number of images per rotation	Image thickness (mm)	0.75 (HQ = 3.0) table travel (mm)	1.5 (HS = 6.0) table travel (mm)
20	4	5	15	30
	2	10		
15	4	3.75	N/A	22.5
	2	7.5	11.25	
10	4	2.5	7.5	15
	2	5		
	1	10		
5	4	1.25	3.75	7.5
	2	2.5		
	1	5		

be used to create images that are 5 mm or greater in thickness. This reconstruction process requires that the scan profile files, or "raw data" files, be available, so in general this must be conducted at or very shortly after the scan-acquisition session is complete. The distance between image centers (image index) can also vary. If the image index is thinner than the image thickness, the images are said to overlap. The ability to create overlapping images without overlapping radiation fields is one of the strong points of all helical scanning. Overlapping images have been shown to increase diagnostic sensitivity and improve the quality of multiplanar and 3D display views (4). This option can allow even busy clinical radiology

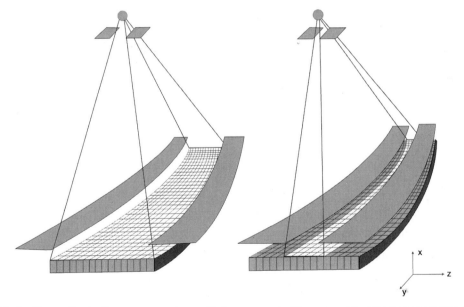

FIG. 2. These illustrations represent a multislice computed tomographic detector geometry. In this case, the slice thickness is determined by a combination of the x-ray beam width (controlled by the pre–patient collimation assembly) and the detector configuration (controlled in some designs by the post–patient collimation assembly). The **(left)** full bank of detectors is set to measure x-ray photons, and **(right)** the collimators are repositioned to accommodate a reduced number of detectors.

areas to quickly provide improved image data for postprocessing activities, such as multi-planar reformat and 3D display (5).

DETECTOR DESIGN AND TERMINOLOGY

The different CT manufacturers have developed various detector configurations, mosaic (General Electric [GE]), adaptive (Siemens, Marconi) and hybrid (Toshiba) (6,7). The available choices of slice thickness and table speed thus vary considerably from one system to the next (Fig. 3). For example, the GE system has detectors with 16 elements of equal size in the z-axis direction, four output channels, and a maximum nominal collimator width of 20 mm (Fig. 4A). Therefore, one, two, or four images can be acquired per tube rotation. If the collimator is set at 20 mm, either two images at 10 mm each or four images at 5 mm each can be acquired. However, images smaller than 5 mm cannot be retrospectively reconstructed using this detector configuration. If the collimator is set at 10 mm, the operator can acquire four images at 2.5 mm each, two images at 5 mm each, or one image at 10 mm and have the ability to reconstruct images as thin as 2.5 mm. The corresponding choices for acquisition parameters are shown in Fig. 4B for Siemens and Philips type MSCT scanners. Toshiba, Siemens, and Philips have implemented an arrangement of detectors of varying size, which can be combined to produce a different pattern of slice thickness options. The available slice thickness choices for acquisition and the resulting available slice thickness options for reconstruction are shown for each vendor in Tables 1 and 2.

The main concept to remember is that the thinnest slice thickness that can be reconstructed depends entirely on the combination of slice thickness and table speed used during an examination. Detector elements are often "binned," or added together, to create thicker images. This operation allows very rapid scanning over relatively long distances. However, when the signals that emerge from individual detectors are combined during the acquisition process, they cannot be subsequently separated to form images thinner than this acquisition setting. If thinner images are desired, this must be fully planned before the image-acquisition process.

DEFINITION OF PITCH

Unfortunately, some CT scanner vendors have developed specific nomenclature for key MSCT concepts. The definition of pitch in particular varies with the manufacturer of MSCT scanners. For SSCT, pitch is defined as follows:

pitch (SSCT) = table travel per x-ray tube rotation ÷ image thickness

For example, if the table travel in one x-ray tube rotation is set at 7.5 mm and the image thickness setting is at 5 mm, then

7.5-mm table travel in one rotation ÷ 5-mm slice thickness = 1.5 : 1 or 1.5 pitch.

In MSCT, the slice thickness parameter can mean several different things, depending on what perspective one chooses. We prefer the definition put forward by McCollough and Zink (8), in which pitch is defined as follows:

pitch (MSCT) = table travel per x-ray tube rotation

÷ total active detector width (or x-ray beam collimation)

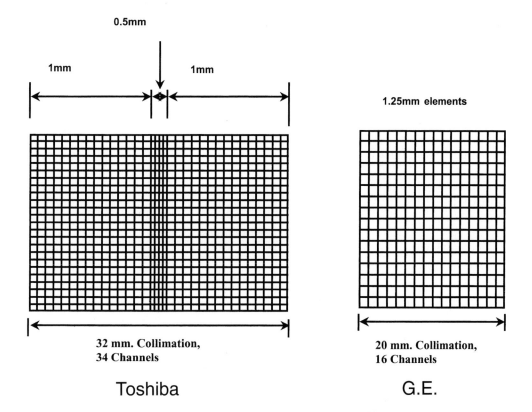

0.5mm

1mm   1mm

32 mm. Collimation,
34 Channels

Toshiba

1.25mm elements

20 mm. Collimation,
16 Channels

G.E.

FIG. 3. The different computed tomographic (CT) scanner vendors have incorporated distinct detector designs for 4 slice. Toshiba **(left)** has implemented a pattern of four rows of small detectors (0.5 mm) surrounded by 15 rows of larger detectors (1 mm). General Electric Medical Systems **(upper right)** has chosen a mosaic of detector elements of all the same size (1.25 mm). Elscint, Siemens, and Philips **(lower right)** all share a common detector pattern, in which two rows of small detectors (1 mm) are surrounded by two rows of slightly larger detectors (1.5 mm), which are surrounded by two more rows of slightly larger detectors (2.5 mm), which are finally surrounded by two more rows of larger detectors (5 mm). In all three designs, the final image slice thickness is defined by both the pattern of detectors used to acquire the projection data and the image reconstruction choice programmed by the operator. These diagrams are related to 4-slice but can be extrapolated to 8-slice, 16-slice, and future developments.

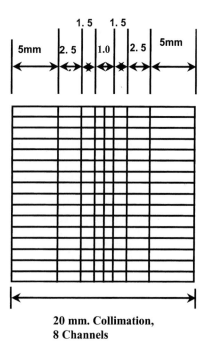

1.5   1.5

5mm   2.5   1.0   2.5   5mm

20 mm. Collimation,
8 Channels

Elscint/Siemens/Philips

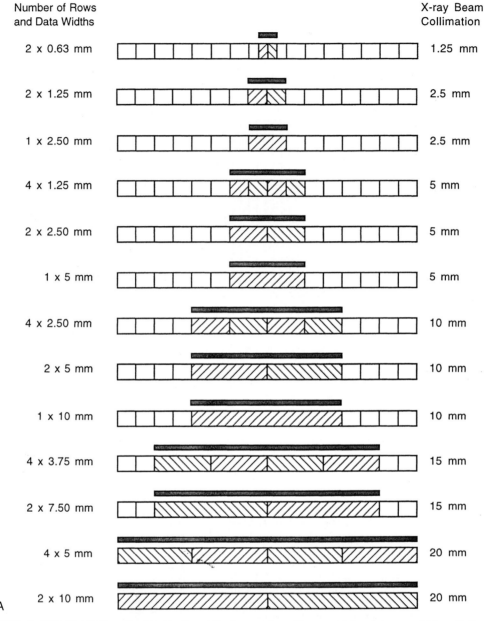

FIG. 4. This illustration represents the detector configuration used for data acquisition **(left-hand column)**, the x-ray beam width (*shaded bar* and **right-hand column**), and the active detectors **(cross-hatched regions)**. **A:** The many options available on the General Electric multislice computed Philips MSCT. **B:** The options available on the Elscient Siemens/Philips type MSCT scanners.

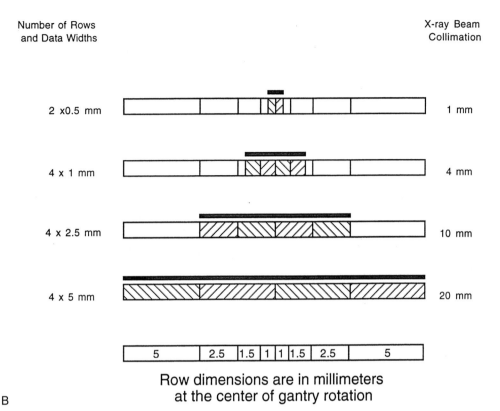

Number of Rows
and Data Widths

X-ray Beam
Collimation

2 x0.5 mm — 1 mm

4 x 1 mm — 4 mm

4 x 2.5 mm — 10 mm

4 x 5 mm — 20 mm

| 5 | 2.5 | 1.5 | 1 | 1 | 1.5 | 2.5 | 5 |

Row dimensions are in millimeters
at the center of gantry rotation

B

FIG. 4. *Continued.*

For example, if the table travel in one x-ray tube rotation is again set at 7.5 mm, and the technologist has requested that four images, each 2.5 mm in thickness, be acquired in each revolution of the x-ray tube, then

7.5-mm table travel in one rotation

$$\div\ (4 \times 2.5\ \text{mm} = 10\text{-mm detector width}) = 0.75 : 1\ \text{or } 0.75\ \text{pitch.}$$

Another way to express the denominator is the overall collimation of the x-ray tube during the scan acquisition. This can always be found by multiplying the number of images to be obtained by the thickness of each image. One manufacturer, GE, has marketed an MSCT scanner that has the unique property of forming images with particularly good image quality at specific pitch values (Fig. 5). Two values of pitch resulted in optimal image quality, so GE has selected two discrete pitch choices instead of a continuous variable pitch parameter on its MSCT units. The two possible pitches are called "high quality" (HQ) and "high speed" (HS). The HQ mode corresponds to a pitch of 0.75 and the HS mode corresponds to a pitch of 1.5, using the definition shown above. We have elected to use this nomenclature in the "Protocol" sections of each chapter with parenthesis indicating that this information is specific to GE equipment—for example, pitch 0.75 (HQ = 3 : 1) and pitch 1.5 (HS = 6 : 1). Additionally, when slice thicknesses are used that can only be achieved by one vendor and not the other, the GE slice thickness is placed in parenthesis—for example, 1 mm (1.25 mm).

GE has chosen to define pitch differently: pitch = table travel per x-ray tube rotation ÷ a single image slice thickness. Thus, in GE terminology, HQ mode corresponds to an image

Helical Pitch and Image Quality

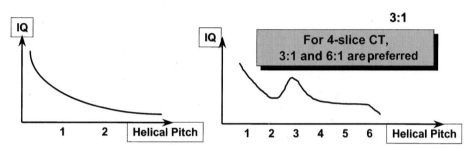

Single Slice CT (SSCT):

IQ deteriorates monotonically as helical pitch increases.

Multi-slice CT (MSCT):

In multi-slice helical CT, certain helical pitches are preferred for optimum IQ.*

FIG. 5. In single-slice conventional computed tomography (CT), image quality in general diminishes as pitch is increased **(left)**. In multislice CT (MSCT), image quality does not change in the same manner, and there are peaks and valleys in the image quality versus pitch plot **(right)**. The location of these peaks represents the high-quality (pitch = 0.75) and high-speed (pitch = 1.5) modes of scanning on the *General Electric Medical Systems scanners.

pitch of 3 : 1 (when four images are acquired per tube rotation, the associated table travel is three times the image width), and HS mode corresponds to an image pitch of 6 : 1 (when four images are acquired per tube rotation, the associated table travel is six times the image width). In terms of the more traditional definition of pitch based on collimation, the HQ mode corresponds to a collimator pitch of 0.75 : 1, and the HS mode corresponds to a collimator pitch of 1.5 : 1. This issue has been examined in more detail elsewhere (9).

Table 2 gives some basic examples of collimator settings, image widths, and the table travel associated with HQ and HS pitches. The expression we will use is pitch = 0.75 (HQ = 3 : 1) or pitch = 1.5 (HS = 6 : 1) (Table 2).

X-RAY AND HEAT PRODUCTION

The concepts of focal spot tracking and "flying focal spot" can best be understood in the context of x-ray production within an x-ray tube. In modern x-ray tubes, an electric current is passed through a tungsten filament, causing the filament to increase in temperature. The heating of the filament causes thermionic emission of electrons into a cloud about the filament. The free electrons are accelerated across the evacuated x-ray tube by placing a large voltage (potential) across the cathode and anode. A massive rotating disk made of a conductive alloy onto which a tungsten focal track is inlaid acts as the anode, or positive electrode. The filament acts as the cathode, or negative electrode. These free electrons, being of like charge, tend to repel each other and therefore tend to diverge as they drift away from the filament. To counteract this mutual repulsion, electrostatic focusing is executed via a focusing cup, into which the filament is recessed. The potential applied to the focusing cup is more negative than the filament, forcing the electrons to converge onto a small area of the anode and form the focal spot.

Typical potentials or voltages used in CT range from 80 to 140 kilovolt peak (kVp), causing the free electrons to accelerate rapidly across the vacuum and collide with the tungsten focal track. Approximately 99% of the electron interactions with the anode will produce heat while about 1% will produce x-rays. One mechanism of interaction is electrodynamic braking of high-speed electrons by the nuclei of the tungsten atoms. The electrons are slowed and their trajectories are bent when they pass near a positively charged nucleus, causing release of some of their kinetic energy in the form of photons of varying energies ranging from infrared radiation to x-rays, depending on the magnitude of the force exerted on the electron. When the magnitude of the retarding force is large, x-rays are produced. These x-rays are known as "bremsstrahlung" (or "braking") radiation. At intermediate magnitudes, lower energy photons are produced ranging from ultraviolet down to red. At still lower magnitudes, the vast majority of photons produced are infrared, thereby causing local heating of the focal track and bulk heating of the anode disk. Another mechanism of interaction is electron–electron collisions. Sometimes, an incoming electron will knock another electron from an inner shell of the tungsten atom, leaving a vacancy. This vacancy will be filled by an electron from another shell farther from the nucleus of the atom. Outer shell electrons have more energy than inner shell electrons, and the excess energy resulting from this movement has a discrete value. X-rays arising from this mechanism are known as characteristic radiation and compose a small fraction of the x-ray spectrum emitted from the anode.

The x-rays formed in the anode of an x-ray tube are emitted in all directions. However, we typically wish to use only those x-rays emitted in a particular direction and exclude the remainder of the x-rays. Therefore, the tube is surrounded by a housing, which absorbs unwanted radiation and contains a port through which the useful portion of the x-ray emission is permitted to pass and is further shaped with the use of a collimator assembly. In CT, the beam is very narrow in the z-axis direction (the direction of table travel), so the collimators must be properly positioned between the focal spot and the detector array.

Heating of the anode causes thermal expansion of the disk, resulting in slight changes in its shape. This expansion and deformation causes the focal spot to drift relative to the collimator assembly and the fixed x-ray detectors mounted across the gantry from the x-ray tube. This drift of the focal spot must be corrected to produce high quality images. GE has developed a focal spot tracking algorithm, which corrects for the drift resulting from thermal expansion of the anode by moving the collimator assembly, resulting in realignment of the beam with the detectors. With the use of such a correction algorithm, the beam can be more tightly collimated to the active detector elements in MSCT, which also reduces the radiation dose associated with a given set of scan parameters.

FLYING FOCAL SPOT

"Flying focal spot" is a technique used by one manufacturer to increase the number of unique views through an object. As seen in Fig. 6, at a single position of the x-ray tube and detector, the CT scanner acquires a fan-shaped series of projection lines of data. One projection line of data is the signal received by a single detector element, and it corresponds to the total attenuation suffered by the x-ray beam along the path from the focal spot to the detector element in question. Along the direction of the detector arc, some scanners have as many as 800 detector elements. For a single focal spot location on the anode, a detector of this type would be able to collect 800 projection lines of data per gantry position. The "flying focal spot" concept doubles the number of projection lines per gantry position by using electrodynamic lenses

A B

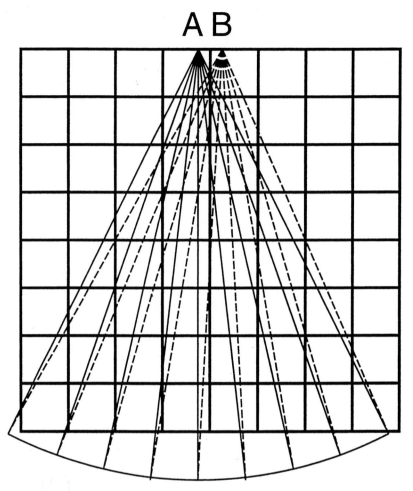

FIG. 6. X-rays emanate from two locations *(A, B)* on the anode disk. Each location gives rise to a unique set of x-ray projection lines through the scanned object (*solid and dashed rays*).

in the x-ray tube to steer the electron beam onto a new location on the anode. This new location then constitutes a new starting point for a second set of 800 projection lines of data. In Fig. 6, the first set of projection lines are labeled "A," and the second set of projection lines are labeled "B." Each set of projection lines traverses the object along slightly different paths, thus giving the reconstruction algorithm a more complete understanding of the internal structure of the object. It is important to note that the movement of the focal spot in this "flying focal spot" technique occurs within the image plane (x–y plane), whereas the focal spot tracking corrects for unwanted motion in the z-axis direction. Another point that must be made is that focal spot tracking can be done in conjunction with the "flying focal spot" technique.

DOSE

It has been generally recognized that the specific drawback of implementing a MSCT scanner is the increase in radiation exposure delivered to the patient (8,10,11). There are many reasons why the dose is higher when using a MSCT scanner compared with an otherwise equivalent conventional SSCT scanner. When deploying a detector pattern with multiple elements in the z-axis, it is necessary that the radiation be uniform over all of the detectors that are active for any given acquisition (7). Thus, the penumbra of the radiation beam must fall outside of the active detector elements (Fig. 7). Although sophisticated focal spot tracking systems have improved this overshoot significantly, some spillover may always be necessary in these scanners.

Smaller detectors, which improve spatial resolution, require a higher dose to maintain a given signal to noise ratio (SNR). Due to the smaller size of the individual segments, the milliamperes per rotation must be increased to maintain a given SNR. Also, due to the gaps between the segments of the detector separating detector elements into different cells, the overall absorption efficiency of the detector is reduced, resulting in a higher noise content in the image; therefore, the milliamperes per rotation must be increased to compensate for the reduction in efficiency.

Another common reason for an increase in patient dose is that the distance from the x-ray tube to the detector is often decreased, which causes an increase in radiation exposure due to the inverse square law.

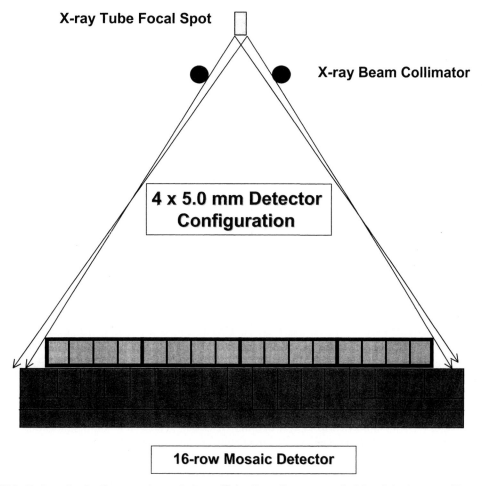

X-ray Tube Focal Spot

X-ray Beam Collimator

4 x 5.0 mm Detector Configuration

16-row Mosaic Detector

FIG. 7. In order for the x-ray beam to be sufficiently uniform over all of the detectors used in an acquisition, the x-ray beam (*arrows*) must overshoot the detector edges. The proportion of overshoot varies with the number of detectors activated. When using a large number of active detectors, the proportion of extra radiation to the beam collimation width is the smallest. The relative proportion of the overshoot is largest when using the fewest detectors, for example, four rows by 1.25 mm for this detector design. The above figure is an example for a 4-slice machine but may be extrapoled for 8-slice and 16-slice machines.

TABLE 3. *Factors affecting computed tomography dose*

Beam geometry	Operating parameters
Focal-spot size	kV(p)
Pre–patient collimation	mA
Source to detector distance	Time per rotation
Detector size	Filtration
Absorption efficiency of detectors	Rotation angle
Geometric efficiency of detectors	Scan-field size
Penumbra	Collimation
Post–patient collimation	Slice thickness and spacing
Scanner generation	Number of adjacent slices
Shape of attenuating filters	Imaging parameters (change milliamperes with pixel size or convolution filter)
Beam quality	Special scan techniques

Many factors associated with beam geometry and operating parameters that affect the CT dose are listed in Table 3. Some aspects of the beam geometry of MSCT scanners are different from those of otherwise comparable SSCT scanners. Although the manufacturers control the factors associated with beam geometry, several of the operating parameters (primarily the milliamperes per rotation, detector configuration, collimator setting, and pitch) can be manipulated by the user to reduce the dose while maintaining adequate image quality.

The conceptualization of dose in CT can be somewhat counterintuitive. If an abdomen scan produces a skin dose of 2 rad for one slice, it produces a skin dose of 2 rad over the length of the scan regardless of the number of slices. Dose is the energy absorbed in a medium per unit mass of the medium. This is the same as the concept of a concentration of a material. For example, if 10 mL of 5% saline was poured into a jar and 90 mL of 5% saline was added to it, the *concentration* of the saline remains at 5% with the increase in volume. Therefore, although additional contiguous slices in CT do not alter the measured dose to the patient, they do alter the biological effect by subjecting a larger volume of tissue to that dose.

Historically, the image thickness and the collimator settings have been directly related to each another. Therefore, the habit has been developed of associating the dose with a particular image thickness. With the advent of multiple image acquisitions for each tube rotation, it is necessary to associate the dose with a particular collimator setting and pitch, rather than with a particular image thickness. For a given pitch, narrower collimator settings will produce a higher dose than wider collimator settings (if kVp and mAs are held constant) due to the greater percentage of beam overlap arising from the greater number of rotations of the tube to cover the same length on the patient. For example, 20 contiguous images that are reconstructed at 5 mm thick can be acquired with three different detector configurations: (a) four simultaneous images of 1.25 mm, resulting in a collimator setting of 5 mm and 20 tube rotations; (b) four simultaneous images at 2.5 mm, resulting in a 10-mm collimator setting and 10 tube rotations; or (c) four simultaneous images at 5 mm, resulting in a 20-mm collimator setting and 5 tube rotations. The final images are all 5 mm; however, the dose for the 5-mm collimator setting will be much higher than that for the 20-mm collimator setting for a given pitch. Therefore, in MSCT, dose *cannot* be associated with image thickness; it *must* be associated with the collimator setting and pitch (as well as kVp and mAs per rotation).

There are several parameters used to describe the dose and/or potential for biological effects in the patient. The CT dose index (CTDI) accounts for the dose from the primary beam plus the scatter contribution from adjacent slices to a distance of seven times the slice thickness (collimator setting) in each direction from the center of the scan plane. This is determined from thermoluminescent dosimeters (TLDs) placed along the central axis of the phantom and is exceedingly tedious, expensive, and subject to error. A related descriptor of CT dose, and one that is much easier to acquire, is the $CTDI_{100}$. This notation is used to indicate that the estimate of CTDI was acquired in a phantom using a pencil-shaped ionization chamber with an active length of 100 mm. The 100-mm chamber length can only collect exposure data for the primary and scatter radiation over a distance of ± 5 cm from the center of the scan plane, resulting in an underestimate of the CTDI for collimator settings larger than 7 mm.

The CTDI represents the dose to the central plane of a cylindrical volume composed of 14 slices, with 7 on either side of the central plane. In reality, there is less scatter contribution at the beginning and end of the scanned volume. The multiple scan average dose (MSAD) is the average dose over the central slice of an examination consisting of multiple slices. (The term "slice" is used in this discussion to represent the collimator setting.) In axial mode, the MSAD is defined as

$$MSAD = (T/I) * CTDI,$$

where T is the slice thickness (collimator setting) and I is the table increment between scans. Therefore, in axial scans, the MSAD accounts for the effects of slice overlap or the presence of a gap between slices. In helical mode, the MSAD is defined as

$$MSAD = (1/pitch) * CTDI,$$

where pitch is defined as the table travel per rotation divided by the collimator setting. The MSAD is generally reported as the "patient dose" and overestimates the dose to the areas at the beginning and end of the scan volume. For contiguous slices less than 7 mm, the MSAD equals the CTDI.

A term for expression of patient CT dose, required in Europe and gaining acceptance in the United States, is the dose length product (DLP):

$$DLP = (MSAD) * (slice\ width\ in\ cm) * (number\ of\ slices\ in\ the\ scan\ volume)$$

Again, the term "slice" refers to the collimator setting and not to the image thickness. The DLP is based on the concept of dose to the scanned volume but also gives an indication of the relative biological risk associated with different detector configuration, pitch, and length of scan volume. For example, an abdomen scan produces a dose of 2 rad to the skin whether the number of slices is 1, 5, or 20, and so on. However, for a 1-cm slice width (10-mm collimator setting, regardless of the number of reconstructed images), one slice produces a DLP of 2 rad-cm, five contiguous slices will produce a DLP of 10 rad-cm, and twenty slices will produce a DLP of 40 rad-cm.

The DLP and the MSAD are concepts based on the definition of CTDI. The CTDI, in turn, is defined for a measurement performed in a cylindrical phantom of uniform acrylic, with dimensions of 32-cm diameter by 16-cm depth for body scan protocols, and 16-cm diameter by 14-cm depth for head scan protocols. For the body phantom, the central axis dose is usually approximately half the dose at 1 cm below the surface, whereas the dose distribution for the head phantom is fairly uniform. In reality, the patient is constructed quite differently, having a typically ellipsoid shape filled with organs of varying density. Therefore, the CTDI should be used as an *index* of dose for purposes of comparing various protocols on a given scanner or a given protocol on different scanner types, rather than representing the actual dose to the patient. To illustrate this point, consider the example used previously of the abdomen scan protocol that results in a surface dose of 2 rad to the body phantom. For the phantom, the central axis dose will be about 1 rad. For a large patient having a roughly circular cross section with a diameter larger than 32 cm, the skin dose will be higher and the central dose lower than that of the phantom.

For the more slender patient with the elliptical cross section and a width no greater than 32 cm, the skin dose will be lower and the central dose higher than the phantom. The presence of bones, fat, air, and internal organs results in uneven attenuation of the x-ray beam and a resulting nonuniform distribution of dose within the patient. Therefore, one must remember that the terms CTDI, MSAD, and DLP represent an index of dose in a standard phantom.

PEDIATRIC APPLICATIONS

The increase in image acquisition speed associated with the implementation of MSCT systems has had particularly strong benefits for pediatric CT scanning. Probably the most advantageous benefit to applying MSCT scanners to pediatric cases is the decrease in patient motion, which can eliminate the need for sedation in almost all children (12,13). This has enormous benefits for these patients, their families, and their clinic visit logistical pathway. In addition, a single injection of intravenous (IV) contrast can be used for all anatomic locations: head and neck, as well as chest, abdomen, and pelvis (13). Optimizing split injections is no longer necessary for these small patients. At the University of Texas M. D. Anderson Cancer Center, pediatric technique factors (kVp and mAs) for MSCT are based primarily on the field-of-view (FOV) parameter. This allows a more consistent application of technique and avoids the pitfalls associated with age or height- and weight-based factors. (We have found that the variability of body size and body shape in our pediatric population confounds attempts at standardizing protocols when based on age, height, or weight.) As long as the FOV is increased appropriately as the child grows, using this parameter to set the technique factors should provide for adequate and fairly consistent image quality in pediatric populations.

Another application for MSCT scanners in pediatric settings is the acquisition of relatively thin CT images at very low milliamperes (such as around 40 mA), reconstructed into thicker more routine images. This approach can be implemented to limit radiation dose substantially and produce images of excellent image quality.

Although there is an increase in radiation dose associated with the use of MSCT systems compared with SSCT, the quality and consistency of the images acquired with MSCT scanners has vastly decreased the number of images requiring a second exposure (retakes). Overall, the trade-off for radiation dose, sedation, and image quality easily justifies this application.

AUTOMATED SCAN-ASSIST FEATURES

MSCT scanners come equipped with a variety of scan-assist features. Most units have optional features that permit the monitoring of an anatomic structure such as the aorta for the presence of iodinated contrast medium. When a desired level of iodine enhancement has been reached, the scanner will start a spiral run. One vendor calls this feature CARE Bolus (Siemens); another calls it SmartPrep (GE), and these are referred to in the literature under the generic term computer-automated scan technology. Issues for the prospective buyer to be mindful of are the delay between the level of enhancement desired and the onset of scanning. This time should be as short as possible. Current scanners can do this procedure in as little a few seconds, somewhat more if the detection slice is at a different z-axis location than the start location of the exam.

PITCH AND IMAGE QUALITY

The advent of MSCT scanning has reopened the issues of how pitch affects image-quality parameters such as noise, in-plane contrast, and spatial resolution, as well as z-axis contrast and spatial resolution. The issue of noise as pitch increases has not changed from single-row spiral CT scanning to multirow CT scanning. The reason for this is that the underlying physics and mathematics of cross-sectional image reconstruction have not changed. The mathematics of cross-sectional image reconstruction dictate that to build an image, projections must be collected over 180 degrees of gantry rotation plus the fan angle of the x-ray beam (in most cases, the fan angle is about 45 degrees) or about 225 degrees of projection data.

Image noise is the random speckling seen in an image of a known uniform object such as water phantom. It is measured by calculating the standard deviation from a population of pixels within a region of interest (ROI). This random speckling has its roots in the statistical fluctuations in the number of x-rays that strike a detector per unit time, as well as the electronic noise in the detector system. It was stated earlier that reconstruction algorithms need a fixed number of projections to reconstruct an image. Pitch affects how these projections are distributed in the spiral pattern of x-ray delivery about the patient; pitch does not affect the number of projections used in the reconstruction algorithm. A potentially helpful way to understand the effect of pitch on projections is to visualize a coil of wire being pulled apart at its two ends. As the coil is stretched, the number of turns of wire *along any unit length* along the long axis of the coil decreases, but the total number of turns does not decrease. When CT scanners reconstruct images, they are looking for about two thirds of a turn's worth of projection data to form an image and will move along the z-axis until that criterion is satisfied. *This is why noise is unaffected by pitch;* it is only the number of projections needed and not their z-axis distribution that affects image noise.

Image quality can, in part, be broken down into contrast resolution and spatial resolution. Contrast resolution is the ability of an imaging system to detect a single structure that varies only slightly from its surroundings. An example of this type of object is a liver lesion surrounded by healthy liver tissue. Spatial resolution is the ability of an imaging system to distinguish two small closely spaced objects that vary greatly from their surroundings. Two 1-mm diameter iodinated arteries that are separated by 1 mm or small bone fragments in a crushed vertebral body are both examples of this type of imaging challenge. The invention of helical CT and now MSCT has opened up the discussion of contrast and spatial resolution not only in the imaging plane, but also along the z-axis.

Contrast resolution is by its nature a noise-limited phenomenon. Less noise in an image creates fewer distractions, which permits low-contrast objects to be recognized as being different than their surroundings. Contrast resolution in the x–y plane decreases as pitch increases in SSCT scanning. The effect of increased pitch in SSCT is to broaden the slice-sensitivity profile (SSP) because of the scanner's need to have a complete set of projections for image reconstruction. This requirement forces the scanner to look to either side of the image location along the z-axis to find a suitable number of projections. Projections required to form an image migrate further from the image location as the pitch increases. Some of these projections may not pass through the low-contrast object being sought. The z-axis interpolator then is used to bring these "distant" data into consideration for image reconstruction. The end result of this is an undersampling of the object. Projections not piercing the object of interest because they are too far away from the image plane are forced into the reconstruction by the z-axis interpolator. These distant projections do not represent information on the object but are included in the final image, thereby decreasing the contrast of the target object as it appears in the image. This sometimes give the impression of motion artifact or blurring in the image.

In MSCT scanning, this does not happen because as the pitch increases, at least one of the multiple rows of detectors passes in the x–y image plane that contains the object (Fig. 8). Projection data from different detectors might be called on to accurately reconstruct the object as

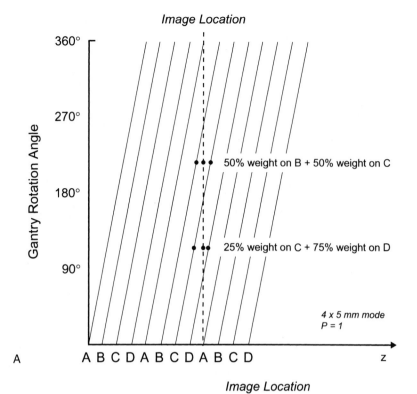

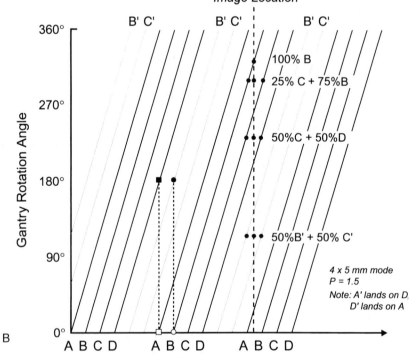

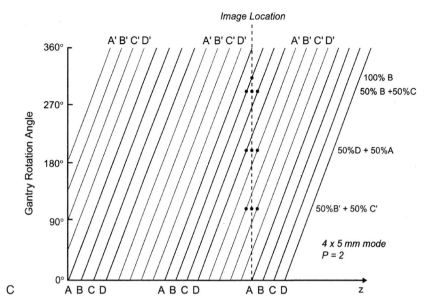

FIG. 8. A: The data-collection scheme for a multislice computed tomographic (MSCT) scanner operated in a four-row by 5-mm detector configuration and a table travel speed of 20 mm/rotation (pitch =1, contiguous helical data). The slanted lines represent the detector rows as they orbit the patient and the table traverses. Each row is labeled *(A, B, C, D)* and the requested image location *(dashed line)* is indicated. Where the dashed line intersects the slanted lines, no data interpolation is needed. Where the dashed line falls between the slanted lines, z-axis interpolation is required. The interpolation weight is proportional to the distance between the dashed line and its nearest slanted line. **B:** This illustration represents the data-collection scheme for an MSCT scanner operated in a four-row by 5-mm detector configuration and a table travel speed of 30 mm/rotation (pitch = 1.5). To complete the data set, 180-degree linear interpolation is used. For example, in the second cluster labeled A, B, C, and D, the signal value of point B at 0 degrees is reflected 180 degrees, thereby generating a data point at B′ and 180 degrees. This process is repeated at every location along lines B and C to create duplicate lines B′ and C′, offset by 180 degrees from the original data. If this process were repeated for line A, duplicate line A′ would fall directly onto line D, adding no new information. Similarly, duplicate line D′ (shifted 180 degrees) would land directly onto line A. The z-axis interpolation then proceeds as previously described (Fig. 8A). **C:** The data-collection scheme for an MSCT scanner operated in a four-row by 5-mm detector configuration and a table travel speed of 40 mm/rotation (pitch = 2). The missing data are generated using the same interpolation as described previously (Fig. 8B), but in this example, duplicate line data are created for all four detector rows A through D *(A′, B′, C′, and D′)*.

pitch increases. However, the chances that projections that lie distant to the imaging plane will be needed to complete a projection data set are rare. Two of the strong points of MSCT scanning are its inherent over sampling of objects and its ability to keep SSPs narrow relative to the requested image slice thickness. The same arguments hold true concerning low-contrast object detection when multiplanar images in x–z (coronal) or y–z (sagittal) planes are considered. Single-row scanning at a high pitch causes z-axis resolution to decrease. MSCT scanning at an increased pitch has little effect on the z-axis resolution (8).

One aspect of helical scanning that has changed considerably is pitch-compensated x-ray output. In SSCT scanning, an increase in pitch results in a decrease in the amount of x-rays penetrating any single cubic centimeter of tissue. This phenomenon permitted pitch to be used as potential dose-lowering tool. Modern MSCT scanners compensate for increased pitch by increasing x-ray output. This is done by automatically increasing the milliamperes as pitch increases. If these adjustments in technique are not changed by the CT technologist, the end result of this adjustment is the same number of x-rays, regardless of the pitch used, penetrating each volume of tissue scanned.

SPATIAL RESOLUTION

The ability of the imaging system to accurately represent very small objects is referred to as its spatial resolution. The objects that are used to evaluate spatial resolution have inherently high contrast, to minimize the influence of noise. The spatial resolution of a CT scanner has two separate components: the scan plane (x–y or "axial") resolution and the z-axis resolution. Both components can independently influence the sharpness of a clinical image.

For MSCT systems, scan plane resolution should be checked during acceptance testing, and periodically thereafter, to ensure that all images acquired during a revolution of the x-ray tube (one, two, or four) are consistent. The scan plane (x–y) resolution can be evaluated by two methods—direct and indirect. The direct method requires scanning a test pattern with objects of varying size, typically air-filled holes or lines. The direct method of scanning test patterns is simple and straightforward but can be subject to observer variability. How the image is magnified, as well as the gray level settings applied, can strongly influence how the patterns are perceived. The indirect method requires scanning a very small test object that represents an impulse function, such as a sub-millimeter metallic bead, or a metal disk with sub-millimeter thickness. The image data from the small test object are then analyzed numerically to describe the resolution characteristics. The indirect methods require more time and effort but are generally free of interobserver subjectivity effects.

The z-axis resolution is directly related to the actual shape of the image plane as observed perpendicular to the scan plane. Thinner slices will produce less partial volume averaging that can compromise the images from the z-axis direction. As in all other x-ray systems, the beam diverges and has a penumbra, so the shape of the image in the z-axis dimension is not truly flat. This is true in axial scanning but is somewhat exaggerated in helical acquisitions due to the interpolation of data in the z-axis direction and the wider collimator settings now permitted. The image thickness can be assessed using an SSP measurement approach described by Davros et al. (16). A small metallic bead is used (it should be no bigger than one tenth of the slice thickness to be evaluated), and helical images are acquired using routine parameters. The image data are then reconstructed at very small intervals (about one tenth of the slice thickness being evaluated). The maximum CT number can then be tracked at the position of the bead for all reconstructed images. The CT number value of the background material is determined (usually this is air), and this value is used for the minimum value of the bead. All other maximum CT values associated with the bead in the intervening images are rescaled between zero (background) and one (maximum of all images). The y-axis is labeled "relative CT number" and will range between zero and one; this value is plotted versus table position. This results in a curve with a minimum at zero, a sharp increase to a maximum value, a variable width plateau (or just a rounded peak), and then a sharp decrease back down to the minimum value (Fig. 9). The width of the SSP plot can be evaluated at half of the maximum value (full width at half maximum [FWHM]), and this is a reliable estimate of the true thickness of an image acquired in helical scan mode. This approach can be applied to axial images in addition to helical images, but the axial images must be acquired at many small table increments, because

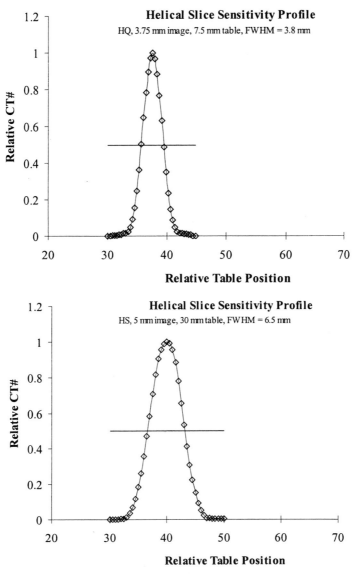

FIG. 9. These plots were generated by scanning a small metal bead with a helical scan protocol and reconstructing images at intervals equal to one tenth of the image thickness. The maximum computed tomography (CT) number for the bead in the image was recorded, and the surrounding air values were set to zero. All intermediate CT numbers were scaled to their relative value between these minimum and maximum values and then were plotted against the table position. This graph yields a description of the slice thickness shape in the z-axis direction and is called the slice sensitivity profile (SSP). Shown **(left)** is a typical SSP for a 3.75-mm thick slice with a pitch of 0.75 and 7.5-mm/rotation table speed. A **(right)** typical SSP for a 5-mm thick slice with a pitch of 1.5 and a 30-mm/rotation table speed is shown.

the data cannot be reconstructed as in a helical acquisition to produce the small intervals needed between images.

For MSCT systems, this z-axis slice thickness parameter should be evaluated for all images acquired during the x-ray tube revolution (one, two, four, etc . . .), to ensure that all images have equivalent z-axis resolution characteristics. This should be evaluated for both helical and axial type scanning modes.

LOW-CONTRAST RESOLUTION

The ability of a CT system to accurately portray in an image small details that have very similar contrast with respect to their background is described as its low contrast resolution. The system noise that is inherent in the imaging chain is primarily responsible for the loss of low contrast resolution in a CT image. This characteristic is generally evaluated by scanning test patterns with varying size and contrast levels. For MSCT scanners, it is important to evaluate all image acquisition modes for consistent low contrast resolution results. Several MSCT quality assurance phantoms have been developed recently and are readily available. These devices include patterns of small cylindrical and/or spherical targets made of material with varying contrast, which allow the evaluation of low contrast resolution for those scan protocols of clinical interest.

RECONSTRUCTION ALGORITHMS

MSCT image reconstruction algorithms are similar to those of SSCT scanner algorithms. These algorithms are applied as part of a two-step process needed to complete the data set and create the cross-sectional images. The first step is to apply a z-axis interpolator to raw projection data. This is done to weight projections nearest the slice location most heavily during the reconstruction phase. It is also done to create a data set that meets the criteria of having a complete set of projections available at the z-axis location for which an image is desired. The second step is to take the weighted projections, appropriately filter them, and back-project them to form an image. The first step in the process is transparent to the user. The CT scanner employs a z-axis interpolator that best suites the scanning parameters chosen. In the second step, the user selects appropriate reconstruction algorithms based on several criteria.

The choice of which image reconstruction algorithm to use depends on the clinical reason for the scan, the body parts being scanned, the age and size of the patient, and personal preference. Scans that involve the detection of soft tissue lesions embedded within soft tissue organs, such as the liver lesions within a healthy liver, are best reconstructed with algorithms that smooth the image and thus suppress the visualization of fine structure noise. Low contrast object detection is a noise-limited process and, therefore, would suffer if an algorithm that increases the visibility of noise were chosen. Modulation transfer functions (MTFs) for soft tissue imaging tend to support low and intermediate line pairs per centimeter (LP/cm) but drop to nearly zero approaching 8 LP/cm (Fig. 10). Algorithms that support higher line pairs per centimeter are often chosen when small high contrast objects are the focus of the scan. Bone fractures and small metallic foreign bodies are examples of scans that would dictate the use of an algorithm that supports higher line pairs per centimeter.

Most vendors have a separate set of algorithms for head scanning. These are provided to compensate for beam hardening that occurs due to the presence of the calvarium. Some vendors also have a separate set of algorithms for use in pediatric scanning. Within the context of a single task, such as finding liver metastases, there is some room for personal preference of one reconstruction algorithm over another. Some vendors supply as many as 10 different algorithms for reconstructing an adult body scan, for instance. In such a spectrum of choices, each successive algorithm incorporates a slightly more fine structure into the image. It becomes the task of the user to determine how much fine structure is needed to pick up edges of objects versus having too much noise in the image. The image noise associated with each reconstruction algorithm is proportional to the area under the MTF curve for that algorithm.

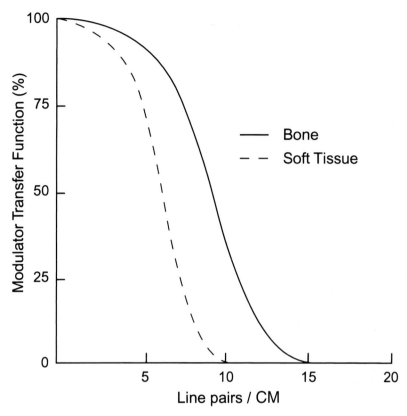

FIG. 10. This illustration represents hypothetical modulation transform function (MTF) curves for two reconstruction algorithms: bone and soft tissue. The bone algorithm, although supporting higher line pairs per centimeter, also allows more noise to be included in the image. This is because image noise is proportional to the area under the MTF curve.

Depending on the vendor, image reconstruction algorithms have different names. Some vendors give them names based on their action on the appearance of the image. Names such as *smooth, standard, bone, or edge* are used. Other venders give them an alphanumeric designation such as "adult body 20" (AB20) and "child head 30" (CH30), in a spectrum of choices ranging from smooth images (low-suffix numbers) to grainy images (high-suffix numbers). Each vendor should be able to supply a graph showing the MTF for each reconstruction algorithm available on its scanner. Comparing these curves from the CT vendor is beneficial to completely understanding the strengths and weaknesses of each reconstruction algorithm.

MSCT scanning requires the use of z-axis interpolation of the projection data to work properly. Different vendors implement different interpolators to accomplish this goal. Generally, the step of engaging a z-axis interpolator is invisible to the user. A good understanding of z-axis interpolation will afford the user a more complete understanding of the imaging sequence along with the clinical limitations z-axis interpolation causes. Z-axis interpolation is necessary for all helical CT scanning because not all of the projections collected are at the exact z-axis location where an image is requested. During helical scanning, the patient is moved at a constant velocity in the z-axis while the x-ray beam orbits in the gantry in the x–y plane. These two motions cause the x-ray beam to trace out a spiral trajectory on the patient's surface. When the scan is complete the raw projection data must be reconstructed to form images. An image in helical scanning can be created anywhere there are projection data. This is not true in conventional axial CT imaging, in which the act of scanning at a z-axis location defines the image location. The issue in spiral scanning becomes one of deciding how to treat projections that pass through the patient at locations that are some distance away in the z-axis direction from where the image is requested. In the past, this weighting procedure was done in a linear fashion using a triangle function (Fig. 11). The apex of the triangle function was placed at the z-axis location where the slice was to be formed. The apex of the function was given a weighting value of 1.0 and the projection that passed through the apex was fully and completely considered in the reconstruction. As the reconstruction algorithm went to either side of the z-axis slice location to find enough projections to form an image, the weighting function decreased to lower values in a linear fashion. Conceptually, this decrease in the weighting function is similar to stating that the farther the projections are from the requested slice location, the less importance will be placed on them. One of the consequences of the linear z-axis interpolation process in single-row scanning was to broaden the SSPs and, thus, broaden the effective image thickness. In today's multirow configurations and with nonlinear z-axis interpolation functions, such as a cosine squared function used for weighting, slice sensitivity broadening has become less of an issue. Incidentally, it is

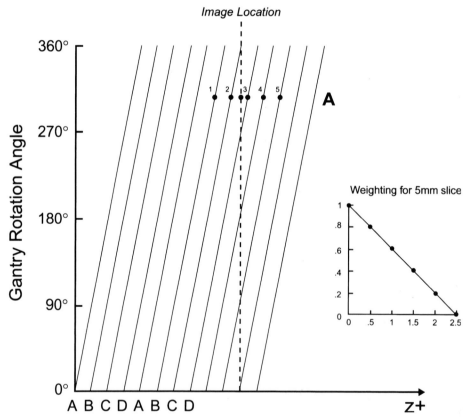

FIG. 11. The data-collection scheme for a four-row by 1-mm detector configuration and a table travel speed of 4 mm/rotation (pitch = 1). To reconstruct an image with a slice thickness of 5 mm, five-point z-axis linear interpolation must be performed. As before, the new image (5 mm thick) is shown (*dashed line*), and the weighting factors are again proportional to the distance from the dashed line to the solid lines (which represent image-projection data paths). These weighting factors are also shown on the plot **(right)**, which illustrates that the maximum distance from the center of the new image location to the real projection data is 2.5 mm.

the z-axis interpolation process that facilitates vendors providing image thicknesses that are non-integer multiples of their detector array sizing. For example, one vendor provides a 3-mm image thickness while scanning in the 4- by 2.5-mm scan configuration. This is done by simply extending the z-axis weighting function to either side of the slice location by 1.5 mm so that the reconstruction algorithm will consider 3 mm of weighted projection data.

CT NUMBER

Because all grayscale values of the CT image are based on the measured attenuation of water, it is critical that CT scanners are frequently monitored and adjusted to accurately reflect this substance. This is typically accomplished by the regular scanning of a quality-assurance phantom.

The ability of the CT scanner to accurately represent a homogeneous object of the same relative contrast as soft tissue is often described as the "uniformity" of the image. A circular water bath is typically scanned using routine acquisition parameters, and the CT number of the water is sampled in several central and peripheral locations using a region-of-interest (ROI) analysis tool. The mean value of the region is used to check the scanner for CT number accuracy (should be very close to zero), and the standard deviation of the mean value reflects the noise of the imaging system. The mean value of water should be quite constant (or "flat") over the entire water bath volume. Typical test criteria require this water value to be within ±4 Hounsfield units (HU) over the entire water volume examined. Noise values will vary considerably with the choice of reconstruction filter (or "algorithm") chosen for the scan set. Standard deviation results will be small (as low as around 2 HU) for options such as "smooth," and high (more than 100 HU) for those choices used to boost image sharpness (e.g., "edge") (17). For multislice helical scanners, all images acquired simultaneously during a single revolution of the x-ray tube should be checked to ensure that the water values are consistent along the z-axis and within the test criteria used for your facility.

The numerical accuracy of pixel values in clinical CT images is generally of interest only when quantification is desired. Applications such as measurement of tissue density (e.g., calcium content in bone or lung nodules) require stringent calibration programs. CT is generally considered to be quite accurate in terms of size depiction; the variability of the measurement method itself (placement of the cursors) is much more prone to error than the imaging methodology. The only factor that would be expected to be different in MSCT is the uniformity in the z-axis direction due to the acquisition of multiple images in each revolution of the x-ray tube. Thus, careful attention to the performance of any measurement in terms of consistent results obtained in the z-axis direction would be warranted for MSCT.

Recent attention has focused on the evaluation of CT numbers of renal cysts (18). One of the characteristics used to classify renal cysts is the increase in the CT number of the cyst region after the injection of IV contrast. Maki et al. (19) has constructed a renal cyst phantom, which incorporates simulated cysts of varying size and shape (cylindrical and spherical) and allows the introduction of increasing contrast in the surrounding background material. This experiment showed that the CT numbers of the simulated cyst areas consistently increased (from a low of 5 HU to a maximum of more than 25 HU) as the background contrast level increased, even though the cyst material itself remained constant. The influence of the background contrast level to the cyst CT numbers was attributed to inadequate correction for beam-hardening errors in the reconstruction process and was consistent for both single-slice helical and axial scanning modes. Although the occurrence of this problem in MSCT systems has not emerged in the literature to date because this phenomenon is consistent for both axial and SSCT scanners, it will likely also affect MSCT images in the same way.

BEAM GEOMETRY

With a shorter source to detector distance and a larger beam angle in the z-axis direction, one would expect the cupping artifact to be more pronounced in the multislice helical images than in single-slice acquisition images, particularly for images acquired using 15- or 20-mm collimator settings. To investigate this potential problem, uniformity images were obtained in axial mode on an MSCT scanner at 10 mm, with one image per rotation and at 5 mm with four images per rotation (20-mm collimator). The set of four 5-mm thick images acquired with 20-mm collimator can be thought of as a series in which the first and last images are located at the exterior of the series (5-mm exterior) and the second and third images are located at the interior (5-mm interior) of the series. Each image was examined for evidence of the cupping artifact. This artifact was not readily apparent in any of the images with the window width and level settings of 100 and 0, respectively. Profiles of the CT numbers across the diameter of the phantom are displayed in Fig. 12. A difference between the profiles of an outer image (5-mm exterior) and an inner image (5-mm interior) from the set of four 5-mm images was expected. However, the CT number profiles show no evidence of the cupping artifact, indicating that the correction algorithm was functioning properly.

INTERPOLATION OR RECONSTRUCTION ARTIFACTS

Third-generation SSCT scanners display concentric ring artifacts when the detectors are improperly balanced. The MSCT scanner uses contributions from each of the four (or more) output channels in the reconstruction of a given image to reduce reconstruction and motion artifacts. Therefore, in the MSCT system, imbalances in the detector segments can be evidenced by the appearance of partial rings in the uniformity images acquired in helical mode. These detector imbalances can appear as conventional ring artifacts in axial mode scan acquisitions. This is the case if the entire detector has failed or is out of balance with neighboring detectors in the x–y plane. If only one or two elements of a detector have failed, the effect will be averaged over all elements (from that detector and neighboring detectors) contributing to the image.

Other artifacts, usually associated with interpolation, are associated with high-contrast objects of high spatial frequency, which lie at an angle along the z-axis. In some cases, this artifact lies near the object (Fig. 13) and appears to radiate away from it. In other cases, the artifact may be some distance from the object and resemble short alternating light and dark bands in a small region. These artifacts are more readily apparent in thinner phantom images acquired with higher pitch (collimator pitch of more than 1.0) or in phantom images retrospectively reconstructed using the edge or similar algorithm. These artifacts have not yet been observed with the clinical images. Other artifacts have been observed in phantom images and are described elsewhere (8). We agree that in our experience, multislice scanners appear substantially less likely to produce clinical images with artifacts present than previous conventional SSCT scanners. We attribute this improvement to the fact that many of the parameters internal to the scanner must be more tightly controlled for the instrument to function, and these tighter specifications in turn produce more reliable clinical images.

PROTOCOL DEVELOPMENT

The scanning parameters that are critical when defining a protocol for MSCT include the following:

- Image thickness and detector configuration, collimation, table speed, interval (spacing between reconstructed images), reconstruction options

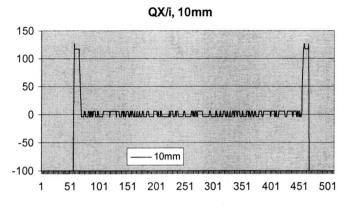

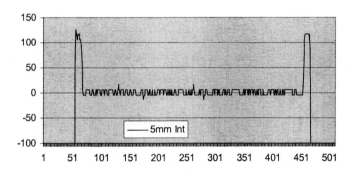

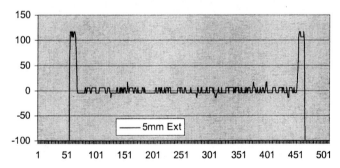

FIG. 12. CT number profiles through the diameter of the phantom image **(top)** for a 10-mm ax-ial scan with 10-mm collimation, an interior image **(center)** from the four-row by 5-mm images acquired in axial mode with 20-mm collimation, and an outer image **(bottom)** of the four-row by 5-mm images acquired with 20-mm collimation. The water values look uniformly flat through-out, which implies that there is no bias in scanner performance among the four images acquired in a single pass.

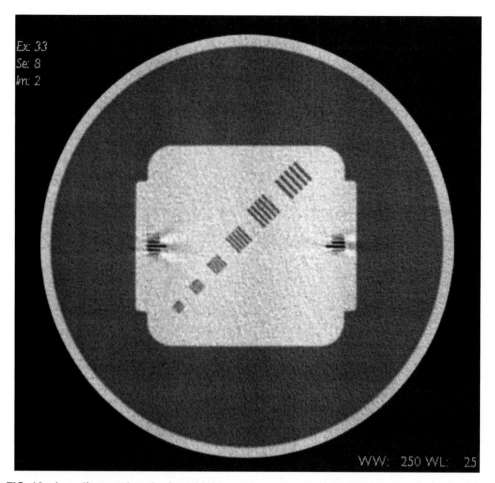

FIG. 13. An artifact produced using a high-pass reconstruction algorithm such as "edge" or "detail" in a high-contrast scan object. Wavelets appear to grow from the horizontal black lines in this example.

- Delay before image acquisition (IV contrast injection parameters)
- Length of acquisition (time); is the breath-hold required feasible for these patients?
- Technique (kilovolts, milliamperes, seconds)
- Reconstruction algorithm
- Scan FOV, display FOV (size of scan and display FOVs)

When transferring scan protocols from a SSCT scanner to the MSCT platform, it is useful to understand the differences in dose for a reference axial scan performed on the two scanners. The reference scan should be carefully selected so that the detector configurations are as identical as possible. For instance, if a 5-mm image is acquired in axial mode on a single-slice CT at 120 kVp and 200 mAs, this can be reproduced on the MSCT with acquisition of a single image of 5 mm in axial mode at the same kVp and mAs. The selection of a single image at 5 mm forces the collimators to the 5-mm setting. The difference in dose can be used to establish the magnitude by which the milliamperes per rotation can be changed to compensate for the differences in scanner geometry and manufacturer. Next, a comparison of image noise (standard deviation of an ROI placed in the water section of the image quality phantom) and low contrast detectability (also in the image quality phantom) can be performed on both scanners, using the adjusted mAs values on the MSCT. Further adjustments to the mAs can enable good matching of the noise and low contrast detection characteristics of the two scanners. The percentage change in mAs from the old to the new scanning platforms can be applied to scan protocols at a given peak kilovoltage and used as a starting place from which the protocols can be further refined.

POSTPROCESSING APPLICATIONS

One of the chief advantages of MSCT scanning is the nearly infinite number of choices available for postprocessing the acquired data sets. A multitude of image reconstruction options are available, which can result in the generation of a very large stack of images that are specifically formulated for optimal visualization using postprocessing tools. In particular, images can readily be produced from an MSCT acquisition with very small intervals (overlapping images), which in turn produce extraordinary images when viewed with 3D display tools. These extremely large image sets can be generated from the same raw data set that were used to produce the clinically interpreted images, so these 3D views can be formed without any additional scanning.

The large image sets can be viewed in many ways, and these choices depend entirely on the hardware and software available at each facility. Reformatted views are often quite helpful; as in magnetic resonance imaging, the axial views alone are sometimes supplemented by information obtained from standard coronal and sagittal sections. Curved reformatted views can also be quite helpful, for example, when following a spinal cord, a curved organ such as the pancreas, or a particular vessel to evaluate stenosis. Surface displays, also called 3D volume renderings, are useful for surgeons, particularly when different tissue types can be displayed with variable levels of transparency. This allows the visualization of several tissue categories in one view and provides valuable information regarding the spatial relation of important anatomic structures.

Of particular interest in MSCT applications is the ability to follow a contrast bolus through the vascular system (14,15). The speed and heat capacity of these systems quite literally allows a scanner to track a bolus of intravascular contrast from its origin to its destination, and images that display the entire vascular system can be readily obtained. Of course, the operators must be able to readily handle the vast amount of images that are required for such a task, but the MSCT scanners are now sufficiently robust to generate these images for the demanding radiologist.

Another particularly strong application for MSCT postprocessing is virtual endoscopy (bronchoscopy or colonoscopy). Extensive image acquisitions can be readily acquired in a short period (typically less than 30 seconds), and these raw data can be reconstructed to form many overlapping images. Data sets of this type can be optimized for surface rendering and then evaluated interactively using "fly-through" software packages available from all vendors of MSCT equipment and by many third-party vendors.

FUTURE DEVELOPMENT

Vendors have expanded beyond the four-slice acquisition and are well into larger detector sampling volumes. We already see equipment that can routinely acquire 8, 16, or more images per rotation of the x-ray tube. The basic concepts in protocol development will, however, remain similar. This will speed the scan process by permitting more coverage for each revolution of the gantry. Also, more and thinner detector rows in the z-axis dimension will allow more data to be collected per gantry rotation. By the end of 2002, there may be 32-channel readout scanners, covering as much as 50 mm per rotation. Complete anatomic coverage of the heart with 0.5 mm slices could come into being. Thinner image thicknesses in the chest, abdomen, and pelvis, 2 mm or less, will become common. This type of scanning will produce hundreds of images per body part and phase. A triphasic liver study with a precontrast and postcontrast pelvis exam may well exceed 800 images.

Several CT scanner vendors have introduced scan times, down to 0.5 seconds per x-ray tube rotation. These scans will further improve image quality for pediatric studies and in trauma departments. The increased speed will also permit higher patient throughput. Higher quality vascular examinations are also feasible. The combination of more slices per tube rotation and faster rotations promises to make an enormous impact on routine CT scanning in the future.

Lung cancer screening programs based on CT images are well suited to MSCT. We believe that a lung CT "screening day" may be feasible, in which only subjects who are part of a lung cancer screening research study are scanned on a high-throughput basis. A single protocol can be established (without IV contrast) and subjects can be positioned, scanned in a single breath-hold (typically in less than 30 seconds), and released, and the cycle then repeated. The task of interpreting these many images is a separate and monumental challenge, and one that we hope will be alleviated by specially designed image display tools.

MSCT is also very applicable to perfusion measurement purposes. Oncologic treatments often target the angiogenesis process, and being able to noninvasively assess the blood flow characteristics that surround specific lesions could be particularly useful in monitoring treatment efficacy. The arterial blood flow measurement, which is required for calibration purposes, is more accurately evaluated with CT than with MRI. Thus, the estimation of blood flow parameters (e.g., blood volume, flow rate, permeability) are readily achievable with MSCT scanners. The primary limitations of MSCT at this date are the limited overall collimation (20 mm in the z-axis direction) and the need for respiratory motion correction for certain anatomic locations during longer data-acquisition time periods (a scan time of more than 2 minutes may become typical for this application).

The use of MSCT images for surgical planning purposes is also beginning to grow. Because such a large volume of tissue can be rendered in exquisite 3D detail, entire surgeries can now be simulated on a patient long before nearing the operating room. Stacks of these CT images can be input to systems that produce accurate 3D plastic models, also very useful for surgical planning (prebending implant plates, for example, can save expensive operating room time). These volume CT data can also be used to develop very detailed 3D radiation therapy treatment plans. Large volume CT data sets can also be very helpful in combination CT–Positron Emission Tomographic scanners; the CT image data are generally used to correct for attenuation differences in the 3D patient tissue patterns for individual subjects.

What lies ahead for MSCT scanning? With this type of scanning just over the technology horizon, new, faster, and more intelligent systems for image transmission and display will be needed. Automated multiplanar reconstruction workstations will probably become common. A 3D treatment of the data will be explored, making obsolete the concept of slice. Finally, flat-panel arrays using cone-beam geometry with cone-beam (z-axis) angles approaching 30 degrees is not unthinkable. In cone-beam helical CT, a flat-panel (or curved panel) detector will be used to collect even larger volumes of data in one rotation of the x-ray tube. This future CT development has the very attractive potential for generating truly isotropic voxels, more like the MRI data-collection process.

What is certain is that MSCT scanning will continue to evolve. It will become faster, offering thinner images; gating technology will help to further arrest motion; gantry rotation speeds will increase; and the physical limits of contrast and spatial resolution will be approached with existing designs and materials. Further advancements will come when materials and designs go to the next level of complexity. What is predictable is that these changes will take place faster than any of us could have imagined only a few years ago.

REFERENCES

1. Knez A., Becker C, Ohnesorge B, et al. Noninvasive detection of coronary artery stenosis by multislice helical computed tomography. Circulation 2000;101(23):e221–e222.
2. Foley WD, Mallisee TA, Hehenwalter MD, et al. Multiphase hepatic CT with a multirow detector CT scanner. Am J Roentgenol 2000;175:679–685.
3. Baum U, Greess H, Lell M, et al. Imaging of head and neck tumors—methods: CT, spiral-CT, multislice-spiral CT. Eur J Radiol 2000;33:153–160.
4. Brink JA, Wang G, McFarland EG. Optimal section spacing in single detector CT. Radiology 2000;214:595–598.
5. Klingenbeck-Regn K, Schaller S, Flohr T, et al. Subsecond multislice computed tomography: basics and applications. Eur J Radiol 1999;31:110–124.
6. Vannier MW. Multislice CT provides unprecedented power. Adv Comp Tomogr December 2000:2–6.
7. Fox SH. An introduction to multislice detector technology. Helical (Spiral) CT Today 2000;6(1):3–4.
8. McCollough CH, Zink FE. Performance evaluation of a multi-slice CT system. Med Phys 1999;26:2223–2230.
9. Silverman PM, Kalender WA, Hazle JD. Common terminology for single and multislice helical CT. Am J Radiol 2001;176:1135–1136.
10. Nelson RC, Silverman PM. "Multislice CT: a new era. Basic technical aspects and clinical capabilities. Helical (Spiral) CT Today 2000;6(1):2–3.
11. Moxley DM, Hazle JD, Shepard SJ, et al. Dosimetry of a new multislice CT scanner: calculated and measured patient doses. Radiology 1999;213(P):284.
12. Pappas JN, Donnelly LF, Frush DP. Reduced frequency of sedation of young children with multisection helical CT. Radiology 2000;215:897–899.
13. Donnelly LF, Frush DP, Nelson RC. Multislice helical CT to facilitate combined CT of the neck, chest, abdomen and pelvis in children. Am J Roentgenol 2000;174:1620–1622.
14. Silverman PM, Roberts S, Tefft MC, et al. Helical (spiral) CT value of an automated computer technique, smart prep for obtaining images with optimal contrast enhancement. Am J Roentgenol 1995;165:73–78.
15. Silverman PM, Roberts SC, Ducic I, et al. Assessment of a technology that permits individualized scan delays on hepatic helical CT.
16. Davros WJ, Herts BR, Walmsley JJ, et al. Determination of spiral CT slice sensitivity profiles using a point response phantom. J Comput Assist Tomogr 1995;19:838–843.
17. Kallender WA. Computed tomography: fundamentals, system technology, image quality, and applications. Munich, Germany: MCD Werbeagentur GmbH, 2000.
18. Bae KT, Heiken JP, Siegel CL, et al. Renal cysts: is attenuation artifactually increased on contrast-enhanced CT images? Radiology 2000;216:792–796.
19. Maki DD, Birnbaum BA, Chakraborty DP, et al. Renal cyst pseudoenhancement: beam-hardening effects of CT numbers. Radiology 1999;213:468–472.

2

Multislice Computed Tomography of the Head And Neck

Ilona M. Schmalfuss* and Anthony A. Mancuso*

*Department of Radiology, Division of Neuroradiology, University of Florida,
Gainesville, Florida 32610

The introduction of multislice computed tomographic (CT) scanners with its additional volumetric acquisition option revolutionized CT imaging. The design of CT study protocols now focuses equally on the acquisition and postprocessing of the available data. For instance, in the past, a sometimes difficult compromise between slice thickness and study duration had to be made. Now, multiple CT images can be obtained simultaneously. This rapid acquisition capability allows for a significant decrease in the examination time when using similar imaging parameters or to decrease the slice thickness at a price of smaller time gain (1).

RAPID ACQUISITION CAPABILITY

It is widely accepted that conventional helical CT, with its rapid data acquisition, reduces, if not eliminates, motion artifacts such as respiratory misregistration seen with conventional CT (2). The ability of the new multislice CT scanners to simultaneously perform multiple slices significantly decreases the scanning time and even further reduces these artifacts (3). Additional reductions in the rotation time to less than 1 second (0.5 to 0.8 seconds depending on the manufacturer) further enhance this beneficial effect. Reduction of motion artifacts is a crucial aspect in imaging of the head and neck region. Swallowing artifacts in particular can cause clinically significant degradation of images in studies of the oropharynx, larynx, and hypopharynx. Respiratory motion may produce gaps in the scanned area, a difficulty most commonly encountered in the larynx (4). Despite this, CT remains the modality of choice for evaluating the larynx, whereas magnetic resonance imaging is optimally used for imaging above this level.

The expected marked reduction in motion artifacts, as well as the decreased necessity for direct coronal imaging in lieu of exceptional high-quality reconstructed images, can also reduce the need for sedation, particularly in pediatric patients. Sedation may still be required if direct coronal imaging is necessary or with subsequent three-dimensional (3D) reconstructions of the region of critical interest, as in patients with craniosynostosis or craniofacial malformation. Any motion during scanning of these patients can result in a nondiagnostic study that will then be repeated and result in additional radiation exposure (5).

There is only one drawback: If the patient moves during the scan, then typically not only one but multiple images are degraded by the motion because four slices and even more in the future are obtained simultaneously. Practically, this is a minor problem because the significantly shorter scanning time makes it easier to coach the patient on avoiding motions during data acquisition.

The rapid acquisition, with its shorter scanning time, also results in a significant reduction of contrast volume.

REDUCED SLICE THICKNESS

Reduction of the slice thickness at the price of lower time gain brings two interesting points. First, it needs to be decided how many images are too many to be looked at and also printed out as hard copy in a nonfilmless department. The threshold will be different between radiologists; suggestions are provided in the protocols.

The second point is more fascinating because it opens an incredible flexibility in data processing. The new multislice CT scanners are capable of obtaining the images with a certain slice thickness and then reconstruct these at a different thickness (6). If the axial imaging mode is used, the reconstructed image thickness is a multiple of the acquisition slice thickness. If the helical multislice mode is used, there are even more options in image thickness reconstructed from the same data set; for example, the scan is performed with 4- $\times$ 1-mm to collimation (four images with a slice thickness of 1.0 to 1.25 mm are obtained simultaneously) and can be reconstructed into a 1.0-, 1.25-, 1.5-, 2.0-, 3.0-, 4.0-, or 5.0-mm slice thickness. This has been referred to as a combiscan (1). Such combiscan scans can significantly decrease artifacts between structures of waste different CT attenuation such as the intrapetrous region. This flexibility brings two major benefits. The narrowed collimation has the advantages of decreased partial volume effects and higher slice sensitivity profiles, resulting in higher quality of reconstructed images (1,3). In addition, if findings are unclear on the images reconstructed at a higher thickness than the acquisition thickness, there is the ability to reconstruct the images at a thinner slice thickness and subsequently perform multiplanar reformations of higher quality than possible with thicker slices. This flexibility has the potential to be beneficial—for example, in patients with floor of the mouth cancer when subtle erosion of the mandible is suggested on the images reconstructed at a thicker slice thickness than the acquisition slice thickness or in patients with low-volume lesions. Reconstruction of the same imaging data set at a thinner slice thickness might avoid additional imaging of the patient.

In summary, a compromise between time saving and flexibility in data processing has to be made. The proposed protocols might have to be modified to some degree for the individual patient and the individual practice.

IMAGING TECHNIQUE

Gantry Angle

In general, the gantry angles used in the multislice CT technique are the same as those used in conventional and helical CT. The head and the portions of the neck and face cephalad to the hard palate are scanned with the gantry angled parallel to the inferior orbital meatal line (IOML). The remainder of the neck and pharynx is studied with the gantry angled parallel to the body of the mandible (Fig. 1). Slightly modified angulation of the gantry around the teeth is sometimes necessary to avoid artifacts from dental amalgam and to ensure coverage of the entire oropharynx and most of the oral cavity without dental artifacts. The coronal scan plane is made as perpendicular to the IOML as possible.

There are some exceptions to these general rules. The examination of the larynx, for example, requires scanning with the gantry angled parallel to the true vocal cords, to avoid distor-

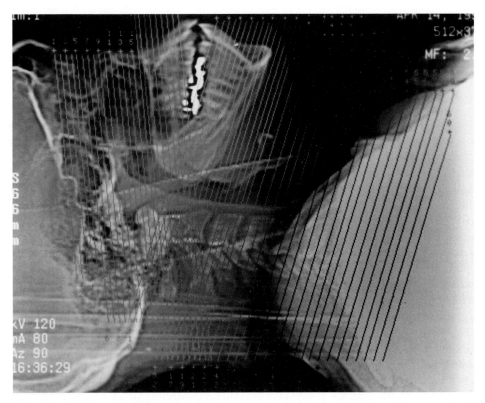

FIG. 1. The lateral scout of the neck demonstrates the different angulation of the computed tomographic images around the teeth to minimize artifacts caused by dental fillings. The overlapping of the images in the oropharynx ascertains coverage of the entire oropharynx without dental artifacts.

tion of anatomic landmarks critical for treatment planning. An inaccurate gantry angle can cause artificial "thickening" of the anterior commissure, indicating more extensive disease in patients with laryngeal tumors than is actually present. False-positive thickening of the anterior commissure may suggest that the patient requires a more extended surgical procedure such as extended vertical partial laryngectomy. Partial volume averaging of the true and false vocal cords with the interposed laryngeal ventricle may result in inability to evaluate the paraglottic fat planes that play a key role in determination of the deep extension inaccessible to the clinical evaluation, and therefore surgical approach, of some laryngeal cancers. Occasionally, the obliteration of these fat planes is the only sign that a lesion is present (7).

The other major exception involves imaging with the multislice CT scanners in helical mode because not all scanners are able to simultaneously obtain multiple slices with the helical scanning technique and the gantry angled to some degree. This is a relatively minor drawback, because such scans can be acquired without any gantry angulation in helical mode and subsequently easily and quickly reconstructed in the desired imaging plane. In addition, it has been already indicated by the manufacturers that all next-generation multislice CT scanners will have the capability to scan with the gantry angled in helical mode.

In the past, neutral position of the gantry was recommended whenever reformations in the coronal or sagittal plane, as well as if 3D reconstructions, were considered. With the significant interval improvement of the computer technique, the differences in processing of the data obtained with or without gantry angulation are negligible. In our experience, there are also no significant differences in image quality. However, because reformations are of better quality using the helical imaging mode, the gantry angle has to be set to 0 degrees for certain CT scanners.

Iodinated Contrast Media

The published experiences regarding multislice CT scanners and contrast administration show a very broad range in total contrast volume, from 75 to 150 mL. Very little is published regarding injection rate and scan delay in this body area. In our experience, only 100 mL of contrast is required for imaging of the head and neck region in the axial plane alone, saving 50 mL of contrast when compared with prior protocols. If direct coronal imaging is necessary, the contrast volume is unchanged with 150 mL, of which 100 mL is used for the axial images and the residual 50 mL for direct coronal imaging, but the vascular enhancement pattern improves because of the increased overall scan speed resulting in better image quality. These doses are specially adjusted for pediatric patients and for adult patients with small body habitus.

For routine brain studies, the injection rate is 0.5 mL per second, with scanning beginning after a 5-minute delay. Evaluation of the extracranial and intracranial vessels and perfusion studies require an injection rate of 3 or 4 mL per second, with a 20-second or no scan delay, respectively.

For most head and neck CT studies, the contrast is injected at 1 mL per second. Sixty milliliters is administered before scanning, resulting in a scan delay of 60 seconds. The remaining volume is injected at the same rate (1 mL per second) without interruption of the injection for reangulation of the gantry for axial imaging. Typically, the entire volume of contrast is given by the time the gantry is reangled and the second set of images is started. If additional direct coronal images are performed, then the contrast administration is interrupted for the time required for repositioning of the patient. If axial images are obtained only from the mid oral cavity or mandible to the thoracic inlet, then the total amount of contrast is administered before scanning at 1 mL per second, resulting in a scan delay of 100 seconds. The suggested injection rate and scan delay result in homogeneous enhancement of the vasculature throughout the entire scan. In addition, the contrast injection is terminated well before the thoracic inlet is reached. This is an important point because significant artifacts that may be caused by the contrast stagnating in the subclavian vein are seen with shorter scan delays. The suggested longer scan delays allow the circulating blood to flush the contrast out of these vessels, which significantly improves the image quality (Fig. 2).

---->

FIG. 2. (A) Axial computed tomographic (CT) image through the thoracic inlet demonstrates significant artifacts (*arrowheads*) caused by the high concentration of contrast in the subclavian vein (*arrows*) on the left side. The study was performed with a 2.5-mm slice thickness after injection of 40 mL of contrast at a rate of 1 mL per second before scan began, followed by continuous injection of 0.7 mL per second with the scan beginning, for a total of 100 mL. Axial CT image **(B)** through the thoracic inlet in a different patient shows significantly less artifacts (*arrowheads*) arising from contrast stasis in the subclavian vein on the left side (*arrows*). This study was also obtained with a 2.5-mm slice thickness and a total of 100 mL of contrast; however, the injection rate was 1 mL per second throughout the scan. A scan delay of 60 seconds was used and the injection was *not* discontinued during gantry reangulation. With this injection protocol, the total contrast was administered by the time the hyoid bone was reached, giving time to dilute the contrast within the subclavian vein by normal blood flow. Nevertheless, excellent and homogenous opacification of the common carotid arteries *(c)* and internal jugular veins *(J)* was seen in the lower neck **(C).**

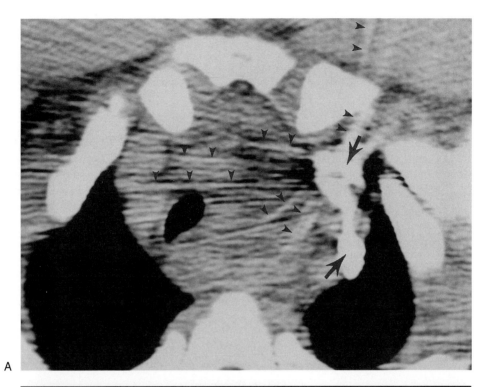

A

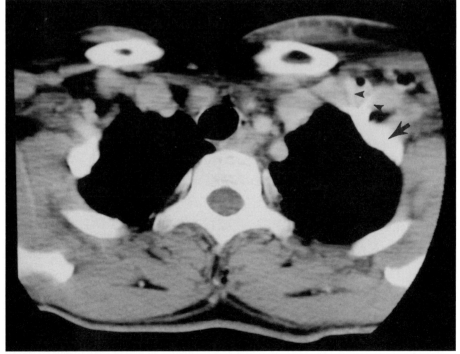

B

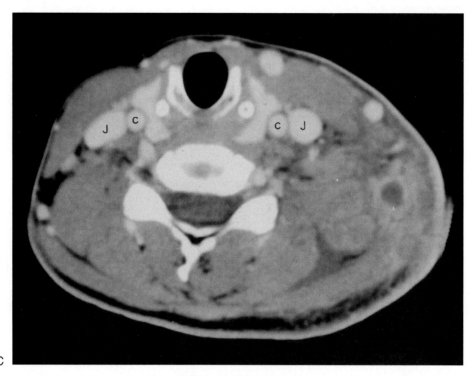

C

FIG. 2. *Continued.*

Acquisition Slice Thickness/Collimation

In general, the best image quality is obtained with the smallest acquisition slice thickness (collimation) as acceptable for a specific clinical setting (within the bounds of low-contrast resolution requirements for the anatomic question) because the image quality of the reconstructed images is higher when the scan is performed with a smaller acquisition slice thickness (collimation). As mentioned previously, this is due to the reduced partial volume effects and better resolution of small objects (1).

The basic slice thickness (collimation) for the different head and neck areas is as follows:

- Head: 2.5 to 3.0 mm through the posterior fossa, 5 mm through the head
- Facial bones, sinuses, mandible, optic nerve: 1.0 to 1.25 mm
- Orbit, neck: 2.5 to 3.0 mm
- Temporal bone: 0.5 to 1.25 mm

Adjustment of the slice thickness may be required for certain indications (see specific protocols).

Pitch

As is known from the single-slice CT scanners, there is a certain slice broadening when using the helical imaging mode with multislice CT scanners. However, in contrast to the single-slice CT scanners, the slice broadening is not significantly dependent on the pitch (6). The choice of pitch is therefore primarily influenced by two factors: scanning time versus need for reconstructions. If the patient, such as a trauma or pediatric patient, is only able to hold still for a very short time, a higher pitch of 1.5 (HS = 6 : 1) is advisable; however, if multiplanar or 3D reconstructions are considered, then a pitch of 0.75 (HQ = 3 : 1) is required for optimal image quality (3). With the latter pitch, there is also significantly less image noise and less pronounced helical artifacts and geometric distortion than that seen with the pitch of 1.5 (HS = 6 : 1) (8).

Tube Current

As previously seen with single-slice CT scanners, imaging of the brain and the thoracic inlet requires markedly more tube current (milliamperes) than the remainder of the head and neck region. These areas are particularly prone to be degraded by beam hardening artifacts caused by the temporal bones and shoulders. Because of the design of the current multislice CT scanners, there is a more pronounced broadening of the slices of the detectors in peripheral location in comparison to the central detectors, resulting in markedly more artifacts caused by high-contrast objects such as bone edges. Therefore, imaging of the brain should be performed at 140 kV and 350 to 400 mA. Through the lower neck and thoracic inlet region, imaging in multislice axial mode may in some cases be preferred over helical mode. The tube current has to be increased to 300 to 350 mA per 2 seconds to optimize image quality (Fig. 3). Because motion artifacts are not common at the shoulder level, helical data acquisition is not as important in this region as it is in the sections through the midpharynx. Children and adults with smaller body habitus are exceptions to this problem.

MULTIPLANAR AND THREE-DIMENSIONAL REFORMATIONS

Multiplanar Reformations

Until now, coronal, sagittal, and oblique reformations have been predominantly used as a default technique in patients who cannot tolerate the position for direct coronal imaging and when the sagittal or oblique plane might add important information related to the planning of treatment. The increased quality of reformations from data sets performed with multislice CT scanners in helical mode (9) justifies elimination of direct coronal imaging for certain indications such as evaluation of sinusitis in nonimmunocompromised patients. It is essential to use a slice thickness (collimation) of usually 1.0 to 1.25 mm and a pitch of 0.75 (HQ = 3 : 1) for optimal quality of reformations. These parameters result in a slice overlap of approximately 25%, significantly reducing the stair-step artifacts that are well known from conventional reconstructions. Reformations may also be used to avoid artifacts from dental amalgam (Fig. 4) (10). If multiplanar reformations are considered, it is also essential to perform the entire image set with the same field of view to avoid nondiagnostic reformatted images (Fig. 5).

Nevertheless, even reformations from data sets performed with multislice CT scanners in helical mode are still suboptimal in comparison with direct coronal imaging. In regions where thin bone lies within the axial plane, reformations of the axial data set may lead to mistaking the thin bone for bone loss or dehiscence on the reformatted images (Fig. 6). This is a particularly important limitation in patients with cerebrospinal fluid leakage, where CT must often detect subtle areas of dehiscence in the skull base, particularly at the cribriform plate. In patients with cancer with suspected subtle bone involvement or in immunocompromised patients, direct coronal imaging might make a critical difference in staging or in the diagnosis of aggressive sinus disease, respectively. Therefore, direct coronal imaging is preferred whenever possible in such situations.

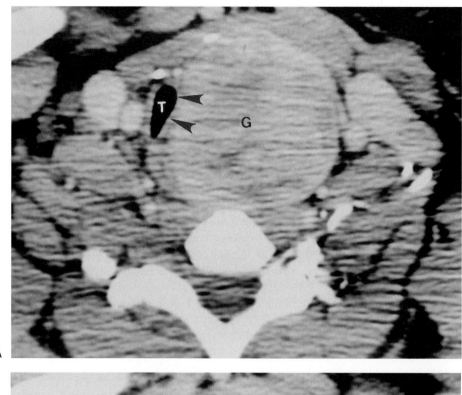

A

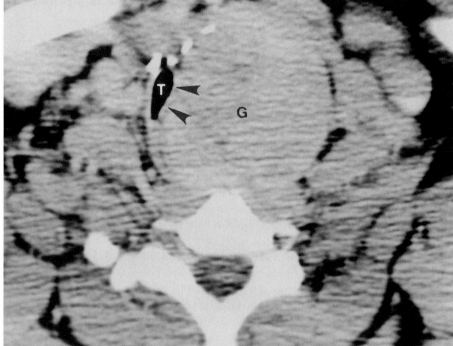

B

FIG. 3. Axial CT images through the lower neck in a patient with large recurrent goiter *(G)* on the left side and significant compression and displacement (*arrowheads*) of the trachea *(T)* demonstrate marked decrease in shoulder artifacts when the kilovolt (peak) was increased from 120 **(A)** to 140 **(B)** by constant milliamperes of 300 per 2 seconds. Even the image through the thoracic inlet **(C)** demonstrates only minimal shoulder artifacts with the higher kilovolt (peak).

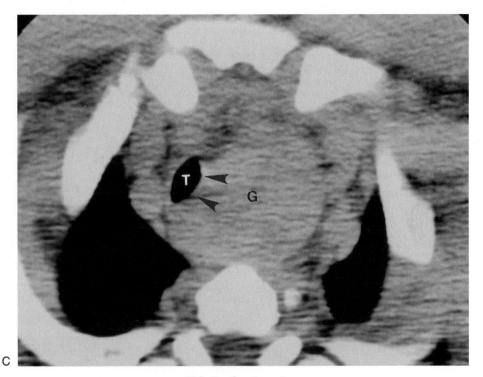

FIG. 3. *Continued.*

Three-Dimensional Display

Three-dimensional display is used most often in evaluating craniofacial abnormalities such as craniosynostosis or facial fractures. It has also been used sparingly for the study of laryngeal or subglottic stenosis, integrity of the ossicular chain, spinal abnormalities, and determination of tumor volume. 3D display is used mainly as an aid in planning surgery, rather than for diagnosis. Multislice CT scanners used in helical mode produce even higher quality 3D images than single-slice helical CT scanners (9). As mentioned already, it is, however, crucial that the data set is obtained with a thin slice thickness (collimation) of usually 1.0 to 1.25 mm and a pitch of 0.75 (HQ = 3 : 1). Artifacts on 3D reformations caused by suboptimal technique in the head region have been described (5). These include the following:

- Boiled egg artifact: This artifact occurs in the high parietal region when data are missing through the last few millimeters of the head. This can be avoided by coverage of the head beyond the vertex.
- Distortion:
  1. Distortion of the head on the 3D display can occur when the available software cannot compensate for the gantry tilt. This can be eliminated by scanning in a neutral position (gantry angle of 0 degrees).
  2. A new distortion artifact called "undulating low-frequency artifactual surface distortion" has been discovered in multislice CT scanners when used in helical mode. This artifact occurs when a subject is scanned off-center. It results in gross distortion of large objects and displacement of small objects (9).
- Threshold selection: The 3D image appearance is dependent on the chosen threshold during reconstructions. For instance, increasing the value will open sutures and enlarge pseudoforamina; decreasing the threshold will mistakenly close the sutures.

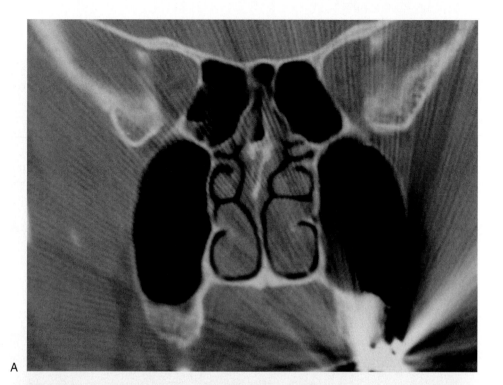

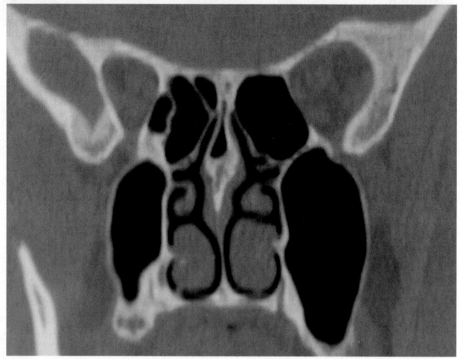

FIG. 4. Direct coronal image **(A)** through the sinuses and nasal cavity is markedly degraded by dental filling artifacts on the left. This can be particularly problematic in patients with a large number of dental fillings. In these patients, coronal reformations from axial images can entirely avoid this type of degradation **(B).** The coronal reformation was performed from axial images acquired at a 1.25-mm slice thickness in helical multislice imaging mode using a pitch of 0.75 (3 : 1) and reconstructed at a 1-mm slice thickness.

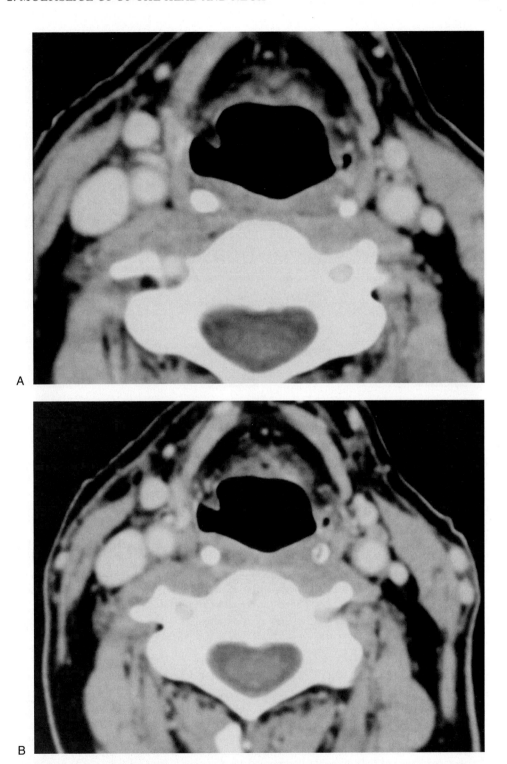

FIG. 5. Axial images through the midneck **(A, B)** in the same patient performed with different field of views but otherwise same scanning parameters were reformatted in the coronal plane. Because of the variation in field of view, the reformatted image in coronal plane **(C)** is nondiagnostic at and around the level of change in the field of view.

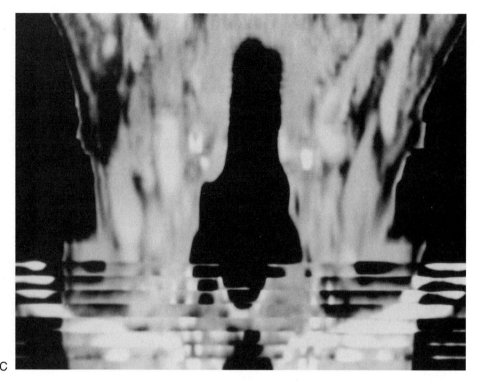

C

FIG. 5. *Continued.*

It is important to note that some of these artifacts also occur in other regions of the head and neck.

Three-dimensional reformations of the larynx, subglottic region, and hypopharynx can provide an endoscopic view through this region and supplement the diagnostic endoscopic examination (11,12). Such 3D images nicely display the areas of luminal narrowing as an airway cast and are therefore complementary to the cross-sectional images. The 3D display does not demonstrate the adjacent soft tissues (11). One group evaluating the value of such postprocessing showed that otolaryngologists ranked the 3D images as more beneficial than radiologists did, usually in bulky masses that precluded definitive direct endoscopic evaluation (12).

Three-dimensional reformations may also be used to display and calculate the volume of pharyngeal and laryngeal cancers. These data have proven useful in selecting treatment and evaluating tumor response to radiation and chemotherapy (13–15).

FIG. 6. Direct coronal image **(A)** through the sinuses and nasal cavity in comparison to coronal reformations **(B)** in the same patient. The reformatted image in the coronal plane **(B)** is of lower anatomic detail than the direct coronal image. The nonvisualization of the cribriform plate (*arrows*) on the right suggested invasive fungal disease in this patient status post–bone marrow transplant. The coronal reformation was performed from axial images acquired at a 1.25-mm slice thickness in helical multislice imaging mode using a pitch of 0.75 (3 : 1) and reconstructed at a 1-mm slice thickness. The follow-up scan **(A)** in direct coronal plane demonstrates progression of the sinus disease (*asterisk*) but no signs of invasive fungal disease because the cribriform plate (*arrows*) turned out to be intact.

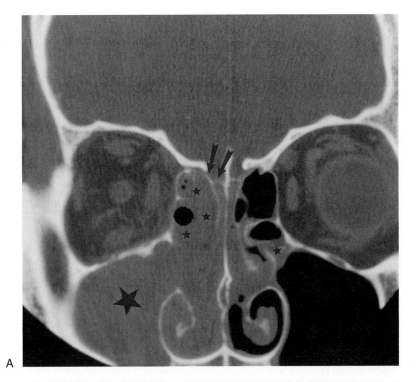

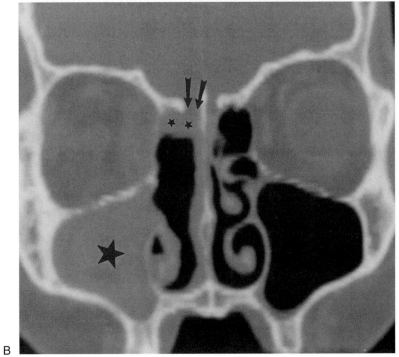

RADIATION EXPOSURE

The radiation dose to the patient is higher at all scan widths in multislice CT scanners than in conventional or single-slice helical CT scanners (8). This is independent of scanning mode; however, the dose increase is more pronounced when the helical scanning mode is used with a pitch of less than 1.0 (less than 4 : 1) because this helical path results in overlapping and interleaved slices, for example, 0.75 (HQ = 3 : 1) (6). The increased radiation dose, however, is partially compensated by decreased frequency of direct coronal images for certain patient population as outline already.

REFERENCES

1. Ohnesorge B, Flohr T, Schaller S, et al. Technische grundlagen und anwendungen der mehrschicht-CT. Radiologe 1999;39:923–931.
2. Mukherji SK, Castillo M, Huda W, et al. Comparison of dynamic and spiral CT for imaging of the glottic larynx. J Comput Assist Tomogr 1995;19:899–904.
3. Lell M, Baum U, Koester M, et al. Morphologische und funktionelle diagnostik der Kopf-Hals-region mit mehrzeilen-spiral-CT. Radiologe 1999;39:932–938.
4. Suojanen JN, Mukherji SK, Wippold FJ. Spiral CT of the larynx. AJNR 1994;15:1579–1582.
5. Craven CM, Naik KS, Blanshard KS, et al. Multispiral three-dimensional computed tomography in the investigation of craniosynostosis: technique optimization. Br J Radiol 1995;68:724–730.
6. Schorn C, Obenauer S, Funke M, et al. Schichtempfindlichkeitsprofile und bildpunktrauschen einer mehrschicht spiral-CT im vergleich zu einer einzelschicht spiral-CT. Rofo Fortschr Geb Rontgenstr Neuen Bildgeb Verfahr 1999;171:219–225.
7. Million RR, Cassissi N. Management of head and neck cancer: a multidisciplinary approach, 2nd ed. Philadelphia: JB Lippincott Co, 1994:431–461.
8. McCollough CH, Zink FE. Performance evaluation of a multi-slice CT system. Med Phys 1999;26:2223–2230.
9. Fleischmann D, Rubin GD, Paik DS, et al. Stair-step artifacts with single versus multiple detector-row helical CT. Radiology 2000;216:185–196.
10. Suojanen JN, Regan F. Spiral CT scanning of the paranasal sinuses. AJNR 1995;16:787–789.
11. Silverman PM, Zeiberg AS, Sessions RB, et al. Helical CT of the upper airway: normal and abnormal findings on three-dimensional reconstructed images. AJR Am J Roentgenol 1995;165:541–546.
12. Silverman PM, Zeiberg AS, Sesseions RB, et al. Three-dimensional (3D) imaging of the hypopharynx and larynx using helical CT: comparison of radiological and otolaryngological evaluation. Ann Otol Rhinol Otolaryngol 1995;104:425–431.
13. Mukherji SK, Mancuso AA, Kotzur IM, et al. Radiologic appearance of the irradiated larynx, Part II: primary site response. Radiology 1994;193:149–154.
14. Pameijer FA, Mancuso AA, Mendenhall WM, et al. Evaluation of pretreatment computed tomography as a predictor of local control in T1/T2 pyriform sinus carcinoma treated with definitive radiotherapy. Head Neck 1998; 20:159–168.
15. Pameijer FA, Mancuso AA, Mendenhall WM, et al. Can pretreatment computed tomography predict local control in T3 squamous cell carcinoma of the glottic larynx treated with definitive radiotherapy? Int J Radiat Oncol Biol Phys 1997;37:1011–1021.

Protocol 1:
HEAD (Fig. 7)

INDICATION:	*Routine*
SCANNER SETTINGS:	kV(p): 140 mA: 350–400
ORAL CONTRAST:	None
PHASE OF RESPIRATION:	Quiet breathing
ROTATION TIME:	1.0 sec
ACQUISITION SLICE THICKNESS:	5.0 mm
PITCH:	0.75–1.5 (HQ = 3:1; HS = 6:1) If the scanner is unable to perform the multislice helical imaging mode with the gantry in angled position, change the gantry angle to 0 degrees and reconstruct the images in the desired plane (see below) or use the multislice axial imaging mode.
RECONSTRUCTION SLICE THICKNESS/INTERVAL FOR FILMING:	5.0 mm/5.0 mm

ANATOMIC COVERAGE:
    SUPERIOR EXTENT:
    INFERIOR EXTENT:
	
	Top of the head
	Foramen magnum

IV CONTRAST:

Concentration:	Low osmolar contrast medium (LOCM) 300–320 mg iodine/mL or high osmolar conrast med (HOCM) 282 mg iodine/mL, 60% solution

Rate:	0.5 mL/sec
Scan Delay:	5 min after start of contrast infusion
Total Volume:	100 mL (minimum catheter size = 22 G)

COMMENTS:

1. **Note:** No contrast if hemorrhage, contusion, craniosynostosis, or hydrocephalus suspected.
2. **DATA RECONSTRUCTION:** Standard
3. **SCAN FIELD OF VIEW (FOV):** Head
4. **SCAN ANGLE:** IOML
5. **SAVE RAW DATA:** Yes
6. **DISPLAY FOV:** 21 cm in adults, less than 19 cm in children
7. Film in bone and soft tissue windows.
8. Consider three-dimensional reformations in patients with craniosynostosis. Change slice thickness to 1–1.25 mm and gantry angle to 0 degrees; use pitch of 0.75 (HQ = 3:1) for optimal quality of three-dimensional reformations.
9. Consider direct coronal images or reformations in coronal plane in patients with abnormalities of the posterior fossa. Change slice thickness to 2.5–3 mm and pitch to 0.75–1.0 (HQ = 3:1–4:1) through the posterior fossa.

FIG. 7. Three-dimensional images of a 10-month-old with a malformed head demonstrate brachycephaly *(B)* secondary to symmetric premature closure of the coronal sutures (*arrowheads*) and to a lesser extent of the lamboid sutures (*arrows*) bilaterally. The frontal fontanel (*open arrow*) remains open. The scan was performed with a 1.25-mm slice thickness using the helical multislice imaging mode with a pitch of 0.75 (3:1) and was reconstructed at a 1-mm slice thickness. With this technique, the three-dimensional images demonstrate no significant artifacts such as those seen with conventional or single-slice helical computed tomographic scanners, for example, squared edges called Lego effect.

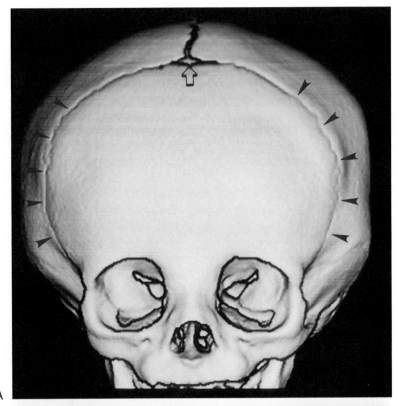

A

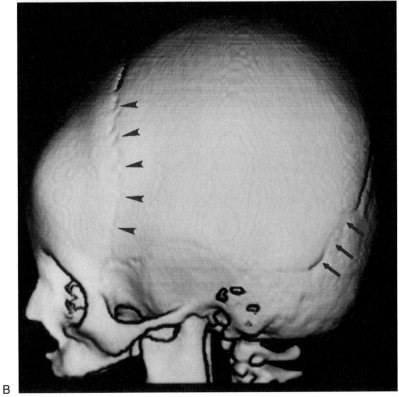

B

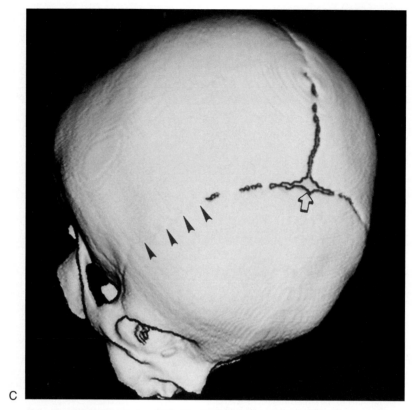

C

FIG. 7. *Continued.*

Protocol 2:
CAVERNOUS SINUS/SELLA (Fig. 8)

INDICATION:	*Suspected microadenoma or macroadenoma of the pituitary gland; mass in cavernous sinus, cavernous sinus thrombosis*
SCANNER SETTINGS:	kV(p): 140 mA: 350–400
ORAL CONTRAST:	None
PHASE OF RESPIRATION:	Quiet breathing
ROTATION TIME:	0.5–0.8 sec through cavernous sinus and sella 1.0 sec through the head
ACQUISITION SLICE THICKNESS:	1.0–1.25 mm through cavernous sinus and sella 5.0 mm through the rest of the head
PITCH:	0.75–1 (HQ = 3:1) through cavernous sinus and sella 1.0–1.5 (HS = 6:1) through the rest of the head If the scanner is unable to perform the multislice helical imaging mode with the gantry in angled position • change for *axial* imaging plane the gantry angle to 0 degrees and reconstruct the images in the desired plane (see below) or use the multislice axial imaging mode • obtain coronal images using the multislice axial imaging mode
RECONSTRUCTION SLICE THICKNESS/INTERVAL FOR FILMING:	2.0–2.5 mm/2.0–2.5 mm from hard palate to superior margin of cavernous sinus 5.0/5.0 mm through rest of the head

ANATOMIC COVERAGE:	*Axial:*	*Coronal*
SUPERIOR EXTENT:	Top of head	Orbital apex
INFERIOR EXTENT:	Hard palate	Dorsum sellae

IV CONTRAST:

Concentration:	LOCM 300–320 mg iodine/mL or HOCM 282 mg iodine/mL, 60% solution
Rate:	1 mL/sec (40-mL bolus) 0.7 mL/sec (60-mL infusion)
Scan Delay:	40 sec
Total Volume:	150 mL (minimum catheter size = 22 G) 100 mL for axial and 50 mL for coronal images

COMMENTS:

1. **DATA RECONSTRUCTION:** Standard
2. **SCAN FOV:** Head
3. **SCAN ANGLE:** *Axial:* Parallel to IOML *Coronal:* Perpendicular to IOML
4. **SAVE RAW DATA:** Yes, bone algorithm through cavernous sinus and sella
5. **DISPLAY FOV:** 21 cm through the entire head, 10 cm through cavernous sinus/sella
6. Film in bone and soft tissue windows.
7. Perform reformations of the axial images in coronal plane if patient unable to tolerate direct coronal imaging. Use a pitch of 0.75 (HQ = 3:1). Reduce the contrast volume to 100 mL.

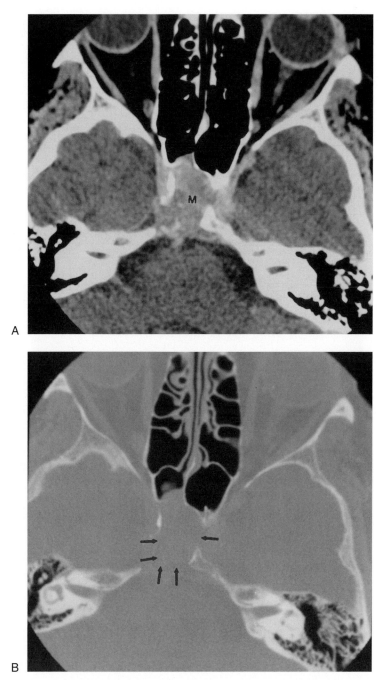

FIG. 8. Axial **(A, B)** and direct coronal **(C, D)** contrasted computed tomographic images through the sella demonstrate a macroadenoma *(M)* of the pituitary gland causing enlargement of the sella and destruction of the lateral and posterior walls (*arrows*). The infundibulum (*white arrowhead*) is displaced to the left. The macroadenoma is extending into the suprasellar cistern (*black arrowheads*) but does not impinge upon the optic nerves (*asterisk*).

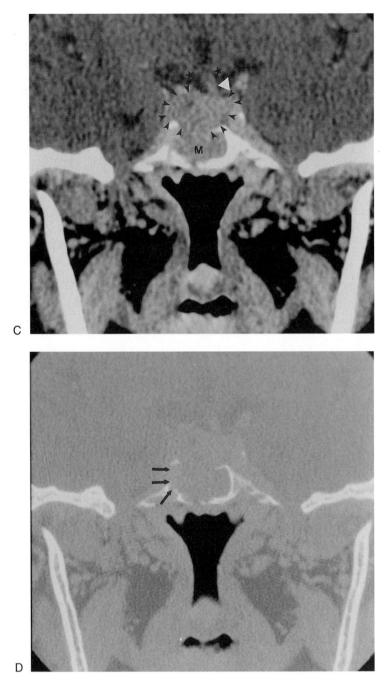

FIG. 8. *Continued.*

Protocol 3:
TEMPORAL BONE WITHOUT IV
CONTRAST (Fig. 9)

INDICATION:	*Evaluation of trauma, congenital abnormalities, localized infectious or inflammatory disease, pulsatile tinnitus with visible middle ear mass on clinical examination, petrous apex mass*
SCANNER SETTINGS:	kV(p): 140 mA: 300–400
ORAL CONTRAST:	None
PHASE OF RESPIRATION:	Quiet breathing
ROTATION TIME:	0.5–1.0 sec
ACQUISITION SLICE THICKNESS:	0.5–1.25 mm
PITCH:	0.75–1.0 (HQ = 3:1–4:1) If the scanner is unable to perform the multislice helical imaging mode with the gantry in angled position • change for *axial* imaging plane the gantry angle to 0 degrees and reconstruct the images in the desired plane (see below) or use the multislice axial imaging mode • obtain coronal images using the multislice axial imaging mode
RECONSTRUCTION SLICE THICKNESS/INTERVAL FOR FILMING:	0.5–1.0 mm/0.5–1.0 mm

ANATOMIC COVERAGE:	*Axial:*	*Coronal:*
SUPERIOR EXTENT:	Top of temporal bone (TB)	Anterior margin of TB
INFERIOR EXTENT:	Tip of mastoid	Posterior margin of TB
IV CONTRAST:	None	

COMMENTS:

1. **DATA RECONSTRUCTION:** Standard
2. **SCAN FOV:** Head
3. **SCAN ANGLE:** *Axial:* IOML
   Coronal: Perpendicular to IOML
4. **SAVE RAW DATA:** Yes, bone algorithm
5. **DISPLAY FOV:** 9–10 cm
6. Film every image in bone and every third image in soft tissue window.
7. Perform reformations of the axial images in coronal plane if patient unable to tolerate direct coronal imaging. Use a pitch of 0.75 (HQ = 3:1).

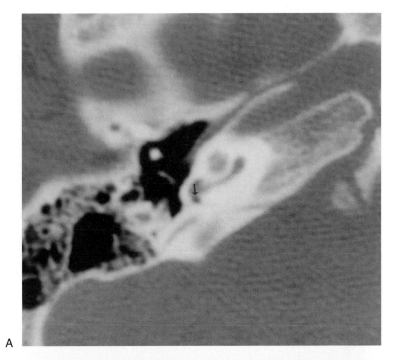

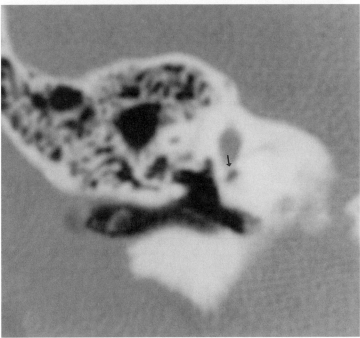

FIG. 9. Axial **(A)** noncontrasted CT image filmed in bone window through the temporal bone demonstrates a smaller than typically seen round window (*arrow*) in a child with sensorineural hearing loss. The direct coronal image **(B)** shows thickening of the round window (*arrow*) and excellent bony detail when compared to the reformatted image in coronal plane **(C).** The reformatted image **(C)** demonstrates fuzzy edges of the various bony structures but better delineates the small size of the round window (*arrow*) since the reformation plane was aligned parallel to the round window itself. The coronal reformation was performed from axial images acquired at 1.25 mm slice thickness in helical multislice imaging mode using a pitch of 0.75 (3 : 1) and reconstructed at 1 mm slice thickness.

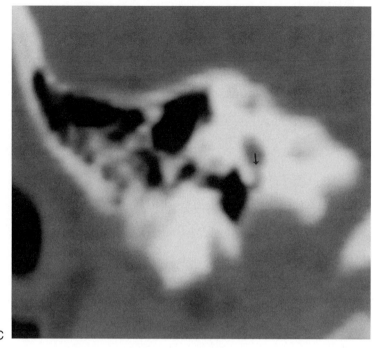

C

FIG. 9. *Continued.*

Protocol 4:
TEMPORAL BONE WITH IV CONTRAST
(Fig. 10)

INDICATION:	*Evaluation of infectious or inflammatory disease suspected to extend beyond the middle ear, pulsatile tinnitus without a visible middle ear mass on clinical examination, malignant tumor of the TB*
SCANNER SETTINGS:	kV(p): 140 mA: 300–400
ORAL CONTRAST:	None
PHASE OF RESPIRATION:	Quiet breathing
ROTATION TIME:	0.5–1.0 sec
ACQUISITION SLICE THICKNESS:	0.5–1.25 mm through temporal bones 5 mm through rest of the head
PITCH:	0.75–1.0 (HQ = 3:1–4:1) through temporal bones 1.0–1.5 (4:1 − HS = 6:1) through rest of the head If the scanner is unable to perform the multislice helical imaging mode with the gantry in angled position • change for *axial* imaging plane the gantry angle to 0 degrees and reconstruct the images in the desired plane (see below) or use the multislice axial imaging mode • obtain coronal images using the multislice axial imaging mode
RECONSTRUCTION SLICE THICKNESS/INTERVAL FOR FILMING:	0.5–1.0 mm/0.5–1.0 mm through TB 5.0 mm/5.0 mm through rest of the head

ANATOMIC COVERAGE:	*Axial:*	*Coronal:*
SUPERIOR EXTENT:	Top of the head	Orbital apex
INFERIOR EXTENT:	Hard palate	Occiput

IV CONTRAST:

Concentration:	LOCM 300–320 mg iodine/mL or HOCM 282 mg iodine/mL, 60% solution
Rate:	1 mL/sec
Scan Delay:	60 sec
Total Volume:	150 mL (minimum catheter size = 22 G) 100 mL for axial and 50 mL for coronal images

COMMENTS:

1. **DATA RECONSTRUCTION:** Standard
2. **SCAN FOV:** Head
3. **SCAN ANGLE:** *Axial:* IOML
   Coronal: Perpendicular to IOML
4. **SAVE RAW DATA:** Yes, bone algorithm through TB
5. **DISPLAY FOV:** 9–10 cm through TB, 19–21 cm through rest
6. Film every image in bone and every third image in soft tissue window through TB and all images in soft tissue through the rest.
7. Perform reformations of the axial images in coronal plane if patient unable to tolerate direct coronal imaging. Use a pitch of 0.75 (HQ = 3:1) and reduce the contrast volume to 100 mL.
8. *Malignant tumors of TB:* Change superior extent to the roof of the orbit and inferior extent to hard palate; obtain coronal images only through the TB; include neck survey (see specific protocol) for evaluation of nodal disease.

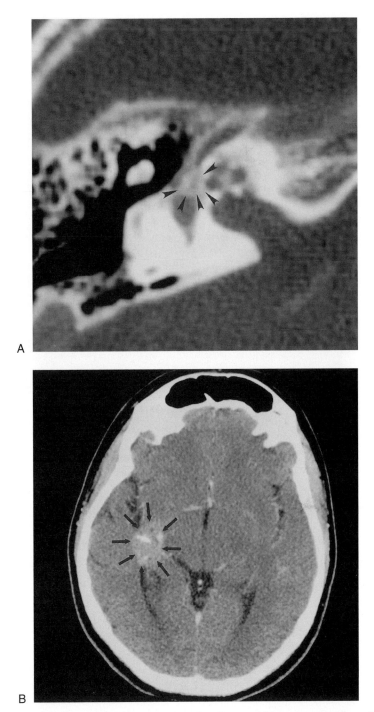

FIG. 10. Computed tomographic (CT) images of a 48-year-old man presenting with pulsatile tinnitus. The axial CT image **(A)** in the bone window demonstrates a focal area of hypodensity at the fenestra ad antrum (*arrowheads*) consistent with a small focus of otosclerosis in the lytic phase. Otosclerosis typically causes hearing loss but not pulsatile tinnitus. The axial **(B)** and coronal **(C)** images performed with contrast over the brain reveal a hypervascular mass (*arrows*) in the mesial temporal lobe on the right, containing large vessels within it. This was confirmed by magnetic resonance imaging to be an arteriovenous malformation—the source of the patient's pulsatile tinnitus.

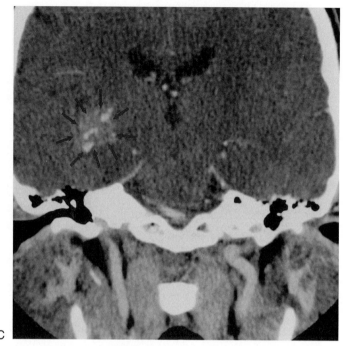

C

FIG. 10. *Continued.*

Protocol 5:
ORBIT (Fig. 11)

INDICATION:	*Trauma, infectious or inflammatory disease, tumor*
SCANNER SETTINGS:	kV(p): 140 mA: 250–350
ORAL CONTRAST:	None
PHASE OF RESPIRATION:	Quiet respiration
ROTATION TIME:	0.5–0.8 sec
ACQUISITION SLICE THICKNESS:	1.0–1.25 mm
PITCH:	0.75–1.5 (HQ = 3:1; HS = 6:1) If the scanner is unable to perform the multislice helical imaging mode with the gantry in angled position • change for *axial* imaging plane the gantry angle to 0 degrees and reconstruct the images in the desired plane (see below) or use the multislice axial imaging mode • obtain coronal images using the multislice axial imaging mode
RECONSTRUCTION SLICE THICKNESS/INTERVAL FOR FILMING:	2.5–3.0 mm

ANATOMIC COVERAGE:	*Axial:*	*Coronal:*
SUPERIOR EXTENT:	Top of frontal sinus	Anterior wall of the frontal sinus
INFERIOR EXTENT:	Hard palate	Dorsum sellae

IV CONTRAST:	**Concentration:**	LOCM 300–320 mg iodine/mL or HOCM 282 mg iodine/mL, 60% solution
	Rate:	1 mL/sec
	Scan Delay:	60 sec

Total Volume:	150 mL (minimum catheter size = 22 G) 100 mL for axial and 50 mL for coronal images

COMMENTS:

1. **DATA RECONSTRUCTION:** Standard
2. **SCAN FOV:** Head
3. **SCAN ANGLE:** IOML
4. **SAVE RAW DATA:** Yes, bone algorithm
5. **DISPLAY FOV:** 15–17 cm
6. Film in bone and soft tissue windows.
7. Perform reformations of the axial images in coronal plane if patient unable to tolerate direct coronal imaging. Change the pitch to 0.75 (HQ = 3:1) and reduce the contrast to 100 mL.
8. *Trauma or endocrine exophthalmus:* No contrast.
9. *Lesion limited to globe:* Change superior extent to roof of the orbit and inferior extent to floor of the orbit; use a reconstruction slice thickness of 1–1.25 mm. Typically, coronal imaging is not necessary.
10. *Retinoblastoma:* Obtain images through the orbit with and without contrast. Use a reconstruction slice thickness of 1–1.25 mm through the orbits. Include imaging through the rest of the head with contrast with a slice thickness of 5 mm and a pitch of 1–1.5 (4:1 − HS = 6:1). Typically, coronal imaging is not necessary.
11. *Varix suspected:* Consider additional scanning with Valsalva maneuver or in prone position.

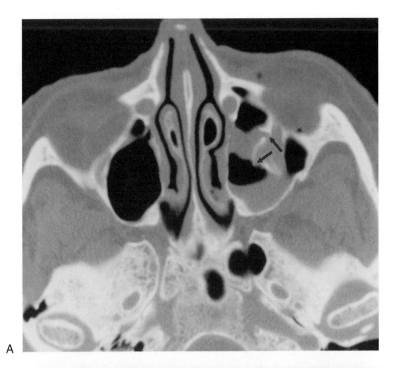

A

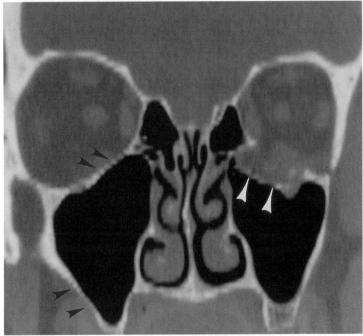

B

FIG. 11. Axial computed tomographic image through the orbit filmed in the bone window **(A)** demonstrates a complex fracture through the floor of the orbit on the left extending across the infraorbital canal (*arrows*). The reformatted images in the coronal plane **(B, C)** better delineate the significant displacement of the fracture fragments (*white arrowheads*) into the maxillary sinus and the prolapse of intraorbital fat (*white arrow*) into the fracture site. There is also a small hematoma (*asterisk*) between the fracture fragments and the inferior rectus muscle *(m)*. The coronal reformation was performed from axial images acquired at a 1.25-mm slice thickness in multislice imaging mode without the helical mode. Notice the mild stair artifacts (*black arrowheads*).

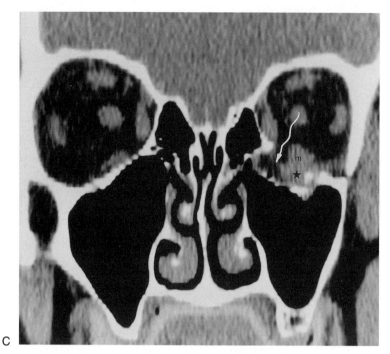

C

FIG. 11. *Continued.*

Protocol 6:
VISUAL PATHWAY (Fig. 12)

INDICATION:	*Suspected inflammatory disease, benign or malignant tumor of the optic nerve, chiasm, optic tracts and/or cortex*
SCANNER SETTINGS:	kV(p): 140 mA: 300–400
ORAL CONTRAST:	None
PHASE OF RESPIRATION:	Quiet breathing
ROTATION TIME:	0.5–1.0 sec
ACQUISITION SLICE THICKNESS:	1.0–1.25 mm through orbits 5.0 mm through rest of the head
PITCH:	0.75–1.0 (HQ = 3:1) through the orbits 1–1.5 (HS = 6:1) through the rest of the head If the scanner is unable to perform the multislice helical imaging mode with the gantry in angled position • change for *axial* imaging plane the gantry angle to 0 degrees and reconstruct the images in the desired plane (see below) or use the multislice axial imaging mode • obtain coronal images using the multislice axial imaging mode
RECONSTRUCTION SLICE THICKNESS/INTERVAL FOR FILMING:	1.0–1.25 mm/1.0–1.25 mm through orbit in axial plane 1.0–1.25 mm/1.0–1.25 mm through the orbital apex and optic canal in coronal plane 2.0–2.5 mm/2.0–2.5 mm through rest of the orbit in coronal plane 5.0 mm/5.0 mm through rest of the head

	Axial:	*Coronal:*
ANATOMIC COVERAGE:		
SUPERIOR EXTENT:	Top of the head	Posterior margin of globe
INFERIOR EXTENT:	Hard palate	Dorsum sellae

IV CONTRAST:

Concentration:	LOCM 300–320 mg iodine/mL or HOCM 282 mg iodine/mL, 60%
Rate:	1 mL/sec
Scan Delay:	60 sec
Total Volume:	150 mL (minimum catheter size = 22 G) 100 mL for axial and 50 mL for coronal images

COMMENTS:

1. **DATA RECONSTRUCTION:** Standard
2. **SCAN FOV:** Head
3. **SCAN ANGLE:** IOML
4. **SAVE RAW DATA:** Yes, bone algorithm.
5. **DISPLAY FOV:** 15–17 cm through orbit; 19–21 cm through head
6. Film in bone and soft tissue windows.
7. Perform reformations of the axial images in coronal plane if patient unable to tolerate direct coronal imaging. Use a pitch of 0.75 (HQ = 3:1) and reduce the contrast to 100 mL.

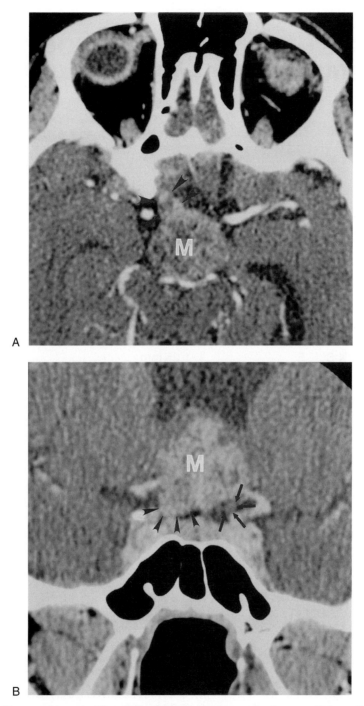

FIG. 12. A 45-year-old man with unilateral visual problems of unknown etiology. The axial **(A)** and direct coronal **(B)** computed tomographic images performed with intravenous contrast demonstrate a large suprasellar mass *(M)* with inhomogeneous enhancement. The mass is extending anteriorly along the right optic nerve (*arrowheads*). The right optic nerve could not be identified as a separate structure. The left optic nerve (*arrows*) is slightly displaced inferiorly by the suprasellar mass. No calcifications were seen within the mass. This mass was resected and a craniopharyngioma was diagnosed on pathologic examination.

Protocol 7:
SINUSES/NASAL CAVITY WITHOUT IV
CONTRAST (Figs. 6 and 13)

INDICATION:

Evaluation of routine infectious or inflammatory disease (e.g., patients with chronic sinusitis being considered for functional endoscopic sinus surgery), congenital abnormalities of the nasal cavity

SCANNER SETTINGS:

kV(p): 120
mA: 200–250

ORAL CONTRAST:

None

PHASE OF RESPIRATION:

Quiet breathing

ROTATION TIME:

0.5–0.8 sec

ACQUISITION SLICE THICKNESS:

1–1.25 mm

PITCH:

0.75–1.0 (HQ = 3:1)
If the scanner is unable to perform the multislice helical imaging mode with the gantry in angled position, change the gantry angle to 0 degrees and reconstruct the images in the desired plane (see below) or use the multislice axial imaging mode.

RECONSTRUCTION SLICE THICKNESS/INTERVAL FOR FILMING:

2.5–3.0 mm/2.5–3.0 mm

ANATOMIC COVERAGE:
    SUPERIOR EXTENT:

Top of frontal sinus

    INFERIOR EXTENT:

Bottom of maxilla

IV CONTRAST:

None

COMMENTS:

1. **DATA RECONSTRUCTION:** Bone
2. **SCAN FOV:** Head
3. **SCAN ANGLE:** No angulation of gantry
4. **SAVE RAW DATA:** Yes, bone algorithm
5. **DISPLAY FOV:** 15–17 cm

6. Film in bone and soft tissue windows.
7. Perform reformations of the axial images in coronal plane perpendicular to IOML.
8. Consider direct coronal images from anterior wall of the frontal sinus to dorsum sellae in patients with suspected small encephalocele or early bone erosion.

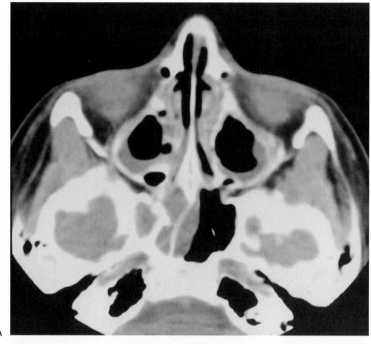

A

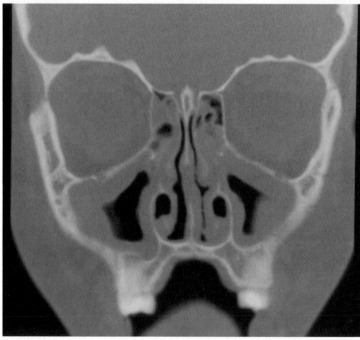

B

FIG. 13. Axial computed tomographic image **(A)** and reformatted image in coronal plane **(B)** demonstrate diffuse mucoperiosteal thickening in all sinuses consistent with pansinusitis secondary to allergic disease. The coronal reformation was performed from axial images acquired at a 1.25-mm slice thickness in helical multislice imaging mode using a pitch of 0.75 (3 : 1) and reconstructed at a 1-mm slice thickness. The bony detail is very good and sufficient for imaging of patients who are suspected of having simple sinus disease. However, if aggressive sinus disease or a malignant process is suspected, direct coronal imaging should be preferred (see also Fig. 6).

Protocol 8:
SINUSES/NASAL CAVITY WITH IV
CONTRAST (Fig. 14)

INDICATION:	_Evaluation of infectious or inflammatory disease suspected to extend beyond the sinuses to the brain or orbits, mucocele, benign or malignant tumor_
SCANNER SETTINGS:	kV(p): 120 mA: 250–300
ORAL CONTRAST:	None
PHASE OF RESPIRATION:	Quiet breathing
ROTATION TIME:	0.5–0.8 sec
ACQUISITION SLICE THICKNESS:	1.0–1.25 mm
PITCH:	0.75–1.0 (HQ = 3:1) If the scanner is unable to perform the multislice helical imaging mode with the gantry in angled position • change for _axial_ imaging plane the gantry angle to 0 degrees and reconstruct the images in the desired plane (see below) or use the multislice axial imaging mode • obtain coronal images using the multislice axial imaging mode
RECONSTRUCTION SLICE THICKNESS/INERVAL FOR FILMING:	2.5–3 mm/2.5–3.0 mm

ANATOMIC COVERAGE:	_Axial:_	_Coronal:_
SUPERIOR EXTENT:	Top of frontal sinus	Nasal tip
INFERIOR EXTENT:	Bottom of maxilla	Dorsum sellae

IV CONTRAST:	**Concentration:**	LOCM 300–320 mg iodine/mL or HOCM 282 mg iodine/mL, 60%

Rate:	1 mL/sec
Scan Delay:	60 sec
Total Volume:	150 mL (minimum catheter size = 22 G)
	100 mL for axial and 50 mL for coronal images

COMMENTS:

1. **DATA RECONSTRUCTION:** Standard
2. **SCAN FOV:** Head
3. **SCAN ANGLE:** *Axial:* Parallel to IOML
   Coronal: Perpendicular to IOML
4. **SAVE RAW DATA:** Yes, bone algorithm
5. **DISPLAY FOV:** 15–17 cm
6. Film in bone and soft tissue windows.
7. Perform reformations of the axial images in coronal plane if patient unable to tolerate direct coronal imaging. Use a pitch of 0.75 (HQ = 3:1). Reduce the contrast volume to 100 mL.
8. *Suspicion for sinus thrombosis:* Include images through the rest of the head with 5-mm slice thickness and a pitch of 1–1.5 (4:1 − HS = 6:1).
9. *Malignant tumors:* Include neck survey (see specific protocol) to evaluate for nodal disease.

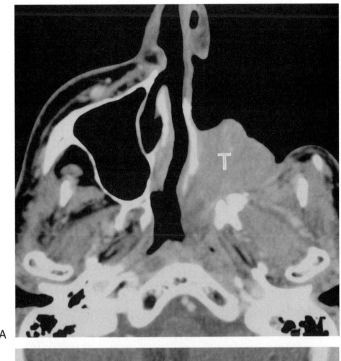

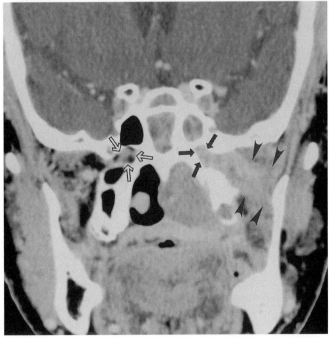

FIG. 14. A 52-year-old man status post–maxillary sinus surgery for cancer presenting with numbness in trigeminal nerve distribution. The axial **(A)** and coronal **(B)** computed tomographic images through the sinuses demonstrate recurrent tumor *(T)* along the posterior aspect of the maxillary sinus on the left side. The tumor extends posteriorly to involve the masticator space (*arrowheads*) and the pterygopalatine fossa (*arrows*) on the left. Notice the obscuration of the fat planes within the pterygopalatine fossa on the left (*arrows*) when compared with the right (*open arrow*). Even more posteriorly, **(C)** gross tumor was seen just beneath and within the oval foramen (*arrowheads*) consistent with perineural tumor spread along V3. The coronal image **(D)** in bone window demonstrates the mild widening of the oval foramen on the left (*arrows*) when compared with the right (*arrowheads*).

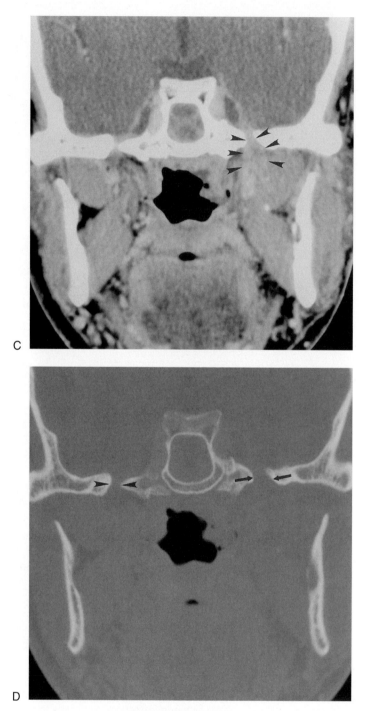

FIG. 14. *Continued.*

Protocol 9:
FACIAL BONES (Fig. 15)

INDICATION:	*Tumor, trauma, congenital*
SCANNER SETTINGS:	kV(p): 120 mA: 250–300
ORAL CONTRAST:	None
PHASE OF RESPIRATION:	Quiet breathing
ROTATION TIME:	0.5–0.8 sec
ACQUISITION SLICE THICKNESS:	1.0–1.25 mm
PITCH:	0.75 (HQ = 3:1)
RECONSTRUCTION SLICE THICKNESS/INTERVAL FOR FILMING:	2.5–3.0 mm/2.5–3.0 mm

ANATOMIC COVERAGE:
  SUPERIOR EXTENT:
  INFERIOR EXTENT:
	
	Top of the frontal sinus
	Bottom of the mandible

IV CONTRAST:	None

COMMENTS:

1. **DATA RECONSTRUCTION:** Standard
2. **SCAN FOV:** Head
3. **SCAN ANGLE:** No angulation of gantry.
4. **SAVE RAW DATA:** Yes, bone algorithm
5. **DISPLAY FOV:** 15–17 cm
6. Film in bone and soft tissue windows.
7. Perform reformations of the axial images in coronal plane perpendicular to the IOML.
8. Consider three-dimensional reformations in patients for surgical facial reconstruction. Perform the data acquisition in standard soft tissue algorithm.

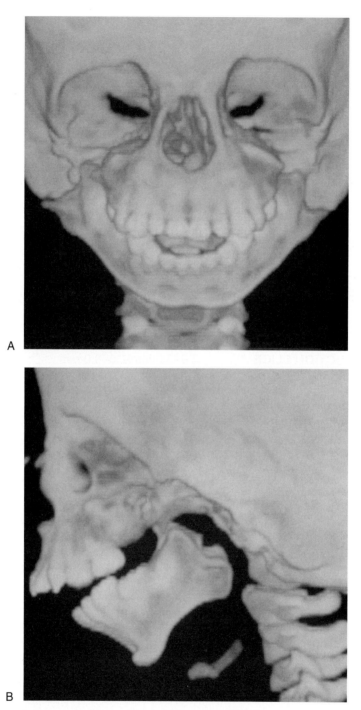

A

B

FIG. 15. Three-dimensional (3D) views in anteroposterior **(A)** and lateral projection **(B)**, as well as coronal reformation image **(C)**, of a patient with Treacher Collins syndrome. The 3D images **(A, B)** very well demonstrate the small midface and the severely hypoplastic mandible. The coronal image **(C)** shows a large defect (*arrows*) in the midportion of the hard palate consistent with cleft palate.

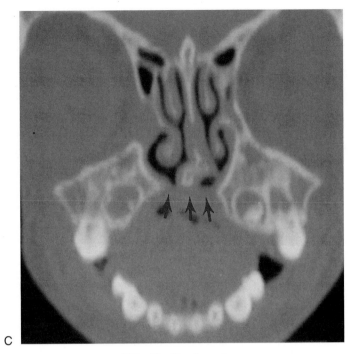

C

FIG. 15. *Continued.*

Protocol 10:
NASOPHARYNX/PARAPHARYNGEAL
SPACE/RETROPHARYNGEAL
SPACE/MASTICATOR SPACE (Fig. 16)

INDICATION:	*Tumor, inflammatory disease, infection*
SCANNER SETTINGS:	kV(p): 140 mA: 250–350 through nasopharynx and skull base 220–260 through upper neck
ORAL CONTRAST:	None
PHASE OF RESPIRATION:	Quiet breathing
ROTATION TIME:	0.5–0.8 sec

**ACQUISITION SLICE
   THICKNESS:**
	1.0–1.25 mm through nasopharynx and skull
	   base
	2.5–3 mm through rest of the neck

PITCH:	0.75–1.0 (HQ = 3:1) through the
	   nasopharynx and skull base
	1.0–1.5 (HS = 6:1) through the rest of
	   the neck
	If the scanner is unable to perform the
	   multislice helical imaging mode with the
	   gantry in angled position
	 • change for *axial* imaging plane the gantry
	   angle to 0 degrees and reconstruct the
	   images in the desired plane (see below)
	   or use the multislice axial imaging mode
	 • obtain coronal images using the multislice
	   axial imaging mode

**RECONSTRUCTION SLICE
   THICKNESS/INTERVAL
   FOR FILMING:**
	2.5–3.0 mm/2.5–3.0 mm

ANATOMIC COVERAGE:	*Axial:*	*Coronal:*
SUPERIOR EXTENT:	Top of sella	Anterior wall of frontal sinus
INFERIOR EXTENT:	Hyoid bone	Dorsum sellae

IV CONTRAST:

Concentration:	LOCM 300–320 mg iodine/mL or HOCM 282 mg iodine/mL, 60% solution
Rate:	1 mL/sec
Scan Delay:	60 sec
Total Volume:	150 mL (minimum catheter size = 22 G) 100 mL for axial and 50 mL for coronal

COMMENTS:

1. **DATA RECONSTRUCTION:** Standard
2. **SCAN FOV:** Head
3. **SCAN ANGLE:** *Axial:* IOML and parallel to the long axis of the mandible (change angle around teeth)
   Coronal: Perpendicular to IOML
4. **SAVE RAW DATA:** Yes, bone algorithm through skull base
5. **DISPLAY FOV:** 16–19 cm
6. Film all images in soft tissue window and only the images through the skull base in both planes in bone window.
7. Perform reformations of the axial images in coronal plane if patient unable to tolerate direct coronal imaging. Use a pitch of 0.75 (HQ = 3:1). Reduce the contrast volume to 100 mL.
8. *Infectious or inflammatory disease:* Continue scanning through the upper chest with slice thickness of 5 mm and a pitch of 1–1.5 (4:1 − HS = 6:1) if retropharyngeal abscess is present or suspected.
9. *Malignant tumors:* Include neck survey (see specific protocol) to evaluate for nodal disease.

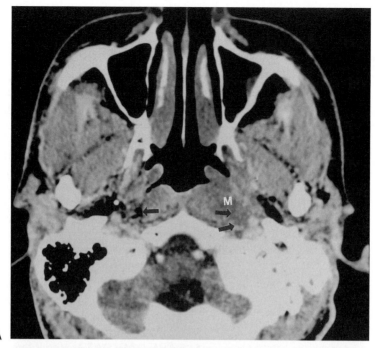

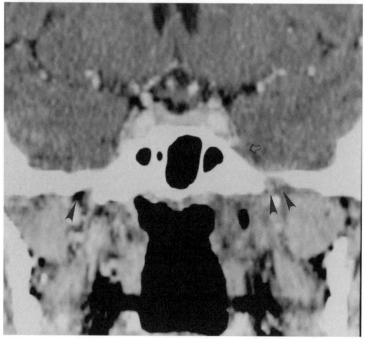

FIG. 16. Axial computed tomographic image **(A)** and reformatted image in the coronal plane **(B, C)** in a patient with persistent nasopharyngeal cancer. The axial image **(A)** demonstrates an infiltrating mass *(M)* in the left nasopharynx with obliteration of the deep fat planes when compared with the right side *(arrow)*. The coronal reformations **(B, C)** also show obliteration of the fat pad *(arrowheads)* below the oval foramen on the left, early invasion of the cavernous sinus on the left *(open arrow)*, and widening of the foramen itself *(curved arrow)*. The coronal reformation was performed from axial images acquired at a 1.25-mm slice thickness in helical multislice imaging mode using a pitch of 0.75 (3 : 1) and reconstructed at a 1.0-mm slice thickness. If gross bony erosions are suspected, coronal reformations are usually sufficient for tumor staging; however, when there is concern of subtle bony erosions, direct coronal images should be preferred.

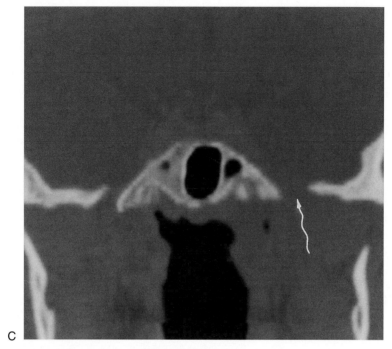

C

FIG. 16. *Continued.*

Protocol 11:
PAROTID GLAND (Fig. 17)

INDICATION:	*Tumor, inflammatory disease, infection*
SCANNER SETTINGS:	kV(p): 140 mA: 250–350 through the maxillofacial area 220–260 through the upper neck
ORAL CONTRAST:	None
PHASE OF RESPIRATION:	Quiet breathing
ROTATION TIME:	0.5–0.8 sec
ACQUISITION SLICE THICKNESS:	1.0–2.5 mm
PITCH:	0.75–1.5 (HQ = 3:1; HS = 6:1) If the scanner is unable to perform the multislice helical imaging mode with the gantry in angled position, change the gantry angle to 0 degrees and reconstruct the images in the desired plane (see below) or use the multislice axial imaging mode.
RECONSTRUCTION SLICE THICKNESS/INTERVAL FOR FILMING:	2.5–3.0 mm/2.5–3.0 mm

ANATOMIC COVERAGE:
   SUPERIOR EXTENT:
   INFERIOR EXTENT:
	
	Bottom of sella
	Hyoid bone

IV CONTRAST:

Concentration:	LOCM 300–320 mg iodine/mL or HOCM 282 mg iodine/mL, 60% solution
Rate:	1 mL/sec
Scan Delay:	60 sec
Total Volume:	100 mL (minimum catheter size = 22 G)

COMMENTS:

1. **DATA RECONSTRUCTION:** Standard
2. **SCAN FOV:** Head
3. **SCAN ANGLE:** IOML and parallel to the long axis of the mandible (change angle around the teeth)
4. **SAVE RAW DATA:** Yes, bone algorithm through skull base
5. **DISPLAY FOV:** 16–19 cm
6. Film all images in soft tissue window and only the images through the skull base in bone window.
7. *Malignant tumors:* Include neck survey (see specific protocol) to evaluate for nodal disease.
8. *With facial nerve palsy:* Include scanning through the TB (see specific protocol).

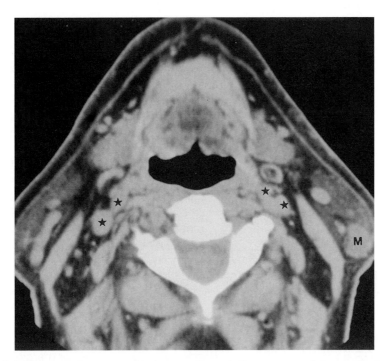

FIG. 17. Axial computed tomographic images through the upper neck in a patient with a benign parotid gland mass *(M)* on the left side. Notice suboptimal enhancement of the vasculature *(asterisk)* at this level. The scan was performed with a total of 100 mL of contrast; however, it was administered at a rate of 1 mL per second with a scan delay of 20 seconds. The scan delay was too short for the injection rate to allow for homogenous and optimal enhancement of the vessels.

Protocol 12:
SOFT/HARD PALATE (Fig. 18)

INDICATION:	*Tumor, inflammatory disease, infection*
SCANNER SETTINGS:	kV(p): 140 mA: :250–350 through the maxillofacial area 220–260 through the upper neck
ORAL CONTRAST:	None
PHASE OF RESPIRATION:	Quiet breathing
ROTATION TIME:	0.5–0.8 sec
ACQUISITION SLICE THICKNESS:	1.0–1.25 mm through nasal cavity, oral cavity and oropharynx 2.5–3.0 through rest of the neck
PITCH:	0.75–1.0 (HQ = 3:1) through the nasal cavity, oral cavity, and oropharynx 1.0–1.5 (HS = 6:1) through the rest of the neck If the scanner is unable to perform the multislice helical imaging mode with the gantry in angled position • change for *axial* imaging plane the gantry angle to 0 degrees and reconstruct the images in the desired plane (see below) or use the multislice axial imaging mode • obtain coronal images using the multislice axial imaging mode
RECONSTRUCTION SLICE THICKNESS/INTERVAL FOR FILMING:	2.5–3.0 mm/2.5–3.0 mm

ANATOMIC COVERAGE:	*Axial:*	*Coronal:*
SUPERIOR EXTENT:	Bottom of sella	Anterior margin of maxilla
INFERIOR EXTENT:	Hyoid bone	Anterior margin of cervical spine

IV CONTRAST:

Concentration:	LOCM 300–320 mg iodine/mL or HOCM 282 mg iodine/mL, 60% solution
Rate:	1 mL/sec
Scan Delay:	60 sec
Total Volume:	150 mL (minimum catheter size = 22 G)
	100 mL for axial and 50 mL for coronal images

COMMENTS:

1. **DATA RECONSTRUCTION:** Standard
2. **SCAN FOV:** Head
3. **SCAN ANGLE:** *Axial:* IOML and parallel to the long axis of the mandible (change angle around teeth)
   Coronal: Perpendicular to IOML
4. **SAVE RAW DATA:** Yes, bone algorithm through hard palate
5. **DISPLAY FOV:** 16–19 cm
6. Film all images in soft tissue window and only the images through the hard palate in bone window.
7. Perform reformations of the axial images in coronal plane if patient unable to tolerate direct coronal imaging. Use a pitch of 0.75 (HQ = 3:1). Reduce the contrast volume to 100 mL.
8. *Malignant tumors:* Include neck survey (see specific protocol) to evaluate for nodal disease.

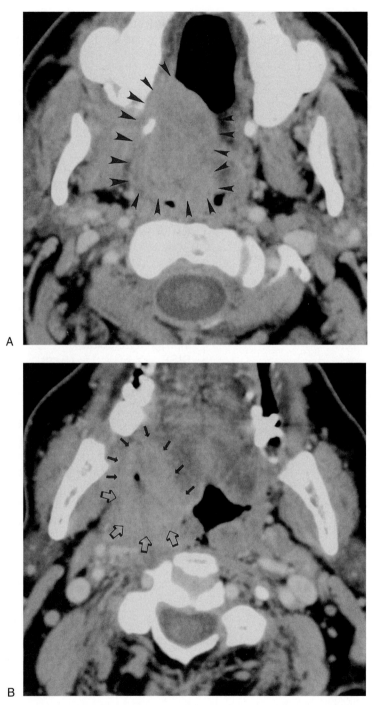

FIG. 18. Axial computed tomographic images through the soft palate and oropharynx demonstrate a large-volume infiltrating mass **(A)** centered in the right soft palate (*arrowheads*) and extending **(B)** inferiorly to involve the tonsillar fossa (*open arrow*) and glossotonsillar sulcus (*small arrows*). The tumor is growing clearly across midline at the level of the soft palate **(A).**

Protocol 13:
OROPHARYNX/ORAL CAVITY/FLOOR OF THE MOUTH (Fig. 19)

INDICATION: *Tumor, inflammatory disease, infection excluding involvement of the soft and hard palates (see separate imaging protocol)*

SCANNER SETTINGS: kV(p): 140
mA: 250–350 through the maxillofacial area
220–260 through the upper neck

ORAL CONTRAST: None

PHASE OF RESPIRATION: Quiet breathing

ROTATION TIME: 0.5–0.8 sec

ACQUISITION SLICE THICKNESS (COLLIMATION): 1.0–1.25 mm through oropharynx
2.5–3.0 mm through rest of neck

PITCH: 0.75–1.0 (HQ = 3:1) through orophaynx
1.0–1.5 (HS = 6:1) through rest of neck
If the scanner is unable to perform the multislice helical imaging mode with the gantry in angled position, change the gantry angle to 0 degrees and reconstruct the images in the desired plane (see below) or use the multislice axial imaging mode.

RECONSTRUCTION SLICE THICKNESS/INTERVAL FOR FILMING: 2.5–3.0 mm/2.5–3.0 mm

ANATOMIC COVERAGE:
SUPERIOR EXTENT: Floor of the orbit
INFERIOR EXTENT: Hyoid bone

IV CONTRAST:

Concentration:	LOCM 300–320 mg \ iodine/mL or HOCM 282 mg iodine/mL, 60% solution
Rate:	1 mL/sec
Scan Delay:	60 sec
Total Volume:	100 mL (minimum catheter size = 22 G)

COMMENTS:

1. **DATA RECONSTRUCTION:** Standard
2. **SCAN FOV:** Head
3. **SCAN ANGLE:** IOML and parallel to the long axis of the mandible (change angle around teeth)
4. **SAVE RAW DATA:** Yes, bone algorithm through mandible
5. **DISPLAY FOV:** 16–19 cm
6. Film all images in soft tissue window and only the images through the mandible in bone window.
7. *Infectious or inflammatory disease in the floor of the mouth:* Coronal reformations perpendicular to IOML through oral cavity might be helpful for delineation of the full extent of disease. If coronal reformations are desired, use a pitch of 0.75 (HQ = 3:1).
8. *Malignant tumors:* Include neck survey (see specific protocol) to evaluate for nodal disease.
9. Obtain images through the mandible with 1–1.25-mm slice thickness in patients with oral cavity tumors and clinical suspicion for mandibular involvement.

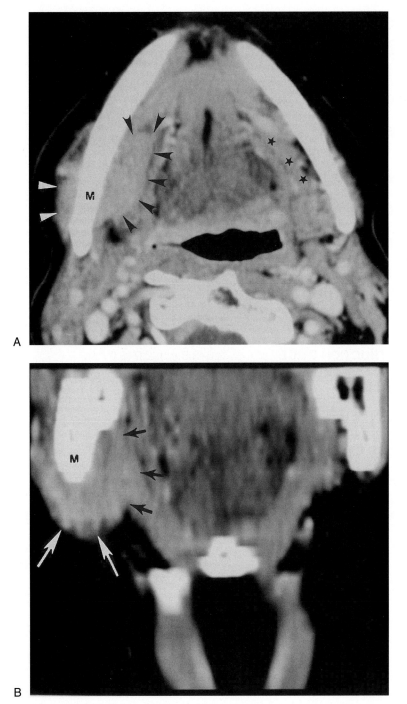

FIG. 19. Axial contrasted computed tomographic image **(A)** through the floor of the mouth demonstrates recurrent floor of the mouth tumor (*arrowheads*) on the right. The tumor involves the mylohyoid muscle (*asterisk* for normal mylohyoid muscle on the left) and grows around the mandible *(M)*. The tumor extension (*arrows*) around the mandible *(M)* is better appreciated on the reformatted images in the coronal plane **(B).** The coronal reformation was performed from axial images acquired at a 1.25-mm slice thickness in multislice imaging mode without the helical technique.

Protocol 14:
MANDIBLE (Fig. 20)

INDICATION:	*Trauma, infection, tumor*
SCANNER SETTINGS:	kV(p): 140 mA: 250–300
ORAL CONTRAST:	None
PHASE OF RESPIRATION:	Quiet breathing
ROTATION TIME:	0.5–0.8 sec
ACQUISITION SLICE THICKNESS:	1.0–1.25 mm
PITCH:	0.75 (HQ = 3:1)
RECONSTRUCTION SLICE THICKNESS/INTERVAL FOR FILMING:	2.0–3.0 mm/2.0–3.0 mm
ANATOMIC COVERAGE: **SUPERIOR EXTENT:** **INFERIOR EXTENT:**	 Temporomandibular joint Inferior margin of mandible
IV CONTRAST:	None

COMMENTS:

1. **DATA RECONSTRUCTION:** Standard
2. **SCAN FOV:** Head
3. **SCAN ANGLE:** No angulation of gantry
4. **SAVE RAW DATA:** Yes, bone algorithm
5. **DISPLAY FOV:** 16–18 cm
6. Film every image in bone and every third image in soft tissue window.
7. Obtain coronal reformations perpendicular to body of the mandible.
8. Consider dental reformations of the mandible.
9. *Infectious and inflammatory process:* Give IV contrast.

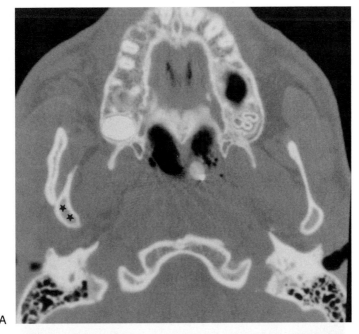

A

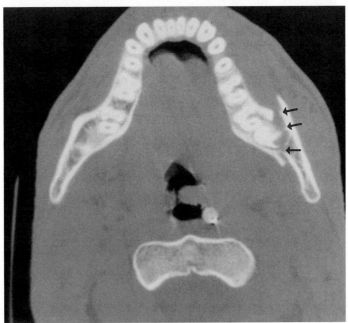

B

FIG. 20. Axial computed tomographic images through the mandible reveal **(A)** a medially displaced fracture fragment secondary to an oblique fracture through the neck of the mandible (*asterisk*) and **(B)** a slightly laterally displaced fracture through the angle of the mandible (*arrows*). The reformatted image in the coronal plane performed without overlap of the adjacent slices **(C)** demonstrates slightly indistinct margins of the bony structures when compared with the reformatted image with some overlap between slices **(D).** Both coronal reformations demonstrate clearly the extent of the fracture and its relation to the teeth (*arrows*); however, the image quality of **D** is better. This subtle difference in image quality might play a crucial role in patients with hairline or chip fractures. Both coronal reformations were performed from axial images acquired at a 1.25-mm slice thickness using multislice imaging mode and a pitch of 0.75 (3 : 1). For part **C**, the axial images were left in a 1.25-mm slice thickness, and in part **D**, the images were reconstructed to 1 mm, resulting in a slice overlap of 0.25 mm on the reformatted image.

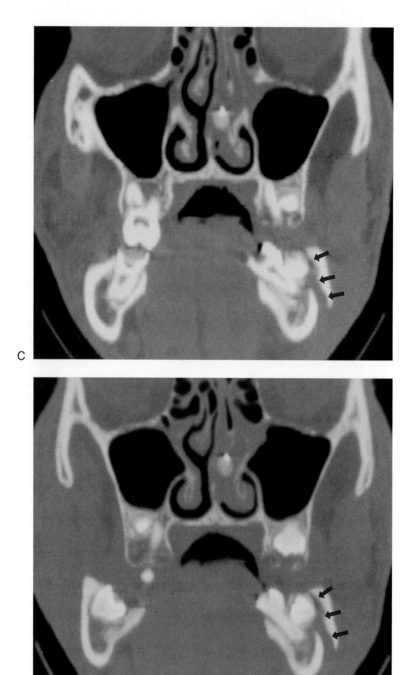

FIG. 20. *Continued.*

Protocol 15:
LARYNX/HYPOPHARYNX (Fig. 21)

INDICATION: *Tumor, trauma, infection*

SCANNER SETTINGS: kV(p): 140
mA: 220–260 upper and mid neck
300 per 2 sec for lower neck and thoracic inlet

ORAL CONTRAST: None

PHASE OF RESPIRATION: Quiet breathing

ROTATION TIME: 0.5–0.8 sec for upper and midneck
2 sec for lower neck and thoracic inlet

**ACQUISITION SLICE
THICKNESS (COLLIMATION):** 1.0–1.25 mm through upper and midneck
2.5–3 mm through lower neck and thoracic inlet

PITCH: 0.75–1.0 (HQ = 3:1) through upper and
midneck
1.0–1.5 (HS = 6:1) through lower neck
and thoracic inlet
If the scanner is unable to perform the
multislice helical imaging mode with the
gantry in angled position, change the gantry
angle to 0 degrees and reconstruct the
images in the desired plane (see below)
or use the multislice axial imaging mode.

**RECONSTRUCTION SLICE
THICKNESS/INTERVAL
FOR FILMING:** 2.0–3.0 mm/2.0–3.0 mm

ANATOMIC COVERAGE:
SUPERIOR EXTENT: Midportion of the body of mandible
INFERIOR EXTENT: Lung apex

IV CONTRAST:

Concentration:	LOCM 300–320 mg iodine/mL or HOCM 282 mg iodine/mL, 60% solution
Rate:	1 mL/sec
Scan Delay:	100 sec
Total Volume:	100 mL (minimum catheter size = 22 G)

COMMENTS:

1. **DATA RECONSTRUCTION:** Standard
2. **SCAN FOV:** Head
3. **SCAN ANGLE:** Parallel to the long axis of the mandible
4. **SAVE RAW DATA:** Yes, bone algorithm through the larynx
5. **DISPLAY FOV:** 10 cm through the larynx, 16–19 cm through the entire scanned area
6. Film all images in soft tissue window and only the images through the larynx in bone window.
7. *Trauma/subglottic stenosis:* No contrast. Consider reformations in coronal and sagittal plane or in three dimensions. If reformations are desired, use a pitch of 0.75 (HQ = 3).
8. *Malignant tumors:* Consider three-dimensional reformations to better determine the relation to adjacent anatomic structures and tumor volume. If three-dimensional reformations are desired, use a pitch of 0.75 (HQ = 3).
9. Change reconstructions' slice thickness for filming to 1–1.25 thin sections from the false vocal cord to the bottom of the cricoid cartilage in patients with small-volume tumors or questionable extent of tumor into the laryngeal ventricle and/or subglottic region.
10. *Vocal cord paralysis:* Extend imaging to the carina with 5-mm slice thickness and a pitch of 1–1.5 (4:1 − HS = 6:1).

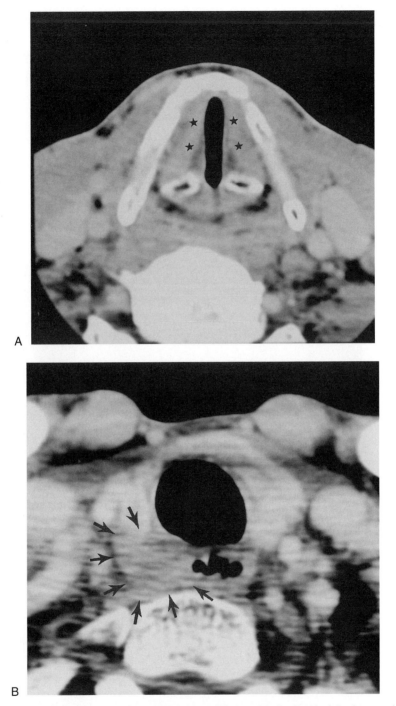

FIG. 21. Axial computed tomographic (CT) image **(A)** through the level of the larynx shows bilateral vocal cord paralysis in the adducted position (*asterisk*). A lower CT images at the thoracic inlet **(B)** demonstrates a mass in the tracheoesophageal groove on the right side (*arrows*). The thyroid gland is slightly obscured by shoulder artifacts but does not reveal any significant abnormalities. The T1 postgadolinium **(C)** and the T2-weighted images **(D)** demonstrate not only the tracheoesophageal groove mass on the right (*arrows*) but also abnormal signal intensity in or adjacent to the posterior aspect of the left thyroid gland (*arrowheads*). This left-sided lesion is best appreciated on the T2-weighted images. Biopsy of these lesions revealed metastatic squamous cell cancer of unknown origin.

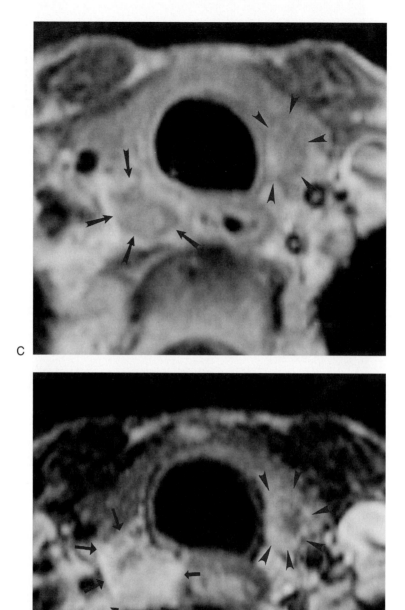

FIG. 21. *Continued.*

Protocol 16:
NECK SURVEY (Fig. 22)

INDICATION:
Neck mass of unknown etiology, lymph node survey, lymphoma, unknown primary, skin cancer, melanoma

SCANNER SETTINGS:
kV(p): 140
mA: 220–260 through upper and midneck
300 per 2 sec through lower neck and thoracic inlet

ORAL CONTRAST:
None

PHASE OF RESPIRATION:
Quiet respiration

ROTATION TIME:
0.5–1.0 sec through upper and midneck
2 sec through lower neck and thoracic inlet

ACQUISITION SLICE THICKNESS:
2.5–3.0 mm

PITCH:
1.0–1.5 (HS = 6:1)
If the scanner is unable to perform the multislice helical imaging mode with the gantry in angled position, change the gantry angle to 0 degrees and reconstruct the images in the desired plane (see below) or use the multislice axial imaging mode.

RECONSTRUCTION SLICE THICKNESS/INTERVAL FOR FILMING:
2.5–3.0 mm/2.5–3.0 mm

ANATOMIC COVERAGE:
SUPERIOR EXTENT:
Top of sella
INFERIOR EXTENT:
Lung apex

IV CONTRAST:

Concentration:	LOCM 300–320 mg iodine/mL or HOCM 282 mg iodine/mL, 60% solution
Rate:	1 mL/sec
Scan Delay:	60 sec
Total Volume:	100 mL (minimum catheter size = 22 G)

COMMENTS:

1. **DATA RECONSTRUCTION:** Standard
2. **SCAN FOV:** Head
3. **SCAN ANGLE:** IOML and parallel to the long axis of the mandible (change angle around teeth).
4. **SAVE RAW DATA:** Yes.
5. **DISPLAY FOV:** 16–19 cm
6. Film all images in soft tissue window.
7. *Skin cancer/melanoma:* Display FOV should include the posterior neck on each slice.

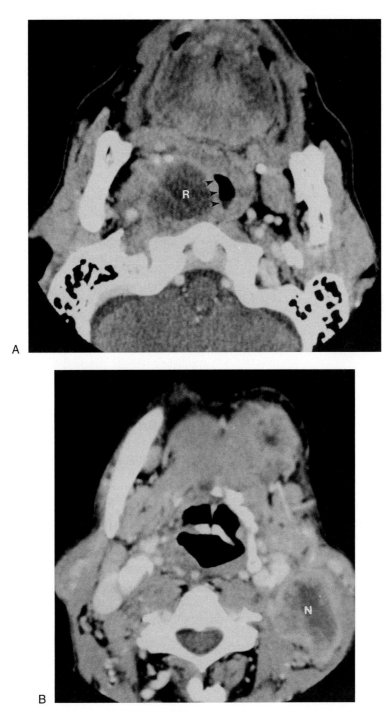

FIG. 22. Axial computed tomographic images through the oropharynx **(A)** and midneck **(B)** show necrotic lymph nodes in retropharyngeal space on the right and group II/III junction node *(N)* on the left. The abnormal retropharyngeal lymph node causes compromise of the upper airway from the right *(arrowheads)*. This patient has known AIDS disease. Biopsy of the midneck lymph showed metastatic squamous cell cancer.

Protocol 17:
SUSPECTED CSF LEAK (Fig. 23)

INDICATION: *CSF otorrhea and/or rhinorrhea*

SCANNER SETTINGS: kV(p): 140
                                 mA: 300–400

ORAL CONTRAST: None

PHASE OF RESPIRATION: Quiet breathing

ROTATION TIME: 0.5–1.0 sec

ACQUISITION SLICE   0.5–1.25 mm
THICKNESS:

PITCH: 0.75–1.0 (HQ = 3:1)
                                 If the scanner is unable to perform the
                                    multislice helical imaging mode with the
                                    gantry in angled position
                                    • change for *axial* imaging plane the gantry
                                      angle to 0 degrees and reconstruct the
                                      images in the desired plane (see below)
                                      or use the multislice axial imaging mode
                                    • obtain coronal images using the multislice
                                      axial imaging mode

RECONSTRUCTION SLICE   0.5–1.0 mm/0.5–1.0 mm
THICKNESS/INTERVAL
FOR FILMING:

ANATOMIC COVERAGE: *Axial:*   *Coronal:*
  SUPERIOR EXTENT: Top of frontal sinus   Anterior margin of
                                                           frontal sinus
  INFERIOR EXTENT: Hard palate   Posterior margin of
                                                           mastoid cells

IV CONTRAST: None

COMMENTS: 1. **DATA RECONSTRUCTION:** Standard
                                 2. **SCAN FOV:** Head
                                 3. **SCAN ANGLE:** *Axial:* IOML
                                    Coronal: Perpendicular to IOML
                                 4. **SAVE RAW DATA:** Yes, bone algorithm

5. **DISPLAY FOV:** 15–17 cm for CSF rhinorrhea, 9–10 cm for CSF otorrhea
6. Film every image in bone window and every third image in soft tissue window.
7. Perform reformations of the axial images in coronal plane if patient unable to tolerate direct coronal imaging. Use a pitch of 0.75 (HQ = 3:1).
8. Consider intrathecal contrast. If intrathecal contrast given and the patient has rhinorrhea, position the patient prone for direct coronal imaging.
9. *CSF rhinorrhea:* Change the inferior extent of scanning in axial plane to midorbit and the posterior extent of imaging in coronal plane to dorsum sellae.
10. *CSF otorrhea:* Change the superior extent of scanning in axial plane to top of sella and the anterior extent of imaging in coronal to anterior margin of the TB.

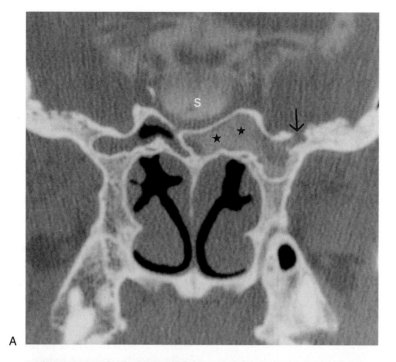

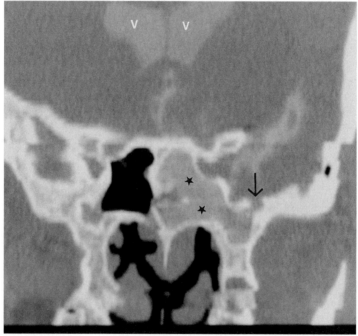

FIG. 23. Direct coronal **(A)** versus reformatted image in the coronal plane **(B)** in a patient with a cerebrospinal fluid (CSF) leak. The study was obtained after injection of intrathecal contrast; notice the contrast in the **(A)** suprasellar cistern *(S)* and **(B)** lateral ventricles *(v)*, respectively, as well as in the left sphenoid sinus (*asterisk*). Both images demonstrate the defect in the superior left lateral aspect of the sphenoid sinus on the left (*arrow*), but the image quality of the direct coronal images is superior to the quality of the reformatted image. Particularly in patients with a CSF leak, it is crucial to perform direct coronal images because areas of thin bone in the plane of the images might be mistaken for a focal defect (see also Fig. 6).

Protocol 18:
CERVICAL SPINE (Fig. 24)

INDICATION:	*Trauma, neck pain, degenerative disease, disc disease, benign or malignant tumor, infectious disease*
SCANNER SETTINGS:	kV(p): 140 mA: 220–240 upper cervical spine 240–260 mid cervical spine 150–200 per 2 sec lower cervical spine
ORAL CONTRAST:	None
PHASE OF RESPIRATION:	Quiet breathing
ROTATION TIME:	0.5–0.8 sec through upper and mid cervical spine 2 sec through lower cervical spine
ACQUISITION SLICE THICKNESS:	1.0–2.5 mm
PITCH:	0.75–1.5 (HQ = 3:1; HS = 6:1)
RECONSTRUCTION SLICE THICKNESS/INTERVAL FOR FILMING:	1.0–2.5 mm/1.0–2.5 mm
ANATOMIC COVERAGE: **SUPERIOR EXTENT:**	One disc space above the level of suspected pathology
INFERIOR EXTENT:	One disc space below the level of suspected pathology
IV CONTRAST:	None
COMMENTS:	1. **DATA RECONSTRUCTION:** Standard 2. **SCAN FOV:** Head 3. **SCAN ANGLE:** No angulation of gantry if multiple levels or the entire cervical spine is imaged; angle parallel to the disc level if only one or two levels are scanned. If the scanner is unable to perform the multislice helical imaging mode with the gantry in angled position, change the gantry angle

to 0 degrees and reconstruct the images in a plane parallel to the disc space or use the multislice axial imaging mode.

4. **SAVE RAW DATA:** Yes, bone algorithm
5. **DISPLAY FOV:** 21 cm in adults, 19 cm in children
6. Film in bone and soft tissue windows.
7. Consider reformations in coronal and sagittal planes.
8. *Infectious disease/tumor:* Consider IV contrast.

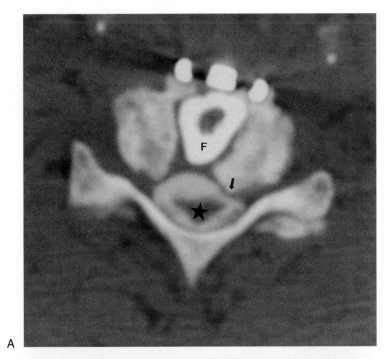

A

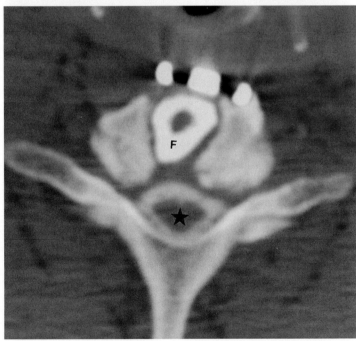

B

FIG. 24. Axial myelo-computed tomographic images in a patient status post–anterior fusion and fibular strut graft *(F)* placement shows **(A)** marked atrophy and deformity of the spinal cord (*asterisk*) at the level of C3-4, when compared with **(B)** the normal size of the cord (*asterisk*). The fibular graft is not bony incorporated yet within the vertebral bodies. Notice also the impingement of the left lateral recess by an osteophyte (*arrow*). The reformatted image in the sagittal plane **(C)** delineates well the alignment of the cervical spine and the relative spinal canal narrowing at the C3-4 level caused by osteophytes (*arrowheads*). The sagittal reformation was performed from axial images acquired at a 1.25-mm slice thickness in multislice imaging mode without helical technique.

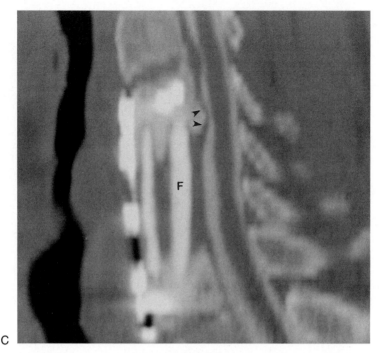

FIG. 24. *Continued.*

Protocol 19:
EXTRACRANIAL VASCULATURE (Fig. 25)

INDICATION:	*Vascular stenosis/occlusion, aneurysm, malformation, trauma*
SCANNER SETTINGS:	kV(p): 140 mA: 300–340
ORAL CONTRAST:	None
PHASE OF RESPIRATION:	Quiet breathing
ROTATION TIME:	0.5–0.8 sec
ACQUISITION SLICE THICKNESS:	1.0–1.25 mm
PITCH:	1.5 (HS = 6:1)
RECONSTRUCTION SLICE THICKNESS/INTERVAL FOR FILMING:	2.5–3.0 mm/2.5–3.0 mm

ANATOMIC COVERAGE:
   SUPERIOR EXTENT:
   INFERIOR EXTENT:
	
	Skull base
	C6 vertebral body

IV CONTRAST:

Concentration:	LOCM 300–320 mg iodine/mL or HOCM 282 mg iodine/mL, 60%
Rate:	3–4 mL/sec
Scan Delay:	20 sec
Total Volume:	100 mL (minimum catheter size = 20 G)

COMMENTS:

1. **DATA RECONSTRUCTION:** Soft tissue
2. **SCAN FOV:** Head
3. **SCAN ANGLE:** None
4. **SAVE RAW DATA:** Yes
5. **DISPLAY FOV:** 15 cm
6. Perform data processing using maximum intensity projection (MIP) technique and display the data in three dimensions and various angles.

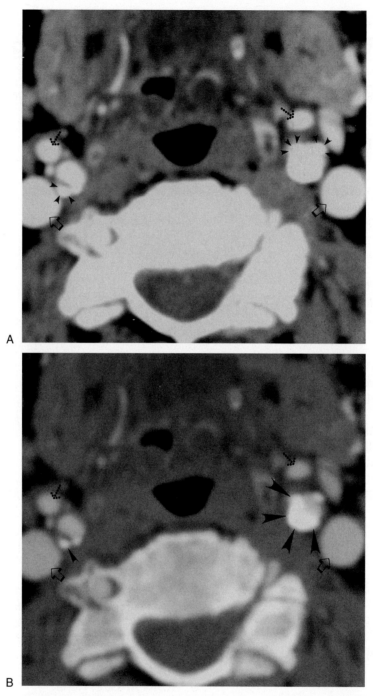

FIG. 25. Computed tomographic angiography source images in the axial plane **(A, B, C)** and oblique sagittal reformation image **(D)** performed through the left carotid bifurcation in a patient with discordant results on Doppler ultrasound examination and magnetic resonance angiography. Parts **A** and **B** are identical images, but windowed differently. One image **(A)** falsely demonstrates a patent lumen of the internal carotid artery bilaterally with small irregularities of the walls, suggesting small ulcerations (*arrowheads*). The internal carotid arteries would be considered as not significantly stenotic.

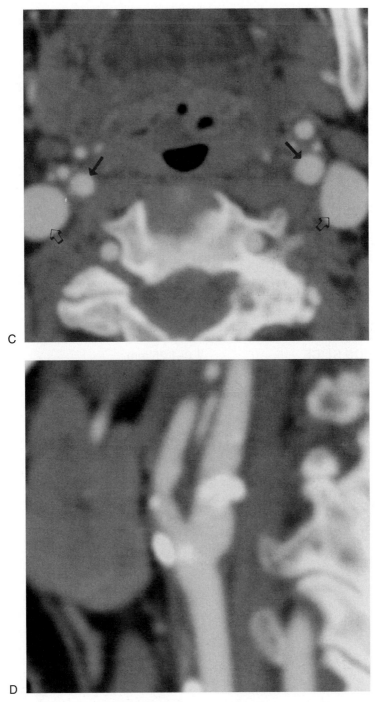

C

D

FIG. 25. *Continued.* Another image **(B)** demonstrates that the wall irregularities are due to dense calcifications within an extensive plaque (*large arrowheads*) on the left, resulting in a stenosis of the lumen of 60%, when compared with the **(C)** normal lumen of the carotid artery proximal to the area of stenosis (*arrow*). On the right, **(B)** the appearance of ulceration within a plaque was due to dense focal calcification (*small arrowhead*). External carotid artery (*dotted arrow* in **A** and **B**); jugular vein (*open arrow*). The reformatted image in the oblique sagittal plane **(D)** through the carotid bifurcation on the left side demonstrates the location of the calcified plaques. The narrowing of the internal carotid artery cannot be determined on this image because of the overlying dense calcifications.

Protocol 20:
INTRACRANIAL VASCULATURE (Circle of Willis/Vertebrobasilar System) (Fig. 26)

INDICATION: *Aneurysm, stenosis, occlusion, vascular malformation*

SCANNER SETTINGS: kV(p): 140
                                   mA: 300–400

ORAL CONTRAST: None

PHASE OF RESPIRATION: Quiet breathing

ROTATION TIME: 0.5–0.8 sec

ACQUISITION SLICE THICKNESS: 1.0–1.25 mm

PITCH: 1.5 (HS = 6:1)

RECONSTRUCTION SLICE THICKNESS/INTERVAL FOR FILMING: 1.25–2.0 mm/1.25–2.0 mm

ANATOMIC COVERAGE:
  SUPERIOR EXTENT: Top of third ventricle
  INFERIOR EXTENT: Skull base

IV CONTRAST:

Concentration:	LOCM 300–320 mg iodine/mL or HOCM 282 mg iodine/mL, 60%
Rate:	3–4 mL/sec
Scan Delay:	20 sec
Total Volume:	100 mL (minimum catheter size = 20 G)

COMMENTS:

1. **DATA RECONSTRUCTION:** Soft tissue
2. **SCAN FOV:** Head
3. **SCAN ANGLE:** None
4. **SAVE RAW DATA:** Yes
5. **DISPLAY FOV:** 15 cm
6. Perform data processing using MIP technique and display the data in three dimensions and various angles.

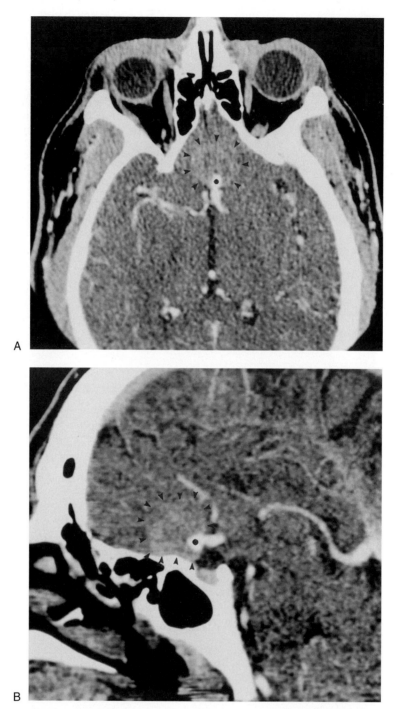

FIG. 26. Computed tomographic angiographic source images in axial **(A)** and their reformation in the midsagittal plane **(B)** demonstrate a large anterior communicating artery aneurysm (*black dot*) pointing anteriorly. Most of the aneurysm is thrombosed (*arrowheads*). The maximum intensity projection image **(C)** shows only the patent portion of the aneurysm (*curved arrow*).

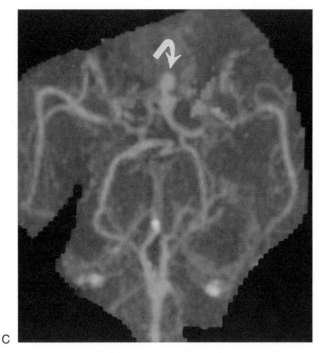

C

FIG. 26. *Continued.*

Protocol 21:
CT PERFUSION (Fig. 27)

INDICATION:	*Suspicion for infarction*
SCANNER SETTINGS:	kV(p): 140 mA: 350–400
ORAL CONTRAST:	None
PHASE OF RESPIRATION:	Quiet breathing
ROTATION TIME:	0.5–1.0 sec
ACQUISITION SLICE THICKNESS:	5.0 mm
PITCH:	NA
RECONSTRUCTION SLICE THICKNESS/INTERVAL FOR FILMING:	5.0 mm/5.0 mm

ANATOMIC COVERAGE:
  SUPERIOR EXTENT:
  INFERIOR EXTENT:
	
	Parietal convexities
	Top of sella

IV CONTRAST:

> **Always perform noncontrast CT scan before perfusion CT.**
>
> | | |
> |---|---|
> | **Concentration:** | LOCM 300–320 mg iodine/mL or HOCM 282 mg iodine/mL, 60% solution |
> | **Rate:** | 4 mL/sec |
> | **Scan Delay:** | None |
> | **Total Volume:** | 100 mL (minimum catheter size = 18–20 G) |

COMMENTS:

1. **DATA RECONSTRUCTION:** Standard
2. **SCAN FOV:** Head
3. **SCAN ANGLE:** IOML
4. **SAVE RAW DATA:** Yes

5. **DISPLAY FOV:** 21 cm
6. Film all images in soft tissue window.
7. Place on each image 6–10 regions of interest bilaterally and symmetrically and regenerate flow curves for each area separately.
8. *Suspicion for infarct in vertebrobasilar distribution:* Change the superior extent to top of sella and the inferior extent to foramen of magnum. Reduce the regions of interest to four to six.

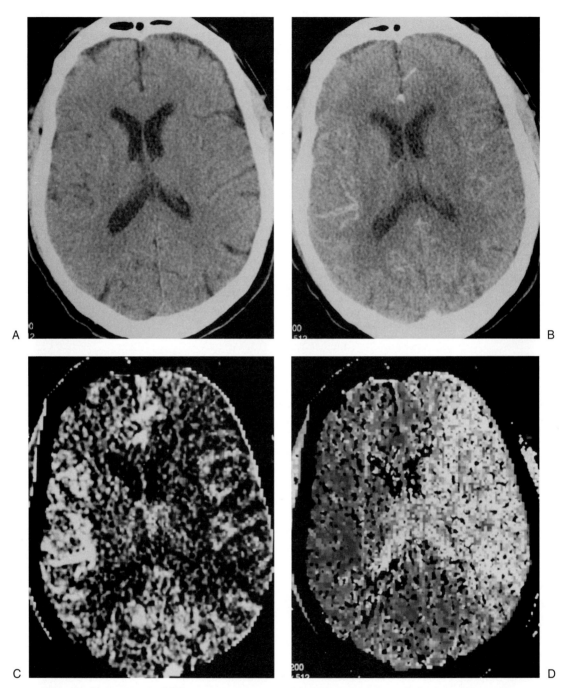

FIG. 27. Noncontrasted **(A)** computed tomographic (CT) image through the head in a patient with right-sided body weakness demonstrates no signs of infarction on the left. The contrasted CT image **(B)** performed as part of the perfusion protocol shows significantly decreased amount of vascular enhancement in the left MCA territory, when compared with the right. The generated blood flow map **(C)** confirms the significantly decreased blood flow to the middle cerebral artery (MCA) territory on the left. The severely delayed mean transit time on the left can be easily depicted on the mean transit time map **(D).**

3

Multislice Computed Tomography of the Chest

Georgeann McGuinness* and David P. Naidich*

*Department of Radiology, Section of Thoracic Imaging, New York University Medical Center, New York, New York 10016

CONVENTIONAL HELICAL TECHNIQUE

Thoracic Imaging Advances

The much anticipated advances in thoracic imaging that were promised with the advent of helical computed tomography (HCT) in the 1980s are established, with helical data acquisition now the standard for all but high-resolution imaging (1). Improvement in longitudinal (z-axis) resolution with conventional HCT, with its ability to acquire contiguous sections with overlapping reconstructions, has proved to be a benefit in CT imaging throughout the body. These rapidly acquired data sets can be obtained without compromising the improved spatial resolution provided by a thinly collimated beam, because a helical pitch of more than 1 allows coverage of relatively large distances with even thinly collimated sections.

In the thorax, however, the most important advance in imaging technique has come through improved temporal resolution attributed to the ability to acquire data during a single breath-hold. Misregistration artifacts resulting from variations in the depth of respiration between scans, as well as respiratory, and to a lesser degree cardiac, motion artifacts, are eliminated. Rapidly acquired scans allow optimization of vascular imaging through precise coordination of the contrast bolus relative to the vascular structures under examination.

The advantages gained through increasing scan speed have been further amplified with the advent of subsecond gantry rotation times (2). With subsecond scanning, the same distance can be covered while further decreasing scan time, diminishing the need for extended breath-hold periods when imaging in the chest or reducing the dose of contrast required without compromising z-axis resolution by increasing the section thickness. Alternatively, the z-axis resolution can be improved by narrowing the section thickness while maintaining the same duration of breath-hold and covering the same distance, if subsecond scanning is employed. Rubin et al. (2) compared 8-mm thick sections obtained with identical parameters except for 1-second gantry rotation versus 0.75-second gantry rotation in 92 patients referred for thoracic CT. These authors evaluated both mediastinal and lung windows at six levels, each for motion artifacts and image noise (which is increased with the decreased patient dose inherent in subsecond scanning), and found image quality subjectively better with shorter scan times for both parameters, particularly in the mediastinum. The primary source of image degradation was motion artifacts from cardiac and vascular structures, rather than noise.

However, with the potential advantages to resolution provided by helical imaging techniques came a huge expansion in possible scan protocols. After initial uncertainty about optimal use of HCT in a given clinical setting, acceptable scan protocols have been developed (3), with the additional flexibility provided by HCT, allowing studies tailored to ever more specialized indications. Variables that need to be considered for helical scanning include collimation, pitch, breath-hold period, field of view (FOV), reconstruction interval, rate and volume of intravenous (IV) contrast administration, reconstruction algorithm, and radiation dose.

It is important when planning HCT protocols to incorporate the fact that although the reconstruction interval, reconstruction algorithm, and FOV can be changed after acquisition of the volumetric data set, it must be done in a timely fashion because limitations in short-term memory capacity preclude retention of the volumetric data indefinitely. Other parameters such as pitch and collimation cannot be altered retrospectively, so they mandate detailed prospective consideration when planning an examination. In general, when planning conventional helical chest CTs, one determines the optimal beam width by considering the size of the structures to be evaluated, and the pitch is calculated to correspondingly provide appropriate anatomic coverage. These parameters anticipate sequential viewing of axial sections representing the thickness of the collimator beam as the primary viewing mode, although overlapping reconstruction and thinner sections are planned if volumetric or multiplanar-reformatted viewing is anticipated.

MULTISLICE TECHNIQUE

Impact on Imaging Principles, Protocol Planning, and Interpretive Approach

Although some of the same basic premises we familiarly apply to HCT apply to multislice CT (MSCT), using an MSCT scanner requires adjustments to the radiologist's conceptual approach to acquisition, preprocessing and postprocessing of data, and image viewing and analysis. Resolution in general continues to benefit from thinner sections using a larger pitch compared with thicker sections using a smaller pitch, when covering the same anatomic volume. This is particularly important in the assessment of small anatomic structures, such as airways, small pulmonary arteries, or the lung parenchyma. In addition, the benefit to be gained from overlapping reconstruction applies up to approximately 25% to 50% of the slice thickness, with little benefit to be gained from overlap beyond that degree.

A paradigm shift in approach is catalyzed, however, by realization that the volume of scan data is dramatically enlarged, with significantly more potentially thinner images obtained at a significantly faster rate, compared with conventional single-detector HCT. Traditional familiar sequential viewing of hard-copy axial images is neither practical nor optimal when approaching these huge volumes of scan data. Sequential viewing of such a volume of axial images is cumbersome and time consuming and underappreciates the capacity for detailed multiplanar reconstructions (MPRs) and three-dimensional (3D) reconstructions. Ongoing technologic advances allow the acquisition of sub-millimeter sections, resulting in isotropic or near-isotropic voxels of data, which potentially provide 3D reconstructions without distortion. These developments presage the abandonment of conventional analysis of traditional axial images in favor of detailed volume-rendered formats (4).

With the simultaneous irradiation of four or more rows of detectors, four times as much data are acquired per gantry rotation using MSCT. This significantly expands options, compared with conventional HCT; if slice collimation is maintained, the same z-axis distance is covered far more quickly and anatomic coverage can be extended, if desired. If thinner slice collimation is chosen, the table speed can remain the same, and from this scan data, thinner or thicker sections can be retrospectively reconstructed. The choice of the detector set is determined by the probable primary viewing mode but incorporates flexibility for potential retrospective variation in the slice thickness as the need arises. For instance, if the clinical indication for an examination is an abnormal radiograph, a survey examination with 5- to 7-mm thick sections is typically appropriate. However, accepting that the "radiographic abnormality" may represent a small nodule requiring detailed characterization with thin sections, the detector set chosen may be four 1.25- or four 1-mm detectors, even though it is planned that the images will initially be viewed with a 5- or 7-mm slice thickness with a 1-mm overlap. These thin detectors are implemented to allow reconstruction of contiguous thin sections if needed retrospectively, obviating a second high-resolution acquisition through the region with thin collimation, which had been usual with HCT. With these data, targeted reconstructions can be generated through the focal region of interest (Figs. 1 and 14). Not only does this represent an improvement in time and convenience to both the patient and the radiologist, but it also decreases cost, anxiety, and the radiation dose to the patient.

A final added advantage to be gained from MSCT in the thorax includes further reductions in artifacts related to cardiac motion and/or arterial pulsation, partly because of an increase in the table travel distance during each cardiac cycle, but more significantly through the capacity for prospective triggering of scan acquisition to the diastolic portion of the cardiac cycle, or retrospective cardiac gating (Fig. 12) (5). Schoepf et al. (5) evaluated the lung parenchyma in the region adjacent to the border of the left side of the heart, with three 1-mm thick sections obtained with subsecond (0.75-second) scans either with prospective cardiac gating during diastole or without gating. These studies were performed in 35 consecutive patients with interstitial lung disease and were evaluated for cardiac motion, respiratory motion, diagnostic value, spatial resolution, and overall improvement by three readers. Electrocardiographic (ECG) gating reduced cardiac motion ($p < .05$) but did not affect respiratory motion or improve the diagnostic value of the scans in the experience of these authors (5).

For purposes of clarity, the remainder of this chapter is divided into a discussion of specific applications of MSCT in the thorax, followed by detailed scan protocols. Vascular applications are discussed first, including the use of MSCT to diagnose pulmonary emboli (PE) and aortic disease. Next, evaluation of the airways, both central and peripheral, are discussed, followed by approaches to the evaluation of focal lung disease and diffuse interstitial lung disease. Use of MSCT in the setting of thoracic trauma is also discussed. Finally, the application of MSCT as a screening tool for early lung cancer detection is reviewed.

VASCULAR DISEASE

Intravenous Contrast Administration

There are varied clinical indications for the IV injection of iodinated contrast, which can be broadly grouped into two categories. The first is a focused evaluation of vascular structures such as the aorta, pulmonary arteries, or abnormal parenchymal vascular structures, such as vascular malformations. The second category is the use of vascular opacification to differentiate normal vascular mediastinal and hilar structures from pathologic conditions. Lung cancer staging, detection of lymphadenopathy, and differentiation of normal vascular structures such as pulmonary arteries from lymph nodes, in our judgment, all require routine IV contrast administration.

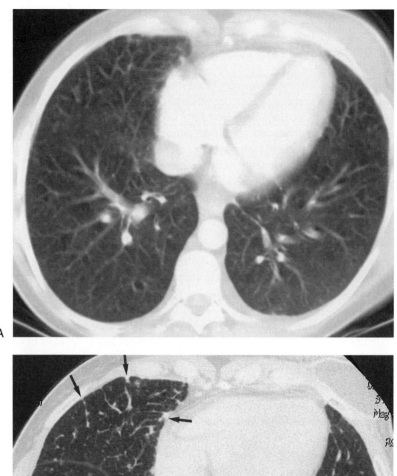

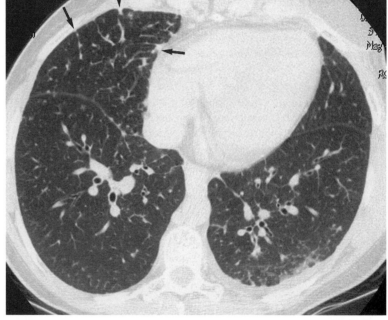

FIG. 1. Thoracic survey examination in a 42-year-old woman with breast cancer. **A:** Axial image obtained with 4- by 1-mm collimation, but reconstructed with 7- by 6-mm images, demonstrates the absence of discrete lung nodules. Subtle increased reticulonodular markings are suggested, however, in the middle lobe. **B:** Because of the suggestion of unsuspected interstitial disease, high-resolution 1-mm thick sections were retrospectively reconstructed through this region, confirming nodular thickening of interlobular septa (*arrows*) characteristic of lymphangitic dissemination of tumor. The ability to incorporate high-resolution imaging into a routine survey examination without follow-up imaging not only is convenient but also diminishes cost and radiation exposure to the patient.

Because MSCT acquisition is minimally four times as fast as HCT, further refinements in strategies for contrast material optimization have become possible, requiring that particular attention be paid to the volume, rate, and concentration of administered contrast. Foremost among these is the reduction in the required volume of contrast media necessary. The possible advantages of reduced administration of contrast volume became evident with single-detector HCT, in which as little as 60 mL of 300 mg/mL of contrast has been demonstrated as diagnostically adequate (6) for imaging in the thorax.

Second, faster scan acquisition allows greater rates of injection, with consequent greater coherency of the contrast bolus, resulting in superior temporal and subjective vascular opacification. An important caveat is that faster injections and faster scanning mandate increasingly accurate determination of the delay between the initiation of the injection and scanning; test injections or use of online bolus tracking software, particularly if there are suspected variations in cardiac output, becomes increasingly important.

A second caveat is that rapid injection of a dense bolus of contrast may produce streak artifacts as it passes through the superior vena cava, which may obscure adjacent structures. Reduction in iodine concentration may actually improve arterial enhancement (7) and decrease perivenous streak artifacts. Rubin et al. (7) showed improved visualization of arterial thoracic structures and less venous artifacts when 50 mL of 300 mg iodine/mL was diluted with 50 mL of normal saline, for 100 mL of 150 mg iodine/mL of contrast, as compared with 50 mL of undiluted contrast. Use of diluted contrast may realize significant cost savings, particularly when nonionic contrast is used. This technique is only appropriate when scanning is limited to the thorax, whereas thoracic scans done in conjunction with other examinations will still require 300 mg of iodine/mL.

In summary, the capabilities of MSCT to provide optimal precisely controlled vascular opacification promise to reinforce and expand the field of CT angiography (CTA) that was introduced with the advent of HCT

Pulmonary Embolism

HCT has been enthusiastically promoted as capable of replacing ventilation/perfusion ($\dot{V}/\dot{Q}$) scanning and pulmonary angiography for the diagnosis of PE, and in fact, in the 8 years since its introduction, it has become accepted in most institutions as the initial examination in the evaluation of the patient suspected of having a PE. Data from several studies report sensitivities ranging from 53% to 100% and specificities ranging from 78% to 100% for HCT in diagnosing PE (8–12).

When evaluation is limited to only central or segmental arteries, sensitivity and specificity approach 90% (9). Much attention and discussion has been directed toward the limitations of CT pulmonary angiography (CTPA) in detecting peripheral thromboembolism, however. In a prospective study of patients with moderate-probability $\dot{V}/\dot{Q}$ scans, Goodman et al. (9) found that although CT has a sensitivity of 91% and a specificity of 86% for segmental and larger pulmonary arteries, sensitivity and specificity rates decreased to only 77% and 79%, respectively, when subsegmental emboli, which are reported to occur in 5% to 36% of cases (8,11,12), were evaluated.

Angiography is now generally reserved for select scenarios: cases with a negative CT and high clinical suspicion or high-probability $\dot{V}/\dot{Q}$ scan; or a directed limited pulmonary angiogram focused on a single vessel to evaluate a questionable finding at CTPA. Finally, in those institutions in which $\dot{V}/\dot{Q}$ scanning may still precede CTPA, pulmonary angiography may still be necessary if the CTPA remains equivocal in the face of an indeterminate $\dot{V}/\dot{Q}$ scan, which occurs overall in approximately 30% to 40% of cases. This subset of particularly challenging patients reveals another limitation of CTPA. Within this specific group, using thinner sections, the rate of indeterminate CTPAs is also elevated; Van Rossum et al. (12) recently demonstrated a sensitivity of 82% to 94% and a specificity of 93% to 96% overall for the detection of emboli with volumetric CT. The sensitivity decreased, however, to 67% to 80% when examining only those patients with indeterminate V̇/Q̇ scans.

The advantages of CTPA performed with MSCT, as compared with HCT, again includes improved image resolution through more thinly collimated sections, without compromise in length of coverage. That thinner sections improve analysis of segmental and subsegmental pulmonary arteries was demonstrated by Remy-Jardin et al. (13) while comparing 20 patients studied with 3-mm thick sections obtained with 1-second helical scans at a pitch of 1.7 with 20 patients studied with 2-mm thick sections obtained with 0.75-second helical images at a pitch of 2. The number of adequately depicted segmental arteries in the second group exceeded that of the first group (93% vs. 85%, respectively; $p < .001$), but the most striking difference concerned the subsegmental arteries, in which 61% of the arteries were coded as analyzable with the thinner sections, compared with only 37% of those on the scans with 3-mm thick sections (13). The authors feel these findings should translate to improvement in the detection of segmental and subsegmental clots (13).

MSCT promises additional improvement in all aspects of the CT evaluation of the patient suspected of having PE, including image quality, ability to detect PE, and uniformity of interobserver interpretation. Quanadli et al. (14) compared 2.5-mm thick sections obtained with 1-second rotation technique and a pitch of 1.5 on a dual-detector CT scanner with pulmonary angiography in 157 patients. The effective slice thickness was 2.7 mm, and these images were reconstructed with a 50% overlap, at 1.3-mm intervals. These authors report a sensitivity of 95% and a specificity of 97% for detection of PE with MSCT, using angiography as the reference standard, which improved to 97% and 98% when subsegmental arteries were excluded from the analysis. Even including "inconclusive" CT scans, arbitrarily considered as false-positive or false-negative based on angiography results, the minimal sensitivity was 90%, and the specificity was 94% for the detection of PE at MSCT. Significantly, the overall number of individual clots detected was higher with MSCT (640 emboli vs. 601 emboli), and most interestingly, the number of subsegmental emboli detected at MSCT (92 emboli) was almost double the number detected by angiography (56 emboli). The interobserver variability was less with MSCT ($\kappa = 0.861$) then with angiography ($\kappa = 0.781$). These authors also report a high technical success rate at MSCT, compared with pulmonary angiography (14).

With MSCT, thin collimation is easily employed during a single breath-hold examination, ranging from 1.25- to 2.5-mm sections, and reconstructed with overlap. In the average-sized patient, the thorax can be scanned with a pitch of 1.5 (high speed [HS] = 6 : 1) and 2.5-mm collimation in 10 to 12 seconds; this reduction in scan duration will also reduce motion artifacts, particularly in a potentially dyspneic patient suspected of having PE. In particular, the reduction in cardiac motion artifacts makes vessels adjacent to the heart easier to analyze. This, too, increases confidence in the diagnosis of thromboembolism in small segmental or subsegmental arteries.

There are two general approaches to the administration of IV contrast when evaluation of the pulmonary arteries is targeted. Some investigators favor a "low-concentration/high flow-rate" protocol; with 30% concentration, contrast is administered at 5 to 6 mL per second. This limits potential compromises in the evaluation of the right main and right upper lobe pulmonary arteries from streak artifacts produced by a column of dense contrast in the superior vena cava. Alternatively, we, among others, favor a "standard-concentration/low flow-rate" protocol, using 60% contrast at 3 to 4 mL per second. This may limit the evaluation of more distal subsegmental vessels, which may not be fully opacified by scan time. Both of these approaches employ approximately a 15-second scan delay after initiation of IV contrast, although with the longer infusion period inherent with the slower rate of injection, precise timing is less critical. In most instances, but particularly when there are variations in the patient's cardiovascular physiology, such as cardiac output, timing runs should optimally be performed to eliminate the inconsistencies in circulation time, which are a frequent cause of suboptimal or uninterpretable studies. Bolus tracking, computer-automated scan technology, software may similarly aid in timing the scan delay relative to contrast administration, although in our experience, results are less consistent.

As with HCT, soft-copy workstation interpretation, which allows operator variation of window levels and tracking vessels on sequential images, is advantageous over hard-copy interpretation. MPRs can help differentiate a filling defect in an obliquely oriented vessel from an extravascular structure, such as a lymph node (Fig. 2). Obliquely oriented vessels in the middle lobe and lingula can be particularly problematic to evaluate; MPRs allow transverse and longitudinal evaluation of oblique vessels, which can aid in the detection of intravascular clot (15). Additionally, if image noise from thin sections causes heterogeneous attenuation of the pulmonary arterial tree, the signal to noise ration can be increased by reconstructing images at greater section thickness, as needed.

Accurate interpretation of these examinations mandates attention to examination technique, knowledge of thoracic vascular, bronchial and lymph node anatomy, and recognition of the signs of acute and chronic PEs (9,16). CT signs of acute PE include an intravascular filling defect surrounded by contrast or a filling defect with an acute angle between the filling defect and the vessel wall. This is the most reliable sign. A vessel "cutoff" sign is a less reliable sign; if acute, the un-opacified portion of the vessel will be enlarged. As has been emphasized, the capability to generate MPR images is useful in clarifying equivocal findings on the axial images. For instance, with extensive perivascular adenopathy, distortion and attenuation of vessels from external mass effect can be difficult to differentiate from an intraluminal clot on the axial images but can be readily distinguished with MPR images (Fig. 2). With a chronic clot, the vessel "cutoff" sign will be recognized with a diminished caliber vessel, because a chronic clot shrinks the vessel as it undergoes organization and retraction. Organizing chronic clots may also produce a partial filling defect within the vessel, but in this case, webs, septations, or small recanalized channels may be identified (Fig. 3). Chronic clots may form a smooth obtuse angle with the vessel wall.

Finally, CTPA with MSCT also allows diagnosis of unrelated thoracic abnormalities that may be responsible for symptoms when CTPA is negative for thromboembolic disease. These include pneumonia, cardiac disease, and pulmonary fibrosis.

Computed Tomographic Venography

Patients suspected of having a PE should also be evaluated for possible deep venous thrombosis (DVT), an evaluation that can be combined with CTPA (17). First described by Loud et al. (18), CT venography of the pelvis and legs is performed after investigation of the pulmonary arteries, using the same contrast injection (19). Venous phase imaging of the pelvis and legs has been proven comparable to venous sonography in the evaluation of femoropopliteal DVT (19) and allows visualization of a clot in the inferior vena cava and pelvic veins, areas inadequately assessed sonographically.

Recently, Garg et al. (20) compared HCT venography with leg sonography for accuracy and efficacy in the diagnosis of DVT from the popliteal vein to the common femoral vein. This study was performed in 70 consecutive patients who were undergoing CTPA for suspected PE, using sonography as the reference standard for extremity clot, an admittedly imperfect study

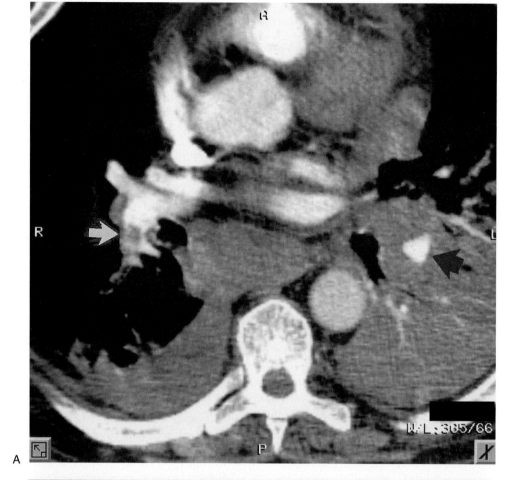

A

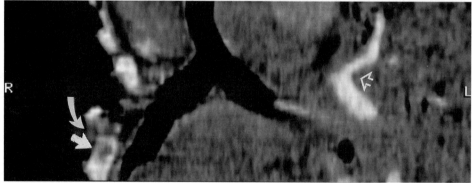

B

FIG. 2. Acute pulmonary embolus in a 63-year-old man with metastatic lung cancer. **A:** This 2.5-mm axial image demonstrates extensive subcarinal and bilateral hilar adenopathy, more severe on the left side. The left lower lobe is collapsed and consolidated, and the left pulmonary artery is narrowed and distorted by tumor encasement (*black arrow*). Only a thin stream of contrast is identified in the interlobar pulmonary artery on the right side (*white arrow*). From the axial images, it is difficult to determine whether this is due to extrinsic compression by tumor or intraluminal clot. **B:** Coronal multiplanar reconstruction image clearly depicts the central filling defect in the interlobar artery on the right side (*white arrow*), diagnostic of acute pulmonary embolus. Adenopathy extrinsic to the vessel (*curved arrow*) is identified. In contrast, encasement, narrowing, and distortion of the left pulmonary arteries by tumor is depicted (*open arrow*), without evidence of internal filling defects. Additionally, tumor extent and relationship to the airways is well demonstrated, including subcarinal and paratracheal adenopathy.

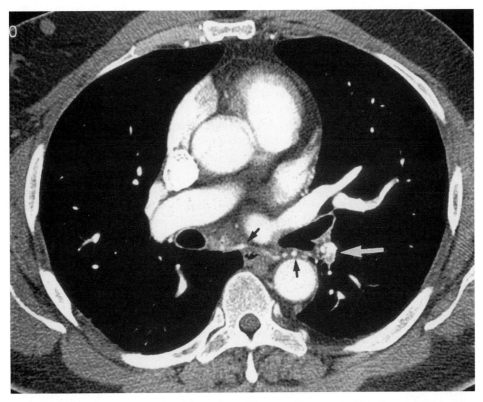

FIG. 3. Chronic thromboembolic disease in a 69-year-old man. A: This 2-mm thick reconstruction depicts a small left pulmonary artery (*arrow*). Eccentric soft tissue filling defects within the vessel represent an organized clot, within which high-density channels of contrast are identified, consequent to recanalization. Note hypertrophic bronchial arteries in the mediastinum (*black arrows*).

design. Compared with sonography, CT venography detected a clot in all 63 patients with DVT (100% sensitivity), but there were two false-positive CT venographic studies (97% specificity), attributed to probable flow artifacts. The authors questioned whether a larger volume of diluted contrast might lessen this phenomenon. CT venography had a 100% negative predictive value and a 71% positive predictive value. CT venography and sonography were deemed equally efficacious in 37% of cases, and CT venography or sonography was considered superior in 36% and 27% of cases, respectively (20). Additionally, although not included in the statistical analysis, a suprainguinal clot was detected in three patients (all with negative leg examinations), and a single patient with either portal vein or subclavian vein thrombus. All five patients with PE at CTPA had positive CT venography and sonography results. These authors conclude that CTPA and venography, combined as a single examination, may be as efficacious as separate CTPA and sonography examinations, particularly in patients under intensive care or obese patients in whom the legs are not easily assessed sonographically.

Aortic Disease

Rapid imaging through a selected region of anatomic interest during the period of high-flow arterial enhancement with IV contrast is the basis for the burgeoning field of CTA. This technique has become an important tool in the assessment of aortic disease, promising to replace conventional angiography in some instances, such as presurgical planning. With conventional HCT, evaluation of the entire aorta was divided into separate studies of the thoracic and abdominal aorta, necessitating sequential administration of contrast, which many times was divided into individual studies performed on different days, due to the high contrast load demanded. MSCT has radically changed our approach to the evaluation of aortic disease (21), allowing evaluation of the aorta during a single breath-hold examination, with the detail allowed by collimation on the order of 2.5 mm and overlapping reconstructions providing reformatted images.

Aortic Aneurysm

The entire thoracoabdominal aorta can be studied during a single breath-hold examination, from the thoracic inlet to the inguinal region, which is usually a 50- to 55-cm area. With a pitch of 1.5 (HS = 3:1) or greater, this can be covered with 2.5-mm collimation in 28 to 30 seconds. Reconstructions with 50% overlap provide data for generation of 3D volume data sets (Fig. 4). Equally importantly, the entire aorta and the iliac arteries can be evaluated with approximately 100 mL of IV contrast, as compared with approximately three times that volume, which was required previously, even with a pitch of 2.

In the thorax, the location, size, extent, and relationship of an aortic aneurysm to the great vessels must be clearly defined for accurate planning of appropriate surgical procedures. Overlapping reconstruction of thin sections reduces volume averaging, which had previously impaired differentiation of calcification, thrombus, and contrast material.

With HCT, the value of MPRs and 3D-reformatted images became apparent in this regard and has become particularly appreciated by the vascular surgical team, oriented to a traditional coronal or sagittal visualization of the aorta. The larger data sets generated with MSCT are further reinforcing deviation away from viewing sequential axial images as the primary approach and emphasizing the value added by MPRs and volumetric renderings.

CTA is also valuable in postsurgical follow-up and ongoing evaluation of stents and grafts. In fact, periaortic leaks around stents or at graft anastomoses are better evaluated with CTA compared with angiography, because extravasation of contrast material, the hallmark of this phenomenon, tends to be a slow-flow leak, which can be missed with conventional angiography (Fig. 5).

Aortic Dissection

HCT is established in most institutions as the initial diagnostic test for the assessment of the patient suspected of aortic dissection (22). Catheter angiography, magnetic resonance imaging (MRI), and transesophageal echocardiography (TEE) are well-recognized, highly accurate alternative means of establishing this diagnosis, but each has drawbacks, which have contributed to the ascendancy of HCT as the initial test in this setting. Catheter angiography carries the attendant morbidity and mortality associated with an invasive procedure and may have limited availability in some institutions. It continues to be valued, however, particularly in its ability to depict coronary artery involvement and aortic valve competency. Patient motion, irregular respirations, or poor ECG gating may degrade MRI image quality, and life support and monitoring devices, if needed, eliminate MRI as an option for critically ill patients. TEE, in combination with transthoracic echocardiography, is highly accurate in making this diagnosis and has the advantage of a portable bedside examination, although 24-hour availability is not provided in many institutions. A well-recognized limitation of this technique is a potential

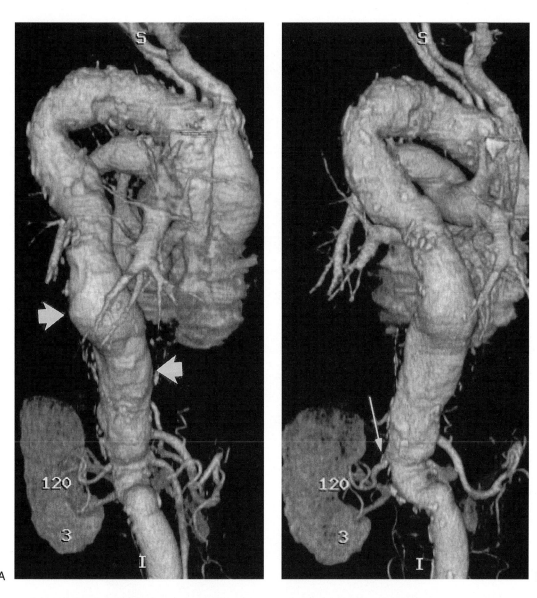

FIG. 4. Distal thoracic and upper abdominal aortic aneurysm. **A:** Three-dimensional recon-struction from volumetric scan data obtained with 2.5-mm collimation during a single breath-hold, from above the aortic arch to the pelvis. Sagittal image depicts tortuosity of the aorta, with extensive atherosclerotic disease and a segment of aneurysmal dilation spanning the lower thoracic and upper abdominal aorta to the level of the celiac axis (*arrows*). **B:** Rotating the im-age slightly to an oblique sagittal position allows identification of the patent left renal artery ori-gin (*arrow*) arising from a point distal to the aneurysm. The patient is status post right nephrec-tomy.

"blind spot" in the ascending aorta, consequent to artifacts from air in the trachea. Sommer et al. (22) recently compared these three modalities and found the sensitivity for the diagnosis of aortic dissection to be 100% in all cases. Specificity was 100% for HCT but 94% for TEE and MRI, respectively (22). HCT, having proved itself as effective as catheter angiography in identifying the site of an intimal tear and the extent of involvement, primary factors in deter-

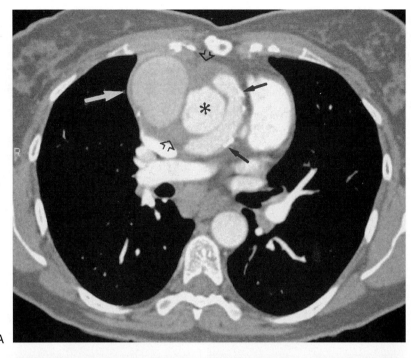

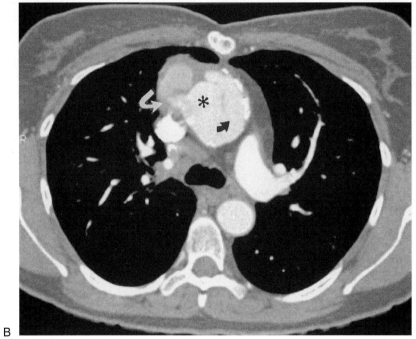

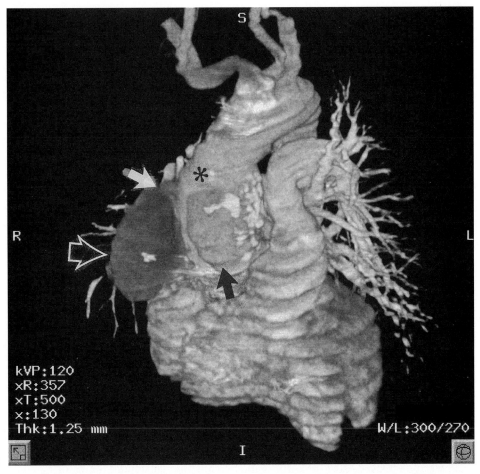

FIG. 5. Pseudoaneurysm formation after inclusion graft placement for an ascending aortic aneurysm. Study was indicated by a dramatic change in the appearance of the chest radiograph. **A:** Axial image obtained with 2.5-mm collimation at a level cephalad to the aortic valve demonstrates contrast-enhanced blood within the endograft lumen (*asterisk*). A crescentic collection of the same density to the left of the graft (*black arrows*) represents perigraft flow, a common occurrence in the potential space created when the native aorta is wrapped around the inclusion graft. Thrombosed blood is also present in the perigraft space (*open arrows*). A partially opacified collection of intermediate density has developed to the right of the ascending aorta, contained by the aortic adventitia (*white arrow*), represents a pseudoaneurysm. **B:** Axial image superior to Fig. 5A demonstrates a wide connection of the graft lumen (*asterisk*) to the perigraft space (*curved arrow*). These channels usually result from partial dehiscence of the suture line. The connection of the graft lumen with the new pseudoaneurysm (*white arrow*) is also demonstrated. Postoperative perigraft flow does not mandate surgical repair, but if there is hemodynamic compromise, symptomatic mass effect, or significant enlargement of a collection, such as in this case, then reoperative repair is indicated. **C:** Three-dimensional reconstruction demonstrates the ascending aortic graft (*asterisk*), the perigraft flow (*black arrow*), and the pseudoaneurysm (*open arrow*) with its connection of the graft lumen (*white arrow*).

mining the prognosis and treatment of the patient, has emerged as the imaging modality of choice for an acutely ill patient (22).

As with single-slice HCT, precontrast sections are obtained, to detect displacement of intimal calcification and high-attenuation aortic wall containing fresh hemorrhage. After administration of contrast, the enhanced resolution of MSCT has made it easier to identify entry tears, fenestrations, or aortic cobwebs and branch involvement. Improved imaging speed provides coverage of the full extent of a potential dissection from the thoracic inlet to the iliac vessels during a single breath-hold and during a single contrast injection. Reconstruction of overlapping images provides multiplanar images, which depict the relationship of intimal flaps to aortic branch vessels more readily than transverse sections alone (23). In fact, reformations in the sagittal or coronal plane of MSCT acquisitions are detailed enough to demonstrate variations in displacement of intimal flaps during the cardiac cycle, which may reveal intermittent occlusion of a true lumen by diastolic expansion of a false lumen. This effect may be hidden at gadolinium-enhanced MR angiography, which averages data obtained throughout a cardiac cycle. The anatomic detail provided could be applied to guide stent deployment, in which accurate preoperative assessment of vessel diameter and tortuosity is essential.

Penetrating Atheromatous Ulcer

Although the clinical presentation may be similar to aortic dissection, characterized by chest or back pain, most penetrating atheromatous ulcers are detected in asymptomatic patients undergoing imaging for another reason. The entity occurs in patients with extensive atheromatous aortic disease, in which ulceration of the atheroma develops and then extends to penetrate the internal elastic lamina into the aortic media (24,25). Blood then leaks into the aortic wall, forming an intramural hematoma, with long-term sequelae including the development of saccular or fusiform aneurysms (26).

Imaging features include a focal collection of contrast material that projects beyond the aortic lumen and may occasionally be multifocal. An intramural hematoma is invariably present, recognized by thickening of the aortic wall, which before the administration of IV contrast, will appear denser than that of the aortic lumen. This blood collection is usually crescent shaped, and although displaced intimal calcifications may be identified, in contradistinction to an aortic dissection, an intimal flap will not be present (24,25) (Fig. 6).

Management generally is conservative, with aggressive antihypertensive therapy as its cornerstone and with surgery reserved for those with an intramural hematoma extending to involve the ascending aorta, those with aortic rupture, pseudoaneurysm, or hemodynamic instability, or those with refractory pain or an enlarging aneurysm (24).

AIRWAY DISEASE

In the past, using conventional HCT, evaluation of the airways entailed an examination divided into various combinations of sequential axial images of varying thickness, to provide sufficient coverage of both central and peripheral airways while providing the resolution necessary for the evaluation of the small airways. This approach is no longer necessary because the entire thorax can be scanned with thin sections during a single breath-hold, and the section thickness appropriate for the region of anatomy under review can then be retrospectively reconstructed. For instance, after obtaining a data set with 1.0- or 1.25-mm collimation, one can perform an evaluation of the trachea with overlapping 3- or 5-mm thick sections (Fig. 7), although detailed evaluation of the hilar airways demands 5- or optimally 3-mm or thinner col-

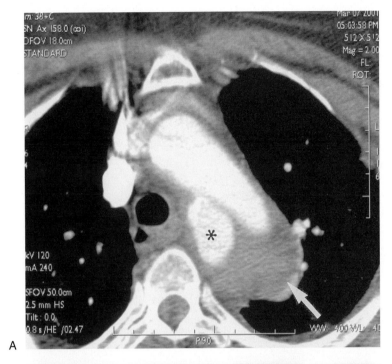

A

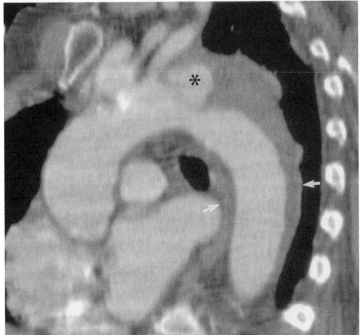

B

FIG. 6. Penetrating atheromatous ulcer. **A:** Axial image obtained with 2.5-mm collimation at the level of the aortic arch depicts a contrast collection (*asterisk*) outside of the aortic lumen, consistent with a penetrating atheromatous ulcer. Low-density material (*white arrow*) represents intramural hematoma. **B:** Sagittal multiplanar reconstruction image better depicts the relationship of the penetrating atheromatous ulcer (*asterisk*) to the great vessels. Anterograde extension of the intramural hematoma (*white arrows*) is creating circumferential thickening of the descending aorta. Calcific atherosclerotic disease is present.

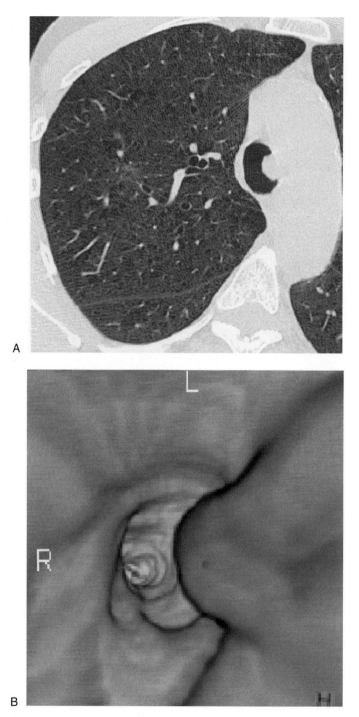

FIG. 7. Central airway lesion: benign cartilaginous tumor. **A:** Axial image obtained with 1-mm collimation demonstrates a nodular density arising from the left wall of the midtrachea. **B:** Internal rendering ("virtual bronchoscopy") simulates the vantage point of an endoscope in the trachea viewing the lesion from above.

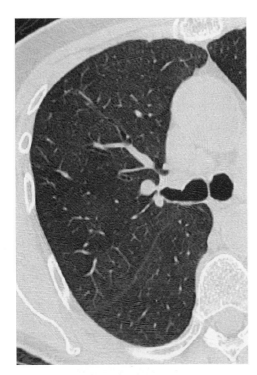 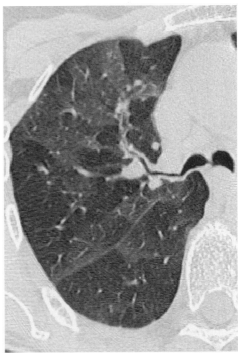

FIG. 8. Central airway disease: dynamic imaging. Axial images of the right lung and carina at inspiration **(left)** and expiration **(right)** demonstrate near-complete collapse of the right upper lobe bronchus and marked narrowing of the main-stem bronchi at expiration. This is consistent with clinically significant tracheobronchomalacia in this 78-year-old woman with shortness of breath. Note that the subtle parenchymal mosaic attenuation pattern on the inspiratory image is accentuated on the expiratory image, confirming regions of air trapping, indicative of small airways disease, as the cause of secondary mosaic perfusion (see also Fig. 9).

limated sections, and high-resolution 1-mm thick sections can be viewed to assess for small airways disease such as bronchiectasis or obstructive small airways disease (Figs. 8 and 9).

Capabilities of MSCT for dynamic inspiratory/expiratory imaging of the airways allow identification of areas of focal or diffuse air trapping or allow physiologic evaluation of the tracheobronchial tree, as may be indicated in such entities as tracheobronchomalacia (Fig. 8). In a study of 13 patients suspected of tracheobronchomalacia, 12 of whom had correlative pulmonary function tests (PFTs) and 6 of whom had correlative fiberoptic bronchoscopy (FOB), airway collapse of more than 75% was identified in 54% at expiration, and collapse of 100% and 50% to 75% was identified in 23% each, respectively, at expiration (27). Significantly, the degree of obstruction as indicated by PFT correlated poorly; all three patients with 100% collapse at MSCT had normal values for the test of forced expiratory volume in 1 second. On the other hand, bronchoscopic findings correlated well in the six patients who underwent FOB, with MSCT underestimating collapse in only one patient. Importantly, volumetric acquisition of data allowed identification of focal areas of malacia in four patients (27), a finding that may be masked on PFTs.

Various reconstruction techniques can now be applied to the huge data sets obtained with thin sections free of respiratory misregistration. These include use of high-resolution MPRs, which are one voxel thick, two-dimensional "tomographic" images, and multiplanar volume reconstructions, which involve the use of average, maximum, or minimum intensity projec-

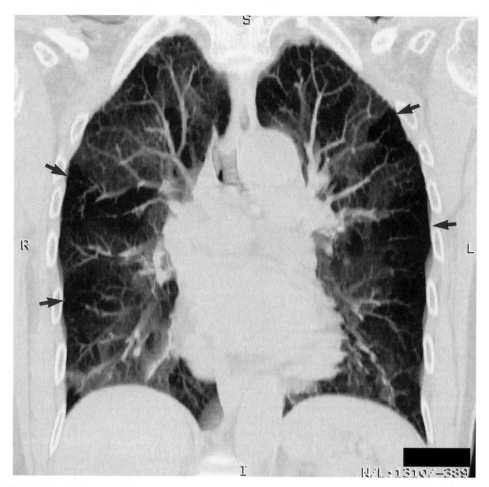

FIG. 9. Small airways disease: dynamic imaging. Coronal multiplanar volumetric reformatted image from scan data obtained with 1-mm collimation during expiration in the same patient as Fig. 8. The lung parenchyma demonstrates a mosaic attenuation pattern, with low-density areas (*arrows*), within which vessels are sparse, representing regions of air trapping. This diffuse pattern of disease is consistent with bronchiolitis obliterans, although this patient also had bronchiectasis identified in selected areas. Disease extent and regional involvement is better appreciated when the entire lung is viewed.

tion imaging. MPRs are easily and quickly reconstructed and may follow any arbitrary straight or curved plane. Curved MPRs along the axis of a bronchus are useful, for instance, in evaluation of bronchial stenoses, such as may occur after lung transplantation or after inflammation, and for localization when planning or following bronchial stent placements. MPRs are also useful in providing detailed visualization of both airways disease and peribronchial/mediastinal extent of disease, for instance, in lung cancer staging (Fig. 2). External renderings with 3D shaded surface displays (SSDs) and internal renderings, popularly termed "virtual bronchoscopy" (Fig. 7), can also be applied to airways evaluation, although in general they add little value over MPRs.

Whether the addition of virtual bronchoscopic images significantly alters diagnoses remains moot. However, these images, which mimic the perspective as seen through an endoscope, may be preferred by pulmonologists accustomed to such vantage points and may in select cases, such as when bronchoscopy is refused or precluded by medical considerations, obviate bronchoscopy (27).

PARENCHYMAL DISEASE

Pulmonary Nodules

Enhanced nodule detection with HCT is well accepted, attributed primarily to improved contrast and spatial resolution provided by overlapping helical reconstructions, which ensure that a given nodule would not be missed due to misregistration artifacts from variations in level of suspended breath and would not "disappear" due to volume averaging with the lung parenchyma. With this technique, even very small nodules are detected. These results promise to be improved with MSCT scanning, in which even thinner sections can be obtained during a single breath-hold, without compromise to anatomic coverage. This is important in cases in which nodule detection is the primary goal, such as an evaluation for metastatic disease, or in lung cancer screening, which is discussed later in this chapter. It is accepted that optimal results require overlapping reconstruction of 20% to 30%.

An important additional advantage to MSCT scans is that use of thin collimation allows routine creation of retrospective reconstructions through detected nodules without the need to rescan patients. The benefits in terms of decreased cost, radiation exposure, anxiety, and effort on the part of both the patient and the radiologist are obvious. This allows easy identification of fat or calcium, if present, and provides the ability to perform a detailed assessment of the morphology of the nodule and accurate size measurements (Fig. 10). From this volumetric data set, considerable research interest is currently directed toward the potential to acquire detailed 3D images of nodules segmented out from the background lung parenchyma on a routine basis. Such data will provide volumetric quantification of nodule size, allowing comparisons of volumetric measurements, rather than the imprecise two-dimensional orthogonal measurements routinely used, in nodule follow-up studies. Although the development of such tools has focused primarily on the field of lung cancer screening, the potential application for such tools includes all oncology patients for whom evaluation of the presence and extent of metastatic disease is clinically significant. In particular, it may be anticipated that the ability to accurately assess subtle temporal changes in the size of lesions as a means of assessing response to therapy will be enthusiastically employed by oncologists.

Diffuse Interstitial Lung Disease

In general, conventional single-detector HCT added little to the high-resolution CT (HRCT) examination technique in the patient being evaluated for interstitial lung disease. HRCT examinations are considered a sampling technique, with large interspace gaps between the thinly collimated sections, so the potential for contiguous volumetric data acquisition has added no significant benefit in most instances.

The use of volumetric HRCT has been described in limited settings, particularly the evaluation of nodular disease. Parenchymal disease may be better characterized and localized relative to the underlying parenchymal anatomy if several thin sections are summed and then viewed using a maximum intensity projection (MIP) reconstruction algorithm. The benefits of this technique have been reported in axial images obtained with conventional HCT (28,29) and can be applied to MPR images (Fig. 11). This postprocessing application is available on most workstations and takes a negligible amount of time to apply. By so doing, the underlying nor-

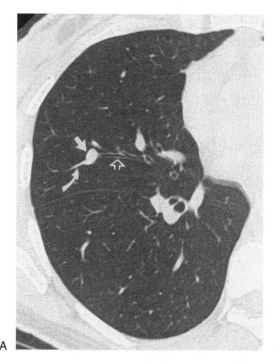

A

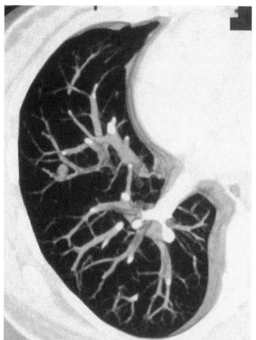

B

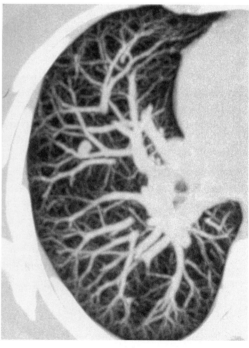

C

FIG. 10. Focal lung disease: solitary pulmonary nodule enhancement study. After scan data are obtained with 1-mm collimation, it can be surveyed with 5- or 7-mm reconstructions to detect focal disease. An identified nodule can then be characterized with targeted 1-mm thick reconstructions **(A)** without the need for follow-up high-resolution imaging. In this case, the relationship of an indeterminate nodule (*arrow*) to the bronchus (*open arrow*) is well demonstrated. Close proximity to a vessel (*curved arrow*) raised the question of whether the density represented a branching vessel or a true nodule. Volumetric reformatted image **(B)** and maximum intensity projection image **(C)** created from 20 mm of volumetric data confirm the abnormality as a nodule abutting a vessel, but independent of the vessel.

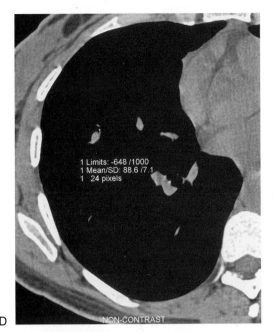
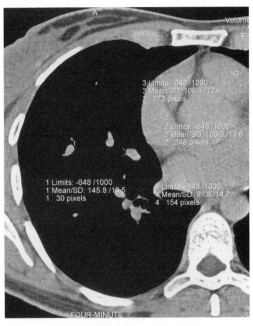

FIG. 10. *Continued.* **D:** This 1-mm targeted axial reconstruction before the administration of intravenous (IV) contrast confirms the absence of calcium within the nodule, and region of interest measurements document its precontrast density as 88.6 Hounsfield units (HU). **E:** Four minutes after the injection of IV contrast, the density of the nodule measures 145.8 HU. Density increases of more than 15 to 20 HU after contrast administration indicate a metabolically active lesion, and the possibility of neoplasm must be considered.

mal lung anatomy, which paradoxically may be difficult to discern with very thin sections in which familiar landmarks may not be well appreciated, is rendered more recognizable. Abnormalities are more readily localized relative to normal vascular, bronchial, and lobular anatomy when these structures become more visible. Small focal abnormalities, such as pulmonary nodules, may also be better appreciated with this technique, because nodules are easily missed on high-resolution thin sections, because they mimic the appearance of small vessels in cross section. With summed thin-section images, spatial resolution is not degraded and the MIP images allow appreciation of vessels as linear and branching structures, as they traverse the thicker summed image, thereby accentuating recognition of small nodules, which are not connected to nearby vascular structures (Fig. 11).

MSCT has the potential to fundamentally change the way HRCT is approached. We routinely obtain our scan data with thin collimation, even when "routine" thick-section contiguous images are indicated. Virtually all dedicated routine thoracic studies, therefore, potentially represent simultaneous high-resolution studies. The volumetric data resulting from this mode of scanning enable the evaluation of HRCT images when and where needed. HRCT examinations can now be easily combined with conventional examinations, which are potentially of importance in many clinical settings that normally require the acquisition of additional HRCT images, sometimes as a follow-up examination. For instance, in the evaluation of the patient with lung cancer, in whom evaluation of the primary tumor, hila, and mediastinum mandates contiguous thicker sections, HRCT images can be reconstructed from the available scan data if the question of lymphangitic spread of tumor (Fig. 1) or drug reaction to chemotherapeutic agents becomes a clinical concern. In patients being consid-

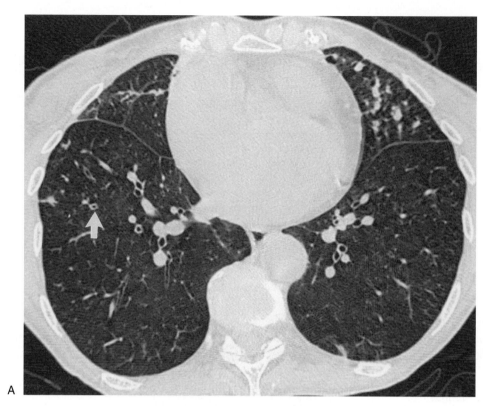

A

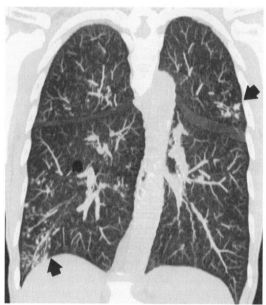

B

FIG. 11. High-resolution computed tomography. **A:** This 1-mm axial image depicts increased nodular and linear markings in the middle lobe, lingula, and anterior right lower lobe. Bronchial wall thickening and mild bronchiectasis is present in the right lower lobe (*arrow*). The pattern and distribution of the nodules is difficult to characterize on thin sections because their relationship to anatomic landmarks such as bronchi and vessels is less readily perceived. **B:** Coronal maximum intensity projection image created from a 15-mm volumetric data set clearly depicts the clustered distribution of the nodules around bronchi, in a classic "tree-in-bud" pattern (*arrows*) consistent with bronchiolar impaction seen in infectious small airways disease. This patient had sputum cultures positive for *Mycobacterium avium* complex.

ered for volume-reduction surgery, HRCT images for evaluation of emphysema can be obtained simultaneously with a survey examination to rule out an associated occult lung carcinoma, which is well known to occur in this population. As is further discussed, a survey examination for a lung nodule with contiguous thicker sections provides data that can then allow high-resolution contiguous thin-section characterization of the nodule, should one be identified. Other potential settings in which combined HRCT and contiguous volumetric imaging are required include the high-resolution evaluation of the lung parenchyma in the patient undergoing CTPA for a possible PE, to detect either parenchymal abnormalities such as mosaic perfusion related to the PE or unrelated abnormalities that may account for the patient's symptoms. In sarcoidosis, the desire to combine the evaluation of the mediastinum and hila for adenopathy with high-resolution evaluation of the lung parenchyma had traditionally resulted in a compromised technique, which can now be optimized without additional time or radiation dose to the patient.

Volumetric data sets obtained in the chest with 1- or 1.25-mm collimation during a single breath-hold can be reconstructed with MPRs, promoting a new approach to the evaluation of the lung parenchyma. All zones of the lung can be evaluated simultaneously, from the apices through the bases, in either the coronal or sagittal dimension. The data either can be paged through sequentially or more appropriately given the large number of images can be moved through with cine mode viewing. Variations in regional disease, including subtle variations in lung attenuation, will be better appreciated with this approach (Fig. 9). The capacity for cardiac gating provides further improvement in HRCT image quality (Fig. 12).

Trauma

The trauma patient is often the most acutely ill patient to present to the radiology suite. Initial imaging studies invariably include a portable chest radiograph, which even with optimal technique is a challenging examination to interpret. In the setting of trauma, a rapid and accurate diagnosis is critical, and examination technique is limited due to patient positioning, overlying instruments, clothing, and occasionally the body habitus and inconsistent exposure technique. MSCT allows rapid and comprehensive screening of the thorax, including evaluation of the mediastinum and aorta, lungs, bronchi, diaphragm, esophagus, spine, and other osseous structures.

Data sets obtained with thin collimation can be reconstructed to evaluate the soft tissue structures (Fig. 13A and B), and again using a bone algorithm for evaluation of the spine and other osseous structures (Fig. 13C and D). Precise timing of contrast administration allows optimal evaluation of the thoracic aorta, and the rapid acquisition of images allows evaluation of the abdomen with the same contrast bolus. MPR images are valuable to assess the course and contour of the aorta and to define its relationship to mediastinal hematoma (Fig. 9C), if present. Imaging during the period of dense intravascular opacification also allows identification of intraluminal thrombus or an intimal flap, if present, which is a less common and often more subtle manifestation of traumatic aortic injury.

Detailed evaluation of the mediastinum also allows identification of mediastinal air, if present, and defines its relationship to the airways, which may aid in localizing the site of a bronchial rupture. MPRs are also useful in this regard and are extremely useful for evaluation of the diaphragm for possible rupture. This is an often missed diagnosis, in part because the diaphragm is generally in the plane of section on axial views and detection of tears or disruption are hence difficult to detect. Herniation of abdominal structures above the diaphragm is more easily appreciated with MPR images.

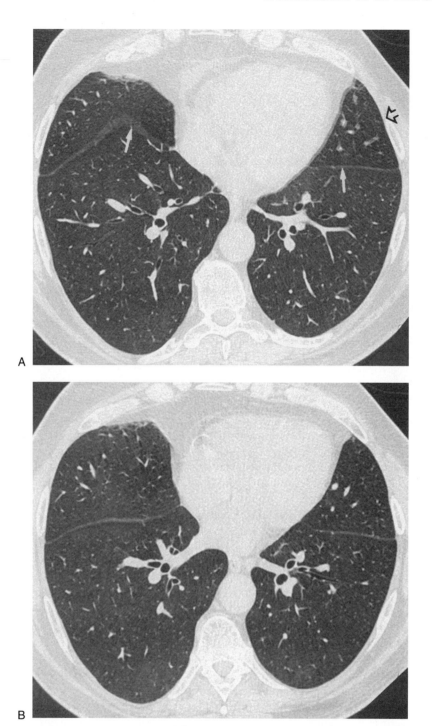

FIG. 12. High-resolution computed tomography: retrospective cardiac gating. **A:** This 1-mm thick section without cardiac gating demonstrates motion artifacts blurring the vessels in the lingula (*open arrow*) and thickening the oblique fissures (*arrows*). Note misregistration artifacts along the border of the left side of the heart. **B:** This 1-mm thick axial section with retrospective cardiac gating shows the motion artifact eliminated. The border of the left side of the heart and the fissures are now sharp.

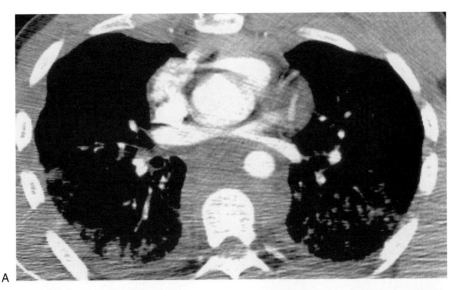

A

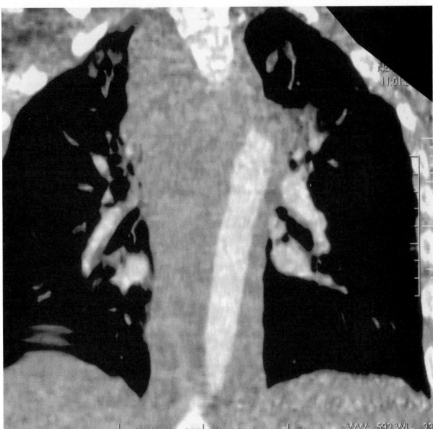

B

FIG. 13. Large mediastinal hematoma in a 25-year-old victim of blunt trauma from a motor vehicle accident. **A:** A 5-mm axial image created from data obtained with 2.5-mm collimation demonstrates a large posterior mediastinal hematoma expanding the paravertebral regions, surrounding the descending aorta, and producing mass effect on the heart. There is also an anterior mediastinal hematoma seen in conjunction with a sternal fracture. **B:** Coronal reconstruction clearly demonstrates expansion of the mediastinum by blood. The aorta is deviated in position, but its size and contour are normal. Because of the large volume of blood in proximity to the aorta, aortography was performed, confirming a normal aorta.

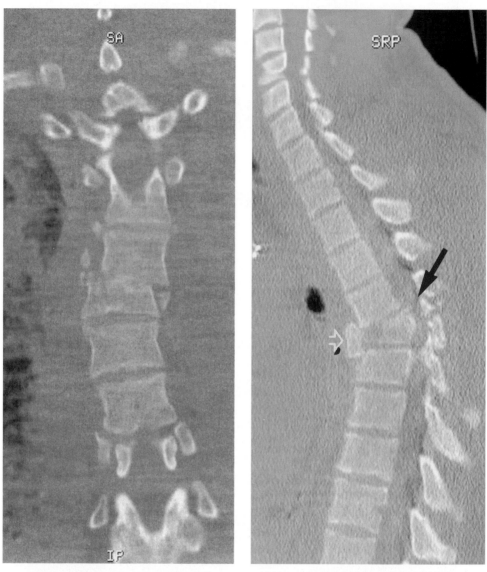

FIG. 13. *Continued.* **C, D:** Detailed evaluation of osseous structures, the diaphragm, and central airways can also be reconstructed from the same data set. In this instance, **(C)** coronal reconstructions demonstrate a compression fracture with displaced fracture fragments in a midthoracic vertebral body. There is lateral subluxation present as well. **D:** Focal kyphosis and the degree of impingement on the osseous neural canal are better appreciated on the sagittal reconstruction (*arrow*). A fracture fragment is displaced anteriorly (*open arrow*).

Lung Cancer Screening

The role of CT in screening for the detection of early lung cancer has emerged as one of the most controversial issues in radiology today. Lung cancer is the leading cause of cancer-related death in both men and women in the United States. Survival statistics are dismal: The overall cure rate remains only 12%, with a 5-year survival rate of 15%. To a degree, this is thought to partially reflect the advanced stage of many lung cancers at presentation.

Routine chest radiography proved sufficiently effective in reducing disease-specific mortality, presumably because of its relative insensitivity in the detection of small tumors. Accordingly, radiologic screening for lung cancer has not been endorsed in the past. Recent studies reporting the potential for low-dose CT screening have incited intense interest in this modality.

In the initial report by Sone et al. (30), of the 5,843 asymptomatic individuals screened with chest radiographs and low-dose CT, 19 cancers with a mean size of 17 mm were detected. In this study, the lung cancer detection rate equaled 0.48% and 0.36% for CT versus chest radiography, respectively (30). Similar results have been reported by Kaneko et al. (31); of the 15 primary lung cancers detected among the 1,369 screened individuals in this series, 11 were visible only at CT. More recently, Henschke et al. (32) used low-dose CT to screen 1,000 asymptomatic smokers in the Early Lung Cancer Action Project (ELCAP). Noncalcified nodules were identified in 233 (23%), 27 (2.3%) of which proved to be malignant. Twenty-six of the 27 proved resectable; in fact, 85% were stage I neoplasms (32).

Despite growing interest and enthusiasm generated by these data, a number of problems relating to single-slice low-dose CT imaging have become apparent. In particular these include limitations in both the sensitivity and the specificity of nodule detection; the necessity for repeated examinations for further nodule characterization, and hence additional cost and radiation dose; and limitations of sophisticated computer-assisted techniques for increasing the ease and accuracy of low-dose CT screening. In each instance, MSCT offers a clear improvement over routine HCT for low-dose imaging for early detection of lung cancer. Once the nodules are detected, coordination of an appropriate management plan for these nodules presents a significant clinical challenge, toward which management algorithms remain in evolution.

The limitation in the sensitivity of low-dose CT in the detection of nodules was emphasized by the study of Kakinuma et al. (33). In this report of 1,443 smokers, studied with a total of 5,418 baseline and follow-up scans, 7 of 22 lung cancers were only identified retrospectively, ranging in size from 4 to 13 mm. Based on these data, these authors concluded that the minimum threshold for accurate identification of nodules was between 7 and 9 mm (33). Similarly, in the ELCAP study, when a conventional-dose diagnostic HCT was later obtained to characterize nodules detected at screening in 188 cases, a total of 31 individuals (16%) proved to have additional nodules. These were missed on the initial scan but could be retrospectively identified (34).

Of equal significance is the problem of specificity and false-positive examination results (30,31,35). In the study by Kaneko et al. (31), only 19 (8.3%) of 228 lesions assessed by HRCT proved to be malignant. More recently in the ELCAP prevalence study, 233 nodules were detected in 23% of the individuals screened, but only 2.7% proved malignant (32). Based on preliminary data from a number of studies presently underway, it is likely that the prevalence of noncalcified nodules among asymptomatic screened individuals may be as high as 50%.

A number of strategies have been employed to accurately characterize pulmonary nodules, to estimate the probability of malignancy. Henschke et al. (35) selected the 133 nodules of 2 cm or less in diameter from the 233 individuals with a baseline CT positive for pulmonary nodules in the ELCAP study for further characterization. Factors assessed included those relating to lung cancer risk such as age, smoking history, and asbestos exposure histories, as well as nodule features such as size, location, shape, and edges. The strongest indicators of malignancy in decreasing order were size, female gender, central location, and smoking history. Only 1% of the nodules 2 to 5 mm in diameter proved malignant; 25% of those between 6 and 10 mm, 33% of those between 11 and 20 mm, and 80% of those between 20 and 45 mm in size proved malignant (35).

These data emphasize that for screening CT to be accepted, improvement in its accuracy and application are required. There is growing interest in computer-aided diagnosis (CAD) as an additional tool. Preliminary work has shown that CAD may be of potential value as a method for both nodule detection and decreasing the time necessary to interpret large data sets (36). It should be noted that efforts in developing CAD have shifted from single-slice to multislice scanners, acknowledging the benefits to be gained from thinner sections, decreased motion, and overlapping reconstructions when applying this tool.

MSCT represents an important improvement in the clinical efficacy and hence potential widespread acceptance of low-dose early detection of a lung cancer. The entire thorax is routinely scanned using thin sections of 1.0 to 1.25 mm during a single breath-hold and can be reconstructed with overlapping sections, as needed. In fact, a section of any slice width desired for routine viewing, such as 5- or 7-mm thick sections, can be reconstructed from the same data set. Then, as needed, target high-resolution images through select regions of interest, such as nodules, can be obtained without the need for additional scans (Fig. 14). By eliminating the need to acquire additional high-resolution scans, a considerable reduction in radiation dose is achieved. Equally importantly, in those instances when the examination isn't reviewed until after the patient has left the department, the ability to retrospectively reconstruct thin sections through select regions of interest obviates having patients return for detailed nodule characterization studies. This significantly reduces the number of follow-up examinations, and hence the overall cost, as well as radiation exposure to the patient. Not to be dismissed is the decrease in attendant anxiety experienced by patients with nodules, particularly those in whom the thin sections reveal occult calcifications, sparing these patients the psychological discomfort of living with an indeterminate lung nodule while waiting for a follow up examination.

A compelling feature of this technique is the ability to perform the examination with significantly reduced tube currents and hence significantly reduced patient exposure dose. Most initial reports used tube currents of approximately 40 to 50 mA and 7- to 10-mm thick sections (30–32). We have found image quality to be adequate with tube currents as low as 10 mA in most cases with 10-mm thick sections at HCT. Preliminary data from our institution using various tube currents show that although the image quality of 7- to 8-mm axial images is adequate in nearly all cases regardless of dose, considerable variation results when these same volumetrically acquired data sets are reconstructed using 1.0- to 1.25-mm thick sections. Accordingly, it is our recommendation to use 20 mA in all cases except for very large patients, for whom adequate images through the lung apices typically require 40 mA.

Finally, as MSCT is applied to low-dose lung cancer screening, it becomes apparent that the ability to generate high-resolution thin CT sections clearly represents an important potential improvement over routine single-slice CT scanners for identifying and characterizing lung lesions (36) (Fig. 15). What is not clear is whether routine axial images are sufficient in themselves for optimal interpretation of these large data sets. Currently only few data are available directly addressing the potential use of alternative viewing techniques, such as sliding MIP images, variable imaging planes, and real-time volumetric rendering techniques. These and other technical improvements should still further enhance the value of MSCT for assessing pulmonary nodules.

As has been mentioned, the capability to obtain 0.5-mm thick sections in some scanners can provide true isotropic voxels, which will allow nodule assessment and volume determinations without distortion. Detection of even subtle interval growth of a nodule in serial examinations is likely to prove the single most important predictor of potential malignancy. As reported by Yankelovitz et al. (37) in a preliminary study of 15 patients with lung nodules, 9 of which proved malignant, it was possible to detect growth in all malignant lesions within 30 days, when comparing serial volume measurements, at a point before nodule growth was evident on

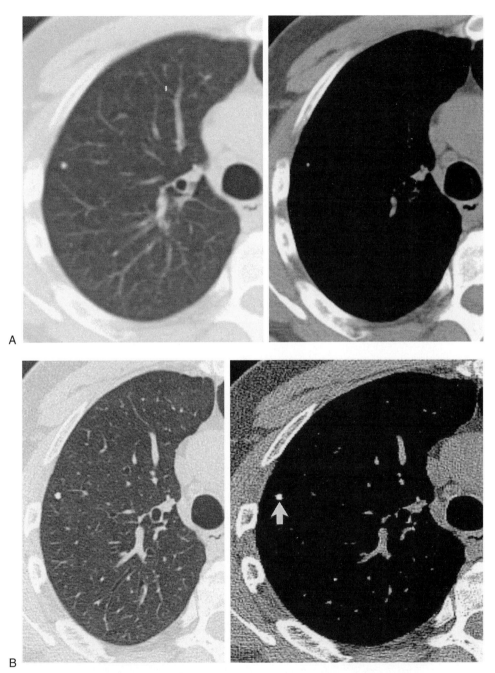

FIG. 14. Early lung cancer detection: computed tomographic screening. **A:** These 7-mm thick axial images of the right lung reconstructed from 1-mm collimated data imaged with wide **(left)** and narrow **(right)** windows reveal a small (approximately 4-mm) nodule in the periphery of the lung (*arrows*). Calcification within the nodule cannot be detected on the 7-mm thick section. **B:** These 1-mm reconstructions from the same data set clearly demonstrate that the nodule is densely calcified (*arrow*). The ability to provide detailed nodule characterization without having to bring the patient back for further imaging decreases radiation exposure, cost, labor, and in many cases, patient anxiety and the need for additional imaging.

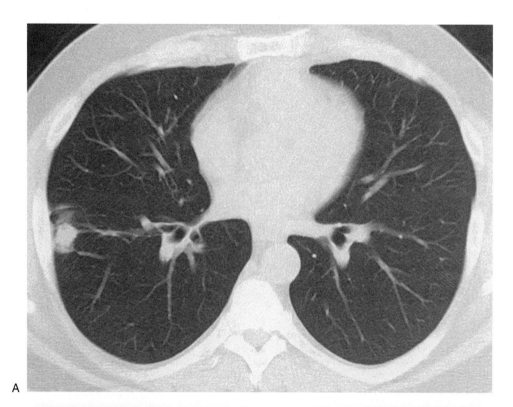

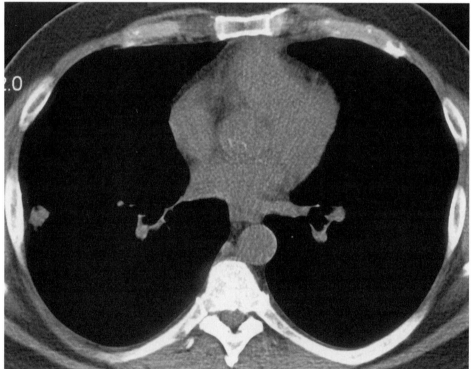

FIG. 15. Early lung cancer detection: screen detected cancer. Axial 1-mm thick sections imaged with **(A)** wide and **(B)** narrow windows demonstrate an unsuspected irregularly marginated nodule in the subpleural right lower lobe in an asymptomatic 60-year-old smoker. This proved to be stage 1A adenocarcinoma.

visual inspection. Hence, tools to allow temporal comparison of nodule volumes, as a means to accurately assess interval change in nodule size, are underdevelopment. These techniques will likely find other applications, such as determining response to chemotherapy of known malignant nodules.

REFERENCES

1. Kalender WA, Seissler W, Klotz E, et al. Spiral volumetric CT with single-breath-hold technique, continuous transport, and continuous scanner rotation. Radiology 1990;176:181–183.
2. Rubin GD, Leung AN, Robertson VJ, et al. Thoracic spiral CT: influence of sub-second gantry rotation on image quality. Radiology 1998;208:771–776.
3. Naidich DP. Helical computed tomography of the thorax. Clinical applications. Radiol Clin North Am 1994;32: 759–774.
4. Rubin GD. Data explosion: the challenge of multidetector-row CT. Eur J Radiol 2000;36:74–80.
5. Schoepf UJ, Becker CR, Bruening ED, et al. Electrocardiographically gated thin-section CT of the lung. Radiology 1999;212:649–654.
6. Costello P, Dupuy DE, Ecker CP, et al. Spiral CT of the thorax with reduced volume of contrast material: a comparative study. Radiology 1992;183:663–666.
7. Rubin GD, Lane MJ, Bloch DA, et al. Optimization of thoracic spiral CT: effects of iodinated contrast medium concentration. Radiology 1996;201:785–791.
8. Goodman LR, Curtin JH, Mewissen MW, et al. Detection of pulmonary embolism in patients with unresolved clinical and scintigraphic diagnosis: helical CT versus angiography. Am J Roentgenol 1995;164:1369–1374.
9. Goodman LR, Lipchik RJ, Kuzo RS. Acute pulmonary embolism: the role of computed tomographic imaging. J Thorac Imaging 1997;12:83–86.
10. Mayo JR, Remy-Jardin M, Muller NL, et al. Pulmonary embolism: prospective comparison of spiral CT and ventilation perfusion scintigraphy. Radiology 1997;205:447–452.
11. Remy-Jardin M, Remy J, Deschildre F, et al. Diagnosis of acute pulmonary embolism with spiral CT: comparison with pulmonary angiography and scintigraphy. Radiology 1996;200:699–706.
12. Van Rossum AB, Pattynama PM, Ton ER, et al. Pulmonary embolism. Validation of spiral CT angiography in 149 patients. Radiology 1996;201:467–470.
13. Remy-Jardin M, Remy J, Artaud D, et al. Peripheral pulmonary arteries: optimization of the spiral CT acquisition protocol. Radiology 1997;204:157–163.
14. Quanadli SD, Hajjam ME, Mesurolle B, et al. Pulmonary embolism detection: prospective evaluation of dual-section helical CT versus selective pulmonary arteriography in 157 patients. Radiology 2000;217:447–455.
15. Remy-Jardin M, Remy J, Cauvain O, et al. Diagnosis of central pulmonary embolism with helical CT: role of two-dimensional multiplanar reformations. Am J Roentgenol 1995;165:1131–1138.
16. Remy-Jardin M, Remy J, Artaud D, et al. Spiral CT of pulmonary embolism: Technical considerations and interpretive pitfalls. J Thorac Imaging 1997;12:103–117.
17. Yankelovitz DF, Gamsu G, Shah A, et al. Optimization of combined CT pulmonary angiography with lower extremity CT venography. AJR Am J Roentgenol 2000;174:67–69.
18. Loud PA, Grossman ZD, Klippenstein DL, et al. Combined CT venography and pulmonary angiography: a new diagnostic technique for suspected thromboembolic disease. AJR Am J Roentgenol 1998;170:951–954.
19. Loud PA, Katz DS, Klippenstein DL, et al. Combined CT venography and pulmonary angiography in suspected thromboembolic disease: diagnostic accuracy for deep venous thrombosis. AJR Am J Roentgenol 2000;174:61–65.
20. Garg K, Kemp JL, Wojcik D, et al. Thromboembolic disease: comparison of combined CT pulmonary angiography and venography with bilateral leg sonography in 70 patients. AJR Am J Roentgenol 2000;175:997–1001.
21. Rubin GD, Shiau MC, Schmidt AJ, et al. Computed tomographic angiography: historical perspective and new state-of-the-art using multi detector-row helical computed tomography. JCAT 1999;23[Suppl]:S83–S90.
22. Sommer T, Fehske W, Holzknecht N, et al. Aortic dissection: a comparative study of diagnosis with spiral CT, multiplanar transesophageal echocardiography, and MR imaging. Radiology 1996;199:347–352.
23. Zeman RK, Berman PM, Soilverman PM, et al. Diagnosis of aortic dissection: value of helical CT with multiplanar reformation and three-dimensional rendering. AJR Am J Roentgenol 1995;164:1375–1380.
24. Kazerooni EA, Bree RI, Williams DM. Penetrating atherosclerotic ulcers of the descending thoracic aorta: evaluation with CT and distinction from aortic dissection. Radiology 1992;183:759–765.
25. Welch TJ, Stanson AW, Sheedy PF, et al. Radiologic evaluation of penetrating aortic atherosclerotic ulcer. Radiographics 1990;10:675–685.
26. Sueyoshi E, Matsuoka Y, Dakamoto I, et al. Fate of intramural hematoma of the aorta: CT evaluation. JCAT 1997;21(6):931–938.
27. Gilkeson RC, Ciancibello LM, Hejal RB, et al. Tracheobronchomalacia: dynamic airway evaluation with multidetector CT. Am J Roentgenol 2001;176:205–210.
28. Bhalla M, Naidich DP, McGuinness G, et al. Diffuse lung disease: assessment with helical CT—preliminary observations of the role of maximum and minimum projection images. Radiology 1996;200:341–347.

29. Remy-Jardin M, Remy J, Artaud D, et al. Diffuse infiltrative lung disease: clinical value of sliding-thin-slab maximum intensity projection CT scans in the detection of mild micronodular patterns. Radiology 1996;200:333–339.

30. Sone S, Takashima S, Li F, et al. Mass screening for lung cancer with mobile spiral computed tomography scanner. Lancet 1998;351:1242–1245.

31. Kaneko M, Eguchi K, Ohmatsu H. Peripheral lung cancer: screening and detection with low-dose spiral CT versus radiography. Radiology 1996;201:798–802.

32. Henschke CI, McCauley DI, Yankelovitz DF, et al. Early Lung Cancer Action Project: overall design and findings from baseline screening. Lancet 1999;354:99–105.

33. Kakinuma R, Ohmatsu H, Kaneko M, et al. Detection failures in spiral CT screening for lung cancer: analysis of CT findings. Radiology 1999;209:61–66.

34. Naidich DP, Yankelovitz DF, McGuinness G, et al. Noncalcified pulmonary nodules missed on low-dose helical CT. Radiology 1999;213:303.

35. Henschke CI, McCauley DI, Yankelovitz DF, et al. Probability of malignancy of small noncalcified nodules detected on low-dose CT of the chest. Radiology 1999;213:303.

36. Naidich DP, Rusinek H. Multislice low-dose CT for early lung cancer detection: current status and future applications. 2000 *(in press)*.

37. Yankelovitz DF, Gupta R, Zhao B, et al. Small pulmonary nodules: evaluation with repeat CT—preliminary experience. Radiology 1999;212:561–566.

Protocol 1:
THORACIC SURVEY (Fig. 1)

INDICATION: *Detection/staging thoracic
                                      neoplasia/adenopathy/complex
                                      pulmonary–pleural disease*

SCANNER SETTINGS: kV(p): 140
                                     mA: 120

ORAL CONTRAST: None

PHASE OF RESPIRATION: Suspended inspiration

ROTATION TIME: 0.5 sec routinely—0.75 for small chests
                                        (0.8 sec)

**ACQUISITION SLICE
   THICKNESS:**   1.0–2.5 mm combined with abdomen

PITCH: Variable, to include thorax in single breath-
                                        hold, usually 4–6 (HS = 6:1)

**RECONSTRUCTION SLICE
   THICKNESS/INTERVAL
   FOR FILMING:**   5.0–7.0 mm/4.0–6.0 mm

RECONSTRUCTION ALGORITHM: Mediastinum − Kernal AB = 40 (standard)
                                     Lung − Kernal AB = 70 (high-frequency E_2
                                        filter)

**ANATOMIC COVERAGE:
   SUPERIOR EXTENT:**   Superior margin of clavicles (above lung
                                        apices)
**   INFERIOR EXTENT:**   Posterior costophrenic sulci (caudal lung
                                        bases) (or adrenal glands)

IV CONTRAST:

Concentration:	High osmolar contrast medium (HOCM) 282 mg iodine/mL (60% solution)
Rate:	2 mL/sec
Scan Delay:	45 sec
Total Volume:	100–125 mL

COMMENTS:

1. 1 or 2.5-mm thick high-resolution images can be reconstructed through focal lesions or lung regions as needed (Fig. 1B), either prospectively or retrospectively.
2. If the study is part of a chest–abdomen–pelvis examination, the 2.5-mm collimation array should be used on the Volume Zoom scanner.
3. 0.75 rotation time is used with the Volume Zoom in small patients. The longer rotation time allows double sampling ("flying focal spot"), which enhances the signal to noise ratio.
4. If radiation exposure is a concern (especially in young patients), the examination may be obtained with a low-dose technique, using 40–80 mA.

Protocol 2A:
PULMONARY EMBOLI (Figs. 2 and 3)

INDICATION:	*Suspicion of acute or chronic thromboembolic disease*
SCANNER SETTINGS:	kV(p): 140 mA: 120
ORAL CONTRAST:	None
PHASE OF RESPIRATION:	Suspended inspiration
ROTATION TIME:	0.5 sec routinely—0.75 for small chests (0.8 sec)
ACQUISITION SLICE THICKNESS:	1.0–2.5 mm
PITCH:	Variable, to include thorax in single breath-hold, usually 4–6 (HS-6:1)
RECONSTRUCTION SLICE THICKNESS/NTERVAL FOR FILMING:	1.0–2.0 mm/2.0–4.0 mm Lung, every other image Mediastinum, each image
RECONSTRUCTION ALGORITHM:	Mediastinum − Kernal AB = 40 (standard) Lung − Kernal AB = 70 (high-frequency E_2 filter)

ANATOMIC COVERAGE:
  SUPERIOR EXTENT:
  INFERIOR EXTENT:
	Entire thorax, caudal to cephalad
	Superior margin of clavicles
	Upper abdomen

IV CONTRAST:

Concentration:	
A. HOCM:	282 mg iodine/mL (60% solution)
B. Low osmolar content medium (LOCM):	150 mg iodine/mL (30% solution)
Rate:	A. 3–4 mL/sec
	B. 5–6 mL/sec
Scan Delay:	Test dose or Bolus Tracking Software; usually about 15–20 sec
Total Volume:	150 mL

COMMENTS:

1. *Test bolus:* image over the pulmonary arteries every 10 sec, following initial test injection of 20 mL of contrast. Base scan delay on time of the image with optimal pulmonary arterial opacification.
2. Protocol 2B uses more dilute contrast at a higher flow rate to prevent streak artifacts from contrast in the superior vena cava.
3. MPRs can be very quickly and easily generated to image vessels along their longitudinal axes. This can be very useful in differentiation between intraluminal clot and extrinsic disease, including possible vascular compression from adenopathy (Fig. 2).

Protocol 2B:
PELVIS/LEG VENOGRAPHY

INDICATION:	*Suspicion of DVT in pelvis or leg veins*
SCANNER SETTINGS:	kV(p): 120 mA: 240
ORAL CONTRAST:	None
PHASE OF RESPIRATION:	N/A
ROTATION TIME:	0.5 sec (0.8 sec)
ACQUISITION SLICE THICKNESS:	5.0–7.5 mm
PITCH:	Variable (HS = 6:1)
RECONSTRUCTION SLICE THICKNESS/INTERVAL FOR FILMING:	5.0–7.5 mm/4.0–6.0 mm

ANATOMIC COVERAGE:
    SUPERIOR EXTENT:
    INFERIOR EXTENT:
	
	Iliac crests
	Tibial plateau

IV CONTRAST:

> No additional contrast when performed in conjunction with the PE study
> **Scan Delay:**   2 min after initial injection

Protocol 3:
THORACIC AORTA (Figs. 4–6)

INDICATION:	*Aortic dissection, aneurysm assessment, penetrating atheromatous ulcer*
SCANNER SETTINGS:	kV(p): 140 mA: 120
ORAL CONTRAST:	None
PHASE OF RESPIRATION:	Suspended inspiration
ROTATION TIME:	0.5 sec (0.8 sec)
ACQUISITION SLICE THICKNESS:	1.0 mm, chest only 2.5 mm, chest–abdomen–pelvis
PITCH:	Variable, usually 4–6 (HS-6:1)
RECONSTRUCTION SLICE THICKNESS/INTERVAL FOR FILMING:	3.0–5.0 mm/2.0–4.0 mm
RECONSTRUCTION SLICE THICKNESS FOR POST-PROCESSING/WORKSTATION:	1.0–2.5 mm/1.0–2.0 mm
RECONSTRUCTION ALGORITHM:	Mediastinum – Kernal AB = 40 (standard) Lung – Kernal AB = 70 (high-frequency E_2 filter)

ANATOMIC COVERAGE:
    SUPERIOR EXTENT:
    INFERIOR EXTENT:
	
	Superior margins of clavicles
	Adrenal glands; continue caudally if disease extends into abdominal aorta

IV CONTRAST:

Concentration:	HOCM 282 mg iodine/mL (60% solution)
Rate:	3–4 mL/sec
Scan Delay:	Use bolus tracking software; usually about 17–20 sec
Total Volume:	150 mL

COMMENTS:

1. Initial noncontrast scans at three levels (aortic arch, mid ascending aorta, distal descending aorta) should be obtained to potentially identify patients with acute intramural hematomas and/or displaced intimal calcifications.
2. Multiplanar reformatted images are very helpful to assist display of the intimal flap, and the true and false lumina.
3. Three-dimensional reconstructions aid presurgical planning for aortic aneurysm repair and are particularly useful in delineating the relationship of the aneurysm to the branch vessels.

Protocol 4:
CENTRAL AIRWAY DISEASE, HILAR EVALUATION (Figs. 7 and 8)

INDICATION:	*Central endotracheal or endobronchial mass, airway patency, stenosis, dehiscence, hilar mass*
SCANNER SETTINGS:	kV(p): 140
	mA: 120
ORAL CONTRAST:	None
PHASE OF RESPIRATION:	Inspiration
ROTATION TIME:	0.5–0.75 sec for small chests (0.8 sec)
ACQUISITION SLICE THICKNESS:	1.0–2.5 mm
PITCH:	Variable, usually 4–6 (HS = 6:1)
RECONSTRUCTION SLICE THICKNESS/INTERVAL FOR FILMING:	5.0 mm/4.0 mm
RECONSTRUCTION ALGORITHM:	Mediastinum − Kernal AB = 40 (standard)
	Lung − Kernal AB = 70 (high-frequency E_2 filter)
ANATOMIC COVERAGE:	
SUPERIOR EXTENT:	Superior margins of clavicles
INFERIOR EXTENT:	Adrenal glands

IV CONTRAST:

Concentration:	HOCM 282 mg iodine/mL (60% solution)
Rate:	3 mL/sec
Scan Delay:	20 sec
Total Volume:	100 mL

Protocol 5:
SMALL AIRWAYS DISEASE (Fig. 9)

INDICATION:	*Bronchiectasis, inflammatory disease, bronchiolitis, mosaic ventilation, air trapping*
SCANNER SETTINGS:	kV(p): 140 mA: 120
ORAL CONTRAST:	None
PHASE OF RESPIRATION:	Inspiration—repeat at expiration as needed
ROTATION TIME:	0.5 sec—0.75 sec for small chests (0.8 sec)
ACQUISITION SLICE THICKNESS (COLLIMATION):	1.0–1.25 mm
PITCH:	Variable, usually 4–6 (HS = 6:1)
RECONSTRUCTION SLICE THICKNESS/INTERVAL FOR FILMING:	1.0–1.25 mm/10.0 mm
RECONSTRUCTION ALGORITHM:	Mediastinum − Kernal AB = 40 (standard) Lung − Kernal AB = 70 (high-frequency E_2 filter)

ANATOMIC COVERAGE:
    SUPERIOR EXTENT:
    INFERIOR EXTENT:
	
	Lung apices
	Adrenal glands

IV CONTRAST:	None

COMMENTS:

1. With the GE Lightspeed, an average 25-cm chest can be imaged in a 26-sec breath-hold. If this cannot be sustained, it's probably best to switch to axial mode, with 1-mm collimation obtained at 10-mm intervals.
2. With the Volume Zoom, an average 25-cm chest, if imaged with a pitch of 5 to 7, can be scanned in approximately 25 to 30 seconds. If the patient is unable to sustain a long breath-hold, the pitch can be increased to 8.

3. Additional images may also be obtained in expiration to detect air trapping if present. This technique should be performed in cases in which a mosaic attenuation pattern of lung parenchymal density is identified, to differentiate airway disease from mosaic perfusion due to primary vascular disease or alveolitis.

Protocol 6:
HEMOPTYSIS (OCCULT AIRWAY DISEASE)

INDICATION:	*Occult airway disease*
SCANNER SETTINGS:	kV(p): 120 mA: 140
ORAL CONTRAST:	None
PHASE OF RESPIRATION:	Inspiration
ROTATION TIME:	0.5 sec—0.75 for small chests (0.8 sec)
ACQUISITION SLICE THICKNESS (COLLIMATION):	1.0–1.25 mm
PITCH:	Variable, usually 4–6 (HS-6:1)
RECONSTRUCTION SLICE THICKNESS/INTERVAL FOR FILMING:	Phase: 1 1.0–1.25 mm/10.0 mm Phase: 2 2.5–3.0 mm/2.0 mm Phase: 3 1.0–1.25 mm/10.0 mm
RECONSTRUCTION ALGORITHM:	Mediastinum − Kernal AB = 40 (standard) Lung − Kernal AB = 70 (high-frequency E_2 filter)
ANATOMIC COVERAGE: **SUPERIOR EXTENT:** **INFERIOR EXTENT:**	*Phase 1:* Superior margins of clavicles 2 cm above carina *Phase 2:* 2 cm above carina Inferior pulmonary veins *Phase 3:* Inferior pulmonary veins Adrenal glands

IV CONTRAST:

Optional **Concentration:**	HOCM 282 mg iodine/mL (60% solution)
Rate:	3 mL/sec
Scan Delay:	20 sec
Total Volume:	100 mL

COMMENTS:

1. This protocol is designed to optimize identification of both endobronchial lesions and bronchiectasis, both potential causes of hemoptysis. It attempts to combine HRCT images with central airway contiguous thin-section imaging. It may be difficult for a given patient to sustain such a lengthy breath-hold. It is also somewhat time and labor intensive for the technician to reconstruct separate sets of images with differing reconstruction parameters.

   With the GE Lightspeed, an average 25-cm chest can be imaged in a 26-sec breath-hold with 1.25-mm collimation. If this cannot be sustained, its probably best to switch to 2.5-mm collimation and get selected axial 1.25-mm thick sections afterward.

   With the Volume Zoom, an average 25-cm chest, if imaged with a pitch of 5 to 7, can be scanned in approximately 25 to 30 sec. If the patient is unable to sustain a long breath-hold, the pitch can be increased to 8.

Protocol 7:
FOCAL LUNG DISEASE (Fig. 10)

INDICATION:	*Solitary pulmonary nodule, arteriovenous malformation*
SCANNER SETTINGS:	kV(p): 120 mA: 240
ORAL CONTRAST:	None
PHASE OF RESPIRATION:	Inspiration
ROTATION TIME:	0.5 sec—0.75 for small chests (0.8 sec)
ACQUISITION SLICE THICKNESS:	Phase: 1 1.0–5.0 mm Phase: 2 (GE Lightspeed scanner) 1.0–1.25 mm
PITCH:	Variable, usually 4–6 (HS = 6:1)
RECONSTRUCTION SLICE THICKNESS/INTERVAL FOR FILMING:	Phase: 1 7.0–7.5 mm/6.0 mm Phase: 2 1.0–1.25 mm/1.0 mm through focal lesions
RECONSTRUCTION ALGORITHM:	Mediastinum − Kernal AB = 40 (standard) Lung − Kernal AB = 70 (high-frequency E_2 filter)
ANATOMIC COVERAGE: **SUPERIOR EXTENT:** **INFERIOR EXTENT:**	*Phase 1:* Superior margins of clavicles Adrenal glands *Phase 2:* (GE Lightspeed scanner) Superior: Above nodule Inferior: Below nodule *Phase 3:* Nodule enhancement studies

IV CONTRAST:

Concentration:	
Phase 1 & 2:	Noncontrast (above)
Phase 3:	HOCM 282 mg iodine/mL (60% solution)
Rate:	2–3 mL/sec
Scan Delay:	1, 2, 3, 4 min postcontrast
Total Volume:	100 mL
Scan Acquisition:	1.25 q 1 mm through nodule

COMMENTS:

1. The nodule enhancement protocol can be modified to assess patients with suspected arteriovenous malformations. Scan acquisition after localization of the lesion should be as follows
   Collimator: 1.0 mm/2.5 mm
   Reconstruction: 2.5–3.0 mm/2.0 mm
   After initial precontrast images are obtained through the lesion, a single acquisition should be obtained 20 sec after a bolus of 100 mL of IV contrast. This allows precise localization, morphologic assessment, and identification of feeding and draining vessels. For smaller malformations, narrower collimation and reconstructions may be necessary.

Protocol 8:
HIGH-RESOLUTION CT (Figs. 11 and 12)

INDICATION: *Characterization of diffuse interstitial lung disease*

SCANNER SETTINGS: kV(p): 140
mA: 120

ORAL CONTRAST: None

PHASE OF RESPIRATION: Inspiration (repeat at expiration as needed)

ROTATION TIME: 0.5 sec—0.075 for small chests (0.8 sec)

ACQUISITION SLICE THICKNESS: 1.0–1.25 mm

PITCH: Variable, usually 4–6 (HS = 6:1)

RECONSTRUCTION SLICE THICKNESS/INTERVAL FOR FILMING: 1.0–1.25 mm/10 mm

RECONSTRUCTION ALGORITHM: Mediastinum − Kernal AB = 40 (standard)
Lung − Kernal AB = 70 (high-frequency E_2 filter)

ANATOMIC COVERAGE:
  SUPERIOR EXTENT: Lung apices
  INFERIOR EXTENT: Adrenal glands

IV CONTRAST: None

COMMENTS:
1. Selected prone images should be obtained in patients with posterior or basilar disease.
2. In patients with a history of asbestos exposure, five to six 1-mm thick sections should be obtained at 15-mm intervals in the prone position, beginning at the lung bases and progressing in a cephalad direction.
3 If a mosaic parenchymal attenuation pattern is detected, additional 1-mm thick sections at 15–20-mm intervals should also be obtained at expiration. This technique allows differentiation of

focal air trapping and secondary mosaic perfusion due to regional hypoxia from primary vascular disease producing mosaic perfusion (such as pulmonary hypertension).

4. This protocol mandates a fairly lengthy breath-hold.

   With the GE Lightspeed scanner, an average 25-cm chest can be imaged in a 26-sec breath-hold. If this cannot be sustained, it's probably best to switch to axial mode, with 1-mm collimation obtained at 10-mm intervals.

   With the Volume Zoom, an average 25-cm chest, if imaged with a pitch of 5–7, can be scanned in approximately 25–30 sec. If the patient is unable to sustain a long breath-hold, the pitch can be increased to 8.

Protocol 9:
TRAUMA SURVEY (Fig. 13)

INDICATION:	*Patient with penetrating or blunt trauma*
SCANNER SETTINGS:	kV(p):140 mA:120
ORAL CONTRAST:	None
PHASE OF RESPIRATION:	Suspended inspiration
ROTATION TIME:	0.5 sec routinely (0.8 sec)
ACQUISITION SLICE THICKNESS (COLLIMATION):	1.0–2.5 mm/2.5 mm combined with abdomen
PITCH:	Variable, to include thorax in single breath-hold (HS = 6:1)
RECONSTRUCTION SLICE THICKNESS/INTERVAL FOR FILMING:	5.0 mm/4.0 mm
RECONSTRUCTION ALGORITHM:	Mediastinum − Kernal AB = 40 (standard) Lung − Kernal AB = 70 (high-frequency E_2 filter)

ANATOMIC COVERAGE:
  SUPERIOR EXTENT:
  INFERIOR EXTENT:
	Superior margins of clavicles
	Adrenal glands

IV CONTRAST:		
Concentration:	HOCM: 282 mg iodine/mi (60% solution)
Rate:	2 mL/sec
Scan Delay:	45 sec
Total Volume:	100–125 mL

Protocol 10:
LUNG CANCER SCREENING
(Figs. 14 and 15)

INDICATION:	*Detection of radiographically occult nodules in an individual at high risk for lung cancer*
SCANNER SETTINGS:	kV(p): 140 mA: 20–40
ORAL CONTRAST:	None
PHASE OF RESPIRATION:	Inspiration
ROTATION TIME:	0.5 sec (0.8 sec)
ACQUISITION SLICE THICKNESS:	1.0–2.5 mm
PITCH:	Variable (HS-6:1)
RECONSTRUCTION SLICE THICKNESS/INTERVAL FOR FILMING:	5.0–7.0 mm/4.0–6.0 mm
RECONSTRUCTION ALGORITHM:	Mediastinum − Kernal AB = 40 (standard) Lung − Kernal AB = 70 (high-frequency E_2 filter)

ANATOMIC COVERAGE:
   SUPERIOR EXTENT:
   INFERIOR EXTENT:
	
	Lung apices
	Adrenal glands

IV CONTRAST:	None
COMMENTS:	1. Contiguous 1-mm thick sections through indeterminate nodules can be reconstructed from the Volume Zoom scan data, targeted to a single lung (FOV of approximately 19 cm). This allows detailed characterization of the nodule without the need for additional scanning.

2. Contiguous 2.5-mm thick images can be generated from the GE Lightspeed data set. Additional 1.25-mm thick collimated sections can then be obtained through the nodule if it proves to be without definite fat or calcium on the 2.5-mm thick sections.

4

Multislice Computed Tomography of the Abdomen and Pelvis

Rendon C. Nelson*, James A. Brink**, and Paul M. Silverman***

*Department of Radiology, Division of Abdominal Imaging, Duke University Medical
Center, Durham, North Carolina 27701
**Department of Radiology, Yale University School of Medicine,
New Haven, Connecticut 06510
***Department of Radiology, Section of Body Imaging, Gerald D. Dodd, Jr.,
Distiguished Chair, Diagnostic Imaging, Department of Radiology, University of Texas M.
D. Anderson Cancer Center, Houston, Texas 77030

Over the past several years, helical CT (HCT) has maintained a very strong presence among diagnostic imaging schemes for the abdomen and pelvis, primarily because images with high in-plane (e.g., 0.5 to 0.7 mm^2) and moderate z-axis (e.g., 5 mm) resolution can be acquired in a reasonably short period. Furthermore, soft tissue, lungs, and bones can all be evaluated effectively. The advantages of multislice CT (MSCT) are perhaps best appreciated in the abdomen and pelvis, where large volume data sets can be acquired covering all or most of the anatomic area of interest in a single and comfortable breath-hold. When designing MSCT protocols, the transition from single to multislice scanners is much more than simply shifting a race car into overdrive (1,2). Various combinations of detector configuration, slice reconstruction thickness, rotation speed, and table speed (i.e., pitch) allow one to build protocols that are not only highly specific to the clinical questions being asked but also more tolerable for the patient. It is particularly advantageous for the multiphasic and CT angiographic examinations commonly employed in this part of the body. This chapter focuses on the fundamental advantages of MSCT in terms of detector configurations, speed, and timing, with emphasis on using advantages to provide superior images of the abdomen and pelvis.

MULTISLICE HELICAL CT SCAN PARAMETERS

The transition from single to MSCT is made possible by the conversion of a one-dimensional row of detector elements to a two-dimensional (2D) array of detector elements as described in Chapter 1. With present hardware and software configurations, up to four slices can be obtained during a single gantry rotation (3,4). The ability to acquire a volumetric data set, more than a limited, fixed set of slices per rotation (e.g., 8, 16, 24, or 32 slices) is currently a major focus of research and development. The ability to acquire very thin sections is also an option, although there are only a few applications for this feature in the abdomen and pelvis.

With most single-slice helical scanners, slices cannot be reconstructed thinner than that acquired. For example, if 5-mm slices are acquired with a pitch of 1.5 (table speed of 7.5 mm/rotation), the minimum reconstruction thickness is 5 mm (2,5,6). With MSCT, one may configure the detector so that slices are acquired thinner than initially reconstructed in case there is a need to return to the raw data to reconstruct thinner slices. For example, if the abdomen is scanned with a 4- by 5-mm detector configuration (four slices per gantry rotation, each 5 mm thick) and a pitch of 0.75 (table speed of 15 mm/rotation), the minimum slice thickness is 5 mm. Alternatively, the abdomen can be scanned with a 4- by 2.5-mm detector configuration and a pitch of 1.5 (identical table speed of 15 mm/rotation) and the slices reconstructed at 5 mm thick, as described in Chapter 1. As long as the raw data are preserved, it is possible to return to the latter data set and reconstruct a slice with a thickness of either 3.75 or 2.5 mm. This feature is particularly useful for characterizing small lesions such as renal cysts or for obtaining high-quality three-dimensional (3D) or multiplanar images (Fig. 1). At least one manufacturer is looking to extend preservation of raw data to the detector row level, so that, in the future, it may be possible to reconstruct slices equal to the thickness of each detector row, regardless of the detector configuration used during initial image reconstruction.

Gantry rotation speeds typically vary from 0.5 to 1.0 seconds. Remember, however, that to achieve adequate signal to noise in the abdomen, the milliamperes must be adjusted, so the number of photons per revolution or milliamperes (milliamperes per rotation) is similar. This adjustment, however, may result in overheating of the x-ray tube, particularly in larger patients. One technique that is very helpful when scanning at faster rotation speeds is to use 140 kV, rather than 120 kV. This alteration allows one to decrease the milliamperes considerably, which in many patients will improve the chance of using a faster rotation speed. The trade-off for using a higher kilovolt is a slight decrease in low-contrast detectability. Furthermore, with some of the faster rotation speeds such as 0.5 seconds, the number of trajectories used in the reconstruction algorithm is less, so aliasing or streak artifacts may be encountered. This is particularly a problem at high-contrast interfaces such as soft tissue and bone. Whether these artifacts affect diagnostic capability has yet to be determined. However, in certain anatomic areas, such as the bony pelvis, where streak artifacts are more inherent, slower rotation speeds may be advantageous.

In the abdomen and pelvis, there are a number of fundamental advantages of MSCT over single-slice helical CT (HCT) and a discussion of both the specific advantages and applications follows. The first advantage is the ability to scan the same anatomic region of interest (ROI) in much less time, using a *similar* slice thickness. For example, on a single-slice scanner, the routine abdomen and pelvis are typically evaluated with 5-mm thick slices at a pitch of 1.5 (table speed = 7.5 mm/rotation). With this protocol, 400 mm of coverage requires 53 seconds, usually broken into at least two different breath-holds. On a multislice scanner, using the 4- by 5.0-mm detector configuration at a pitch of 0.75, 400 mm or the entire abdomen and pelvis can be covered in 20 to 25 seconds, a single and comfortable breath-hold in most patients (7).

The second advantage is the ability to scan the same anatomic ROI in less time using *thinner* slices. For example, rather than scanning the entire abdomen and pelvis with the 4- by 5-mm detector configuration and a pitch of 0.75, the 4- by-2.5 mm configuration can be used with a pitch of 1.5, resulting in the same table speed and acquisition time. However, when the slices are reconstructed with a thickness of 2.5 mm and a reconstruction interval of 1 mm, longitudinal resolution is improved substantially, of great value when 3D imaging is contemplated. This feature will be much more advantageous on scanners with the capability of acquiring more than four slices per rotation.

The third advantage is the ability to achieve much more anatomic coverage in the same acquisition time, using a *similar* slice thickness. For example, on a single-slice scanner using 3-mm thick slices and a pitch of 1.5 (4.5 mm/rotation), 180 mm of anatomic coverage can be achieved in 40 seconds. On a multislice scanner using a detector configuration of 4 by 2.5 mm

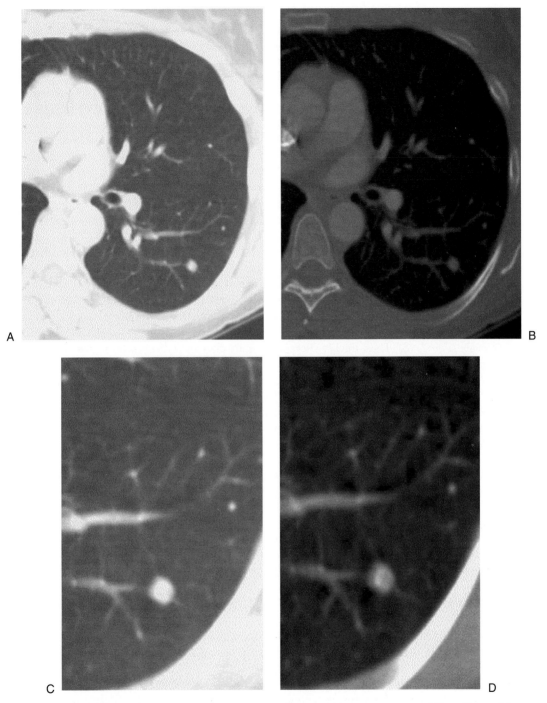

FIG. 1. A 48-year-old woman with breast cancer. Transaxial images with lung **(A)** and bone **(B)** display windows from a multislice computed tomographic scan (slice thickness = 5 mm; table feed = 15 mm/rotation; pitch = 1.5 [HS = 6:1]; and reconstruction interval = 5 mm) reveal a pulmonary nodule in the left lower lobe. Reconstruction of thinner sections **(C, D)** (slice thickness = 2.5 mm; reconstruction interval = 1.5 mm) was possible without rescanning the patient (original slice thickness less than detector group thickness), revealing a small amount of eccentric calcification within the nodule, prompting conservative management.

and a pitch of 1.5 (15 mm/rotation), 600 mm of anatomic coverage can be achieved in 40 seconds. This is particularly useful for scanning the entire thoracoabdominal aorta or aortoiliac region in a single breath-hold. When 2D image review will suffice for diagnosis (as in suspected aortic dissection), it is not necessary to prescribe ultrathin slices because the aorta is a vessel that courses *perpendicular* to the axial plane. It should also be noted that even though 40 seconds is a longer period than many patients can hold their breath, respiratory motion and associated artifacts are considerably less in the lower abdomen and pelvis. Therefore, quiet breathing while scanning in this portion of the body is acceptable.

The fourth advantage is the ability to achieve more anatomic coverage in the same acquisition time using *thinner* slices. In the past, thinner slices always meant less anatomic coverage or more coverage meant thicker slices. With MSCT, it is possible to acquire a data set with thinner slices in less time. For the clinical scenario in which small blood vessels that course *parallel* to the axial plane are being evaluated, such as the hepatic, splenic, and renal arteries, thin slices are advantageous as long as the acquisition is sufficiently short to minimize respiratory motion. On a single-slice scanner using 3-mm thick slices and a pitch of 1.0 (3 mm/rotation), 100 mm of anatomic coverage can be achieved in 33 seconds, a somewhat lengthy breath-hold. On a multislice scanner using a detector configuration of 4 by 1.25 mm and a pitch of 1.5 (7.5 mm/rotation), 200 mm of anatomic coverage can be achieved in 21.3 seconds.

Because so many combinations of slice thickness, pitch, and table speed are available, designing protocols can be confusing. What guidelines determine which combination is optimal? In general, table feeds greater than 15 mm per rotation are prone to artifacts and should be used cautiously (Fig. 2) (8). Thus, thicker slices are usually coupled with smaller pitches (e.g., 4- by 5-mm detector configuration; pitch = 0.75; table speed = 15 mm/rotation), whereas thinner slices are usually coupled with larger pitches (e.g., 4- by 2.5-mm detector configuration; pitch = 1.5; table speed = 15 mm/rotation). The main question to ask for each application is which slice thickness is required to depict potential pathologic processes? For instance, when evaluating the retroperitoneum for hemorrhage, a gross pathologic process, thin slices are not required. Another way of looking at this issue is to ask yourself the following question: What are you willing to miss with the slice thickness you have chosen? For example, when evaluating the liver for focal lesions, thin slices (such as 2.5 mm) will indeed aid in the detection of small lesions on the order of 5 mm or less. The overwhelming majority of these small lesions, however, are benign, even in the presence of a known malignancy, and their detection may not necessarily be advantageous (9). Therefore, 5-mm thick slices may be sufficient in this scenario. For CT angiography (CTA), the choice of slice thickness again depends on which blood vessels are of primary interest. For example, when evaluating the abdominal aorta for aneurysmal dilatation, a long and large-caliber blood vessel that courses *perpendicular* to the axial plane, ultrathin slices are not necessary. When evaluating the hepatic or renal arteries, small-caliber blood vessels that course *parallel* to the axial plane, ultrathin slices are advantageous.

The impact of scan technique on radiation dose must also be considered. For example, when using the General Electric Lightspeed CT scanner (General Electric Medical Systems, Milwaukee, WI), one may consider using the high-speed mode (HS) (pitch = 1.5) for routine body imaging, because the 25% overlap with HQ mode (pitch = 0.75) is replaced with a 50% gap. However, the system software automatically adjusts the scan milliamperes, to obtain comparable levels of image noise, which, in part, offsets this benefit. We have observed a net increase in the dose length product (DLP) of approximately 2% with HS, as compared with HQ mode for our routine abdominal CT protocols (5-mm slice thickness, 4- by 2.5-mm detector configuration) (10). However, our specialized protocols, such as those performed for evaluation of a hepatic, renal, or pancreatic masses, or for suspected aortic dissection, resulted in a 10% to 25% decrease in the DLP when all scan series were performed with HS, as com-

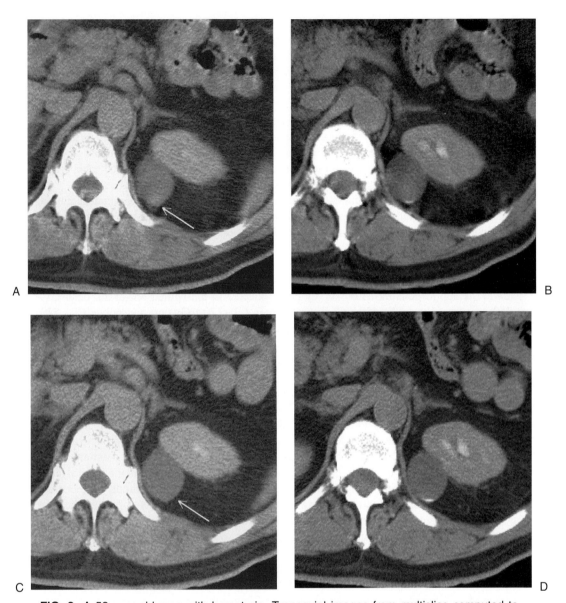

FIG. 2. A 53-year-old man with hematuria. Transaxial images from multislice computed to-mography after intravenous pyelogram **(A, B)** (slice thickness = 5 mm; table feed = 30 mm/ro-tation; pitch = 1.5 [HS = 6:1]) reveal an apparent nodule (*arrow*) along the posterior wall of a left renal cyst. Because images could not be reconstructed with a thinner slice thickness (orig-inal slice thickness = detector group thickness), the patient was rescanned with a reduction in the table feed **(C, D)** (slice thickness = 5 mm; table feed = 15 mm/rotation; pitch = 1.5 [HS = 6:1]). With this reduction in table feed, the apparent nodule disappeared and likely resulted ini-tially from interpolation artifacts related to adjacent calcification in the posterior wall of the cyst.

pared with HQ imaging. This is because our protocols have more instances in which the de-sired scan thickness is set equal to the detector group thickness, and this results in greater slice profile broadening with HS mode than with HQ mode. Greater slice profile broadening results in more photon flux to the detector, which permits a reduction in the x-ray dose without com-promising image noise. However, significant helical artifacts have been observed with HS mode when coupled with a very high table speed (22.5 and 30 mm per rotation), particularly for high-contrast interfaces oblique to the longitudinal axis of the scanner as occur commonly with CTA and CT colonography (Fig. 2) (8,11,12).

Thus, for most imaging applications in the abdomen, HS mode (pitch = 1.5) is favored, so long as interpolation artifacts are not excessive, as may occur when the absolute table feed exceeds 20 mm per rotation. The temporal efficiency of HS mode outweighs the minimal dose increase observed when the nominal slice thickness is greater than the detector group thickness (to preserve the ability to reconstruct images with a thinner slice thickness for problem solving). And, the temporal efficiency is synergistic with the dose benefit observed for specialized applications in which the nominal slice thickness is set equal to the detector group thickness (to maximize longitudinal resolution for a given set of scan parameters).

Regardless of the technique that is chosen, one must be cognizant of the overall radiation dose imparted to the patient. Aside from economic considerations, the only reason not to capitalize on the myriad technical advantages of MSCT is the increase in radiation dose associated with this technology. Both radiologist and technologist alike must monitor the DLP (μGy/cm) for each examination and compare their protocols to established standards. For example, Shrimpton et al. (13) produced the following reference DLP (third-quartile) values for various CT applications based on survey data collected in the United Kingdom: head CT, 1,050 μGy/cm; chest CT, 650 μGy/cm; abdomen CT, 770 μGy/cm; and pelvic CT, 570 μGy/cm (13). Particularly when choosing a narrow slice thickness, one must recognize that high-resolution imaging must be balanced with an effort to reduce tube current to keep the overall radiation dose within reason.

LIVER

Because the liver has a dual blood supply, the hepatic artery and the portal vein, there are several phases of enhancement after the IV administration of a bolus of contrast material. These include the hepatic arterial phase (HAP), the portal venous phase (PVP), and the equilibrium phase. The combination of phases chosen in each patient depends on the clinical situation, although imaging in the equilibrium phase alone is generally contraindicated. During the equilibrium phase, the contrast material in the intravascular component of the extracellular space equilibrates with the extravascular component of the extracellular space, thereby obscuring lesions. It typically required 1.5 to 2.5 minutes to image the entire liver with a conventional incremental CT technique. Consequently, the entire liver is generally not imaged with conventional CT during the optimum postenhancement scanning interval (i.e., the time after achievement of high hepatic enhancement levels but before the onset of the equilibrium phase) (5,6). The relative speed of HCT, including both single and multislice scanners, overcomes this problem; that is, an HCT scanner requires about 20 to 25 seconds to cover the entire liver, whereas an MSCT scanner requires about 4 to 12 seconds, depending on the size of the liver and the gantry rotation speed. Because an HCT scan is completed within a very short scanning interval (i.e., usually less than 30 seconds), a uniphasic injection using a relatively rapid injection rate (e.g., 3 to 5 mL/sec) is most advantageous (14,15). For HCT of the liver, it is generally necessary to use a longer scan delay than that used for conventional incremental CT. However, the optimal scan delay depends on the volume of contrast material and the rate at which it is injected. For most IV contrast injection protocols, a scan delay of 60 to 80 seconds is appropriate. At very rapid rates, such as 5 mL/sec, a delay of 50 to 60 seconds may be employed. For the PVP, lists recommended scan delays for various IV contrast material injection protocols.

TABLE 4.1. *Recommended Scan Delays for Hepatic Computed Tomography*

Volume (mL)	Injection rate (mL/sec)	Delay (sec)
100	1.5	70
100	2	60
100	3	55
125	1.5	85
125	2	70
125	3	60
150	1.5	100
150	2	85
150	3	70
150	4	55
150	5	50
200	1.5	135
200	2	110
200	3	85
200	4	70
200	5	60

Note: Power injection of central lines and Port-A-Cath catheters should be performed at 1.5 mL/sec. The attending radiologist should review the scout topogram or a recent chest x-ray to be sure that the line is in good position. Central venous catheters placed via a peripheral vein should not be power injected. Hand injection is acceptable for these catheters.

In recent years, semiautomated techniques have emerged to determine the adequacy of contrast enhancement during infusion of contrast material intended for a diagnostic scan (e.g., computer-automated scan technology [CAST], SmartPrep, or bolus tracking). These techniques take the "guesswork" out of deciding the optimal scan delay by acquiring a series of low x-ray dose axial images at a predetermined level that is representative of the scan volume (16,17). Once contrast enhancement is deemed adequate (by the operator or by the computer), the acquisition of low-dose axial scans is terminated and the diagnostic scan is initiated. If the axial level for the preliminary low-dose data acquisition (e.g., midliver) is different than the first slice in the helical acquisition (e.g., top of the liver), the table will have to move before initiating the diagnostic portions of the scan. Data have shown this technique to be highly effective, resulting in better contrast enhancement than with the standard fixed-delay approach. For capturing images during the PVP, a threshold of 50 Hounsfield units (HU) above baseline for enhancement has been recommended (16). On single-slice helical scanners, it may be difficult to use these techniques for triggering the HAP primarily because both the triggering algorithm and the acquisition speed are relatively slow. One group has reported improved accuracy in the timing of the HAP with automated triggering (18), although others have had less success with this technique because the time to initiate scanning is so short in comparison to routine scans in which only PVP imaging is desired. On a multislice scanner, however, both the triggering algorithm and the acquisition speed are considerably faster; therefore, these techniques can be reliably used to trigger the HAP on a routine basis. This is particularly advantageous because the timing of the HAP is much more variable than the PVP.

Because of the speed of HCT, one may scan the liver during either the HAP or the PVP of enhancement, or during both phases. Because most metastases are hypovascular compared with normal hepatic parenchyma when imaged during the PVP of enhancement, conventional dynamic incremental hepatic CT scanning protocols were designed to optimize imaging during this phase of contrast enhancement. However, many primary hepatic neoplasms and some metastases are isovascular or hypervascular and can become isoattenuating during the PVP of enhancement. Because of their vascularity, such neoplasms may be better imaged during the arterial phase of hepatic enhancement. However, dynamic incremental scanning requires too much time to image the liver during both the HAP and the PVP. HCT provides the potential to image the entire liver twice, once during the HAP and once during the PVP. The desired arterial phase scan usually begins 25 to 30 seconds after initiation of the contrast injection, although there is considerable variability from one patient to another (19). Dual-phase or biphasic hepatic imaging is used in selected patients who are at high risk for vascular hepatic neoplasms. Studies of patients with hepatocellular carcinoma and various types of hypervascular metastases (endocrine tumors, renal cell carcinoma, melanoma, thyroid cancer, carcinoid) and other particularly endocrine tumors have demonstrated an 8% to 13% increase in lesion detection with dual-phase HCT compared with PVP imaging alone (20–23). In comparisons of dual-phase HCT and dynamic magnetic resonance imaging (MRI), arterial phase MRI has been shown to be slightly superior for hepatic lesion detection (24,25). However, for delayed-phase imaging (more than 180 seconds), HCT was significantly better than MRI for hepatocellular carcinoma (25). Hepatic lesion characterization may also be improved by imaging during the arterial, portal, and equilibrium phases of contrast enhancement (26).

MSCT offers a marked reduction in the time required to image the liver relative to standard single-detector HCT (27). The increased temporal resolution of MSCT has lead some investigators to test the use of an additional phase of hepatic imaging to maximize the sensitivity for small hypervascular tumors such as hepatoma. Foley et al. (28) have piloted the use of an HAP, a "portal venous inflow phase," and a hepatic venous phase for detection of hypervascular primary and metastatic neoplasms. These investigators found that MSCT permitted hepatic imaging with thin slices during these three distinct vascular phases. They found that the portal venous inflow phase is optimal for detection of hypervascular primary and metastatic tumors. This phase is included only during the latter portion of the HAP of a biphasic HCT scan with a single detector row scanner. Due to the speed of MSCT, the entire liver can be imaged during this optimal phase of enhancement, in addition to complete imaging of the liver during the HAP, which is advantageous for quality CT arteriography. Finally, the hepatic venous phase, most commonly referred to as the PVP of a biphasic HCT scan, permits detection of relatively hypovascular tumors, the vast majority of hepatic metastases that would otherwise be poorly imaged during the other two phases.

Similarly, in a relatively large trial, Kadota et al. (29) describe the use of both early (25-second delay) and late (35-second delay) arterial phases for the detection of small (≤3 cm) hepatomas in 97 patients with 109 tumors. The area under the receiver operating characteristic curve was 0.76 for the early arterial phase, 0.81 for the late arterial phase, and 0.87 for the combination of both the early and the late phase. In a similar study of 25 patients with 39 hypervascular hepatomas, Murakami et al. (30) found an increase in sensitivity from 79% to 87% with the addition of an early arterial phase to the standard arterial phase. Further, the positive predictive value rose from 84% to 97% with this addition. Of course, these benefits must be weighed against the costs of the addition scan, both in terms of the radiation exposure for the patient and in terms of the operational costs associated with the examination.

The continuous data acquisition of HCT offers additional advantages for hepatic imaging as compared with standard incremental scanning. These include the potential for improved lesion detection due to elimination of respiratory misregistration, the retrospective reconstruction of images at arbitrary positions along the z-axis, and the production of high-quality multiplanar images. HCT with smaller interscan spacing increases both the number and the confidence of focal hepatic lesion detection. By viewing images of the liver reconstructed at 4-mm intervals (8-mm collimation, 50% overlap), one can detect 7% more lesions in a group of patients with liver metastases, as compared with viewing contiguous images of the same patients reconstructed at 8-mm intervals (31). The detection of additional small lesions, however, is not necessarily useful, because the overwhelming majority of these are benign, even in patients with a known extrahepatic malignancy (32). 3D measurements of the size of liver metastases in patients undergoing cancer treatment have been found to be reproducible with HCT images acquired in a breath-hold and reconstructed with a 25% overlap (33). However, longitudinal resolution is maximized when images are reconstructed with a 60% overlap; higher degrees of overlap are not advantageous (34). Multiplanar reconstructions (MPRs) and 3D displays of the volume-acquired data can be useful in precisely localizing and defining the extent of hepatic tumors before resection. Furthermore, the acquisition of thin slices through the entire liver during the early arterial phase, starting at about 20 seconds, is useful for depicting the hepatic arterial anatomy preoperatively. This may be particularly important in patients who are candidates for intraarterial chemotherapy via an implantable pump. Overall, these advantages make HCT the preferred method over invasive techniques such as CT arterial portography (35,36).

The amount of intravenous (IV) contrast material required for hepatic enhancement may be reduced with HCT. Although the degree of arterial enhancement is predominantly a function of timing and injection rate, peak hepatic parenchymal enhancement during the PVP is predominantly a function of the total contrast media dose. Therefore, the overall percentage decrease in dose with HCT may be less than expected and relatively unaffected by whether single or multidetector-multirow technology is employed. For example, adequate hepatic enhancement has been reported with an iodine dose that is 25% lower than that with conventional CT (15). In thin patients, the potential to reduce contrast dose is more pronounced and a reduction of up to 40% is possible. Contrast material reduction is best achieved when helical scan technology is coupled with automated bolus tracking as a means of determining enhancement adequacy (37).

PANCREAS

After the IV administration of a bolus of contrast material, three phases of pancreatic parenchymal enhancement have been described: the arterial phase (20 to 40 seconds), the pancreatic or parenchymal phase (40 to 60 seconds), and the venous phase (60 to 90 seconds). With HCT, high levels of pancreatic enhancement may be achieved that help accentuate the difference between normal pancreas and tumor or glandular necrosis and permit exquisite definition of arterial and venous involvement by pancreatic disease (38,39) (Fig. 11). Parenchymal enhancement during the pancreatic phase (40 to 60 seconds) of a dual-phase HCT has been reported to be slightly greater than that during the venous phase (60 to 90 seconds) (40,41). No study to date has evaluated all three phase in the same patient. In addition, because of the speed of single-slice HCT (SSHCT) and MSHCT, smaller volumes of contrast material have been shown to produce equivalent or superior peripancreatic vascular opacification compared with conventional CT (39). Furthermore, automated bolus tracking techniques on a multislice scanner have optimized the timing of arterial enhancement. As noted above, however, the degree of enhancement during the venous phase is more predicated on the dose of contrast material, so the percentage reduction in contrast material with HCT may not be substantial. The ability to scan the entire pancreas during arterial enhancement and to reconstruct images at overlapping intervals may improve the ability of CT to demonstrate and stage small pancreatic adenocarcinomas, although this potential benefit of HCT has yet to be demonstrated in a prospective study (42). On a single-slice helical scanner, it may be difficult to scan the entire pancreas with thin slices (e.g., 3 mm) during a comfortable breath-hold. On a multislice scanner, however, the entire upper abdomen can be easily covered with even thinner slices (e.g., 1 to 1.25 mm) during a very comfortable breath-hold. 2D rendering using curved MPRs, and 3D rendering using maximum intensity projection, shaded surface display, or volumetric rendering technique (VRT) may be useful in confirming vascular encasement or invasion. The curve MPR images perhaps are the most useful, because they depict both the vascular lumen and the perivascular soft tissue. This is particularly important because circumferential tumor encasement can occur without luminal narrowing or irregularity.

Because islet cell tumors are typically hypervascular, they should be more conspicuous during the early phases of dual-phase pancreatic HCT. Although this phenomenon has been described anecdotally (38,43), a large prospective study confirming this finding has not emerged. Instead, a small series of 10 patients with 11 surgically proven islet cell tumors has been published, in which dual-phase HCT was performed with a 5-mm slice thickness (44). All tumors larger than 5 mm and one of three lesions less than 5 mm in diameter were detected with dual-phase pancreatic HCT. Two lesions were better seen during the arterial phase, and two lesions were better seen during the parenchymal phase. Thus, the arterial and parenchymal phases may be complementary, and both phases may be necessary to fully evaluate patients with suspected islet cell tumors.

BILIARY TREE AND PORTA HEPATIS

The porta hepatis may be difficult to evaluate with conventional CT because of its complicated anatomy and oblique orientation. With HCT, thin slices can be obtained (e.g., 3 mm) that are reconstructed with at least a 50% overlap. From this data set, curved or straight multiplanar reformations of the porta hepatis can be performed in any plane to optimally depict important vascular, nodal, and biliary structures. With MSCT, very thin slices can be obtained (e.g., 1.25 mm) through the entire liver during a single and comfortable breath-hold. The multiplanar reformations from these data sets are exquisite. Detection of common bile duct stones and strictures may be improved with contrast-enhanced HCT, particularly when an interactive cine display console is used to determine the most beneficial planes for displaying the biliary tree (45).

3D cholangiographic quality images may be produced after the IV infusion or oral ingestion of a biliary contrast agent (46–51). However, with the IV agents, not only is there a significant risk of toxicity, but also the excretion of these agents is decreased in the setting of biliary obstruction. Thus, successful depiction of the biliary tree is impeded in the very population in whom it is most desirable. The oral agents have a much better safety profile, although absorption by the gastrointestinal tract is somewhat unpredictable and excretion into the bile is also diminished by biliary obstruction. However, 2D reformations of the bile duct may be generated from routine helical scans performed with IV contrast material (52). Such images depict the bile ducts as low-attenuation structures against a background of enhancing soft tissue. Such images may be helpful in depicting complex anatomy in the hepatoduodenal ligament, particularly in the setting of invasive gallbladder or pancreatic cancer.

KIDNEY

Small renal masses that are indeterminate by other imaging techniques may be better evaluated with HCT (53,54). As in the liver and pancreas, the lack of respiratory misregistration artifacts and the ability to reconstruct images at different or overlapping intervals diminishes the possibility that a small mass will be either not detected or not characterized. With HCT, the kidneys are typically scanned with 5-mm thick slices during a single breath-hold and are reconstructed at 5-mm intervals. Overlapping reconstructions can be performed when needed.

With MSCT as implemented by General Electric (Lightspeed CT), the detector configuration can be set up to acquire either 4- by 5-mm thick slices with a pitch of 0.75 (HQ = 3:1; 15 mm/rotation table speed) or 4- by 2.5-mm thick slices with a pitch of 1.5 (HS = 6:1; 15 mm/rotation table speed), both during a single and very comfortable breath-hold. The latter configuration, however, is advantageous, because it takes no longer to acquire yet should be more reliable for characterizing small lesions because the slices are narrower in the z-axis. A pseudoenhancement phenomenon whereby the attenuation of water-containing structures such as cysts reveals an increase in attenuation postcontrast has recently been described (55,56). This phenomenon is more pronounced in smaller intraparenchymal cysts compared with larger or exophytic cysts and is more significant on some multislice scanners compared with single-slice helical scanners (57,58).

With helical renal CT, the kidneys may be imaged precontrast, followed by three distinct phases of contrast enhancement: the corticomedullary phase, the nephrographic phase, and the excretory phase. Unlike with the liver or pancreas, noncontrast imaging is critical in the kidneys so enhancement of a lesion can be determined postcontrast. The corticomedullary phase occurs between 30 and 60 seconds, the nephrographic phase between 80 and 130 seconds, and the excretory phase about 3 minutes after the intravascular introduction of contrast material. Although little has been published regarding characterization of known lesions during these phases, one study has shown greater enhancement of renal neoplasms during the nephrographic phase (59), and another has shown limited detection of renal lesions when imaged only during the corticomedullary phase (60). Of 417 lesions detected in 33 patients, 62% were depicted during the corticomedullary phase, whereas 93% were seen during the nephrographic phase. When the nephrographic phase images were added to the corticomedullary phase images, the number of medullary lesions detected increased by a factor of 4.4, whereas the number of cortical lesions increased by a factor of 1.2.

A study by Szolar et al. (61) evaluated the use of multiphasic HCT for the detection and characterization of small (less than 3 cm) renal masses. As suggested in prior studies, the authors found that nephrographic phase images enabled greater lesion detection and better characterization of small renal masses than corticomedullary phase images. However, there are several theoretical advantages of scanning during the corticomedullary phase that argue against discarding it entirely. Tumor vascularity may be better appreciated during the corticomedullary phase (62). Corticomedullary differentiation can be helpful in distinguishing normal variants such as prominent columns of Bertin or dromedary humps from renal masses (59). Subtle asymmetries in the cortical nephrogram that result from renal artery stenosis or ureteral obstruction may be more apparent during the nephrographic phase than during the corticomedullary phase. Thus the cost versus benefit of multiphasic helical renal CT must be elicited in future studies, particularly regarding these theoretical advantages of imaging during the corticomedullary phase of enhancement.

2D and 3D renderings may be helpful in defining certain types of renal abnormalities. 3D reconstructions may provide useful information in the staging of renal cell carcinoma and in planning renal-sparing surgery (i.e., nephrogram sparing) selected patients (63). Multiplanar reformations of dynamic arterial and venous phase CT images in patients with ureteropelvic junction (UPJ) obstruction help identify large crossing vessels at the UPJ before endopyelotomy (Fig. 18) (64). This CT nephrogram and pyelogram can be quite useful. Transaxial renal HCT images, in combination with 3D reconstructions, have been shown to be suitable replacements for IV urography and angiography in the assessment of living renal donors, particularly if the surgery is to be performed with a laparoscope (65).

CT performed without IV contrast material is a suitable substitute for IV urography in many patients with acute flank pain (66,67). Direct visualization of renal or ureteral calculi and secondary signs of stone disease, including hydronephrosis, hydroureter, and perinephric, or peri-ureteral soft tissue infiltration, may be seen in patients with acute renal colic (68). In addition, extraurinary causes of acute flank pain, such as appendicitis, cholecystitis, or diverticulitis, may be revealed when urinary calculi are not responsible for the patient's symptoms. Although the x-ray dose associated with an HCT examination (particularly on a multislice scanner) is greater than that with a tailored IV urogram, the HCT examination is performed much more quickly and does not require IV contrast material.

RECONSTRUCTIONS FOR COMPLEX ANATOMIC RELATIONSHIPS (WORKSTATIONS)

Interpretative difficulties arising from complex anatomic relationships may be clarified with curved or straight multiplanar reformations of HCT data sets. Images targeted to the area of concern that overlap by at least 50% may be reconstructed retrospectively from the raw projection data. Multiplanar images reconstructed from these images may be useful, for example, in determining the site of origin of large abdominal masses or in localizing peridiaphragmatic abnormalities to the abdomen, diaphragm, or thorax (69).

Recently, investigators have evaluated use of HCT to detect colon polyps (70,71). Preliminary data correlating CT colonography with endoscopic colonoscopy suggest that the noninvasive technique is quite good at detecting polyps larger than 10 mm. Although progress is being made, this technique still has the following requirements: a bowel preparation, the intraluminal insufflation of a considerable amount of gas via a rectal tube, imaging in both the supine and the prone position, and lengthy periods of post–acquisition processing and review. Some advocate the use of 2D reformations to "straighten" the colon, whereas others suggest performing 3D perspective volume or surface rendering to fly through the colon simulating colonoscopy using various workstations. These workstations, along with picture archiving and communication system (PACS), will undoubtedly become more widely used in radiology as MSCT scans generate larger and larger data sets.

GENERAL COMMENTS

1. For HCT examinations of the abdomen, respiration should be suspended, although quiet breathing is tolerable when scanning the pelvis. Prolonged breath-holding can be facilitated by preliminary coaching and by hyperventilating the patient with three or four deep breaths in rapid succession just before beginning the HCT scan. These considerations, of course, are less of a problem on a multislice scanner.

2. In general, on a single-slice scanner use, a pitch of 1.0 to 1.5 (i.e., table increment per gantry rotation equal to 50% or greater than the beam collimation). In some cases, it will be necessary to use a pitch of 2.0 to cover the entire volume of interest. On a multislice scanner, acquiring up to four slices per rotation, use a pitch of 1.5 (HS = 6:1; i.e., table increment per gantry rotation 50% greater than the beam collimation or the width of all four slices combined), so long as the absolute table increment per gantry rotation is not excessive (i.e., greater than 20 mm per rotation).

3. CAST, a generic term for automated bolus tracking, may be used to determine the delay time for initiation of hepatic imaging. For triggering the PVP, position three ROIs in the periphery of the liver parenchyma away from blood vessels. Initiate scanning when at least two of the three ROIs reach 50 HU of enhancement. For triggering the HAP, position an ROI in the descending thoracic aorta, at the same level as the initial slice through the liver (so the table will not need to move or index once the scan is triggered). HAP imaging should commence

about 5 to 7 seconds after the aorta first enhances.

4. On a single-slice scanner, automated bolus tracking should not be used to trigger the arterial phase in dual-phase HCT examinations of the liver or pancreas or in CTA applications. This is not necessarily true on a multislice scanner. For CTA, position the ROI in or around the aorta at the same level as the top or initial slice of the helical acquisition and commence the scan immediately after the aorta begins to enhance.

5. FOV: Most abdominal examinations should be reconstructed with an FOV targeted to, at least, the abdominal wall, except for patients with a history of melanoma or other abnormalities in the subcutaneous tissues. For these cases, the FOV should be increased to include the entire abdominal circumference. In extremely large patients, a second image reconstruction targeted to the abdominal wall may be required. In these instances, re-review of the HCT data may be performed retrospectively. Some specialized protocols may call for an FOV targeted to the structure of interest such as the pancreas, kidney, or aorta.

6. Oral contrast material: Abdominal and abdominal–pelvic CT patients are given 600 to 800 mL of oral contrast material to drink 45 to 60 minutes before their examination, and an additional 200 mL just before scanning. Either water-soluble contrast solutions or barium solutions may be used, depending on the clinical indication for the examination, as well as several technical and environmental factors. Dilute water-soluble contrast may be preferred for outpatients to increase bowel motility and promote uniform bowel opacification. Water-soluble contrast material is also given to postoperative posttraumatic patients in whom bowel perforation or leakage is a possibility. Dilute barium may be preferred for routine inpatients, largely because of the ease of contrast delivery to the patient floors and to avoid the increase in bowel motility associated with water-soluble agents.

Regardless of the initial oral contrast material chosen, patients may be given a large cup of water to ingest immediately before their abdominal CT scan. This is better tolerated by the patients than another cup of contrast material and may provide better definition of the wall of the stomach and duodenum, particularly if IV contrast material has been administered.

REFERENCES

1. Brink JA. Spiral CT angiography of the abdomen and pelvis: intervention applications. Abdominal Imaging 1997;22:365–372.
2. Brink JA, McFarland EG, Heiken JP. Helical/spiral computed body tomography. Clin Radiol 1997;52:489–503.
3. Hu H, He HD, Foley WD, et al. Four multidetector-row helical CT: image quality and volume coverage speed. Radiology 2000;215:55–62.
4. Hu H. Multislice CT: scan and reconstruction. Med Phys 1999;26:5–18.
5. Foley WD. Dynamic hepatic CT. Radiology 1989;170:617–622.
6. Heiken JP, Brink JA, McClennan BL, et al. Dynamic contrast-enhanced CT of the liver: comparison of contrast medium injection rates and uniphasic and biphasic injection protocols. Radiology 1993;187:327–331.
7. Killius JS, Nelson RC. Logistic advantages of four-section helical CT in the abdomen and pelvis. Abdominal Imaging 2000;25:643–650.
8. McCollough CH, Zink FE. Performance evaluation of a multi-slice CT system. Med Phys 1999;26:2223–2230.
9. Schwartz LH, Gandras EJ, Colangelo SM, et al. Prevalence and importance of small hepatic lesions found at CT in patients with cancer. Radiology 1999;210:71–74.
10. Cuomo FA, Brink JA. Radiation dose with multidetector row CT: comparison of high and low pitch scanning strategies for abdominal imaging (Abstract). Radiology 2000;81:505.
11. Fleischmann D, Rubin GD, Paik DS, et al. Stair-step artifacts with single versus multiple detector-row helical CT. Radiology 2000;216:185–196.
12. McCollough CH, Bruesewitz MR, Zink FE, et al. CT colonography (CTC) using a multislice scanner: optimization of scan acquisition parameters (Abstract). Radiology 1999;213(P):97.
13. Shrimpton PC, Jones DG, Hillier MC, et al. Survey of CT practice in the United Kingdom, part 2: dosimetric aspects. London: Chilton, 1991. Vol NRPB-R249.
14. Foley WD, Hoffman RG, Quiroz FA, et al. Hepatic helical CT: contrast material injection protocol. Radiology 1994;192:367–371.

15. Brink JA, Heiken JP, Forman HP, et al. Hepatic spiral CT: reduction of dose of intravenous contrast material. Radiology 1995;197:83–88.
16. Silverman PM, Roberts S, Tefft MC, et al. Helical CT of the liver: clinical application of an automated computer technique, SmartPrep, for obtaining images with optimal contrast enhancement AJR Am J Roentgenol 1995;165:73–78.
17. Kopka L, Funke M, Fischer U, et al. Parenchymal liver enhancement with bolus-triggered helical CT: preliminary clinical results. Radiology 1995;195:282–284.
18. Kopka L, Rodenwaldt J, Fischer U, et al. Dual-phase helical CT of the liver: effects of bolus tracking and different volumes of contrast material. Radiology 1996;201:321–326.
19. Frederick MG, Paulson EK, Nelson RC. Helical CT for detecting focal liver lesions in patients with breast carcinoma: comparison of noncontrast phase, hepatic arterial phase, and portal venous phase. J Comput Assist Tomogr 1997;21:229–235.
20. Oliver JH III, Baron RL, Federle MP, et al. Detecting hepatocellular carcinoma: value of unenhanced or arterial phase CT imaging or both used in conjunction with conventional portal venous phase contrast-enhanced CT imaging. AJR Am J Roentgenol 1996;167:71–77.
21. Baron RL, Oliver JH III, Dodd GD III, et al. Hepatocellular carcinoma: evaluation with biphasic, contrast-enhanced, helical CT. Radiology 1996;199:505–511.
22. Hollett MD, Jeffrey RB, Nino-Murcia M, et al. Dual-phase helical CT of the liver: value of arterial phase scans in the detection of small malignant hepatic neoplasms. AJR Am J Roentgenol 1995;164:879–884.
23. Bonaldi VM, Bret PM, Reinhold C, et al. Helical CT of the liver: value of an early hepatic arterial phase. Radiology 1995;197:357–363.
24. Oi H, Murakami R, Kim T, et al. Dynamic MR imaging and early-phase helical CT for detecting small intrahepatic metastases of hepatocellular carcinoma. AJR Am J Roentgenol 1996;166:369–374.
25. Yamashita YY, Mitsuzaki KM, Yi T, et al. Small hepatocellular carcinoma in patients with chronic liver damage: prospective comparison of detection with dynamic MR imaging and helical CT of the whole liver. Radiology 1996;200:79–84.
26. Van Leeuwen MS, Noordzij J, Feldberg MAM, et al. Focal liver lesions: characterization with triphasic spiral CT. Radiology 1996;201:327–336.
27. Schoepf UJ, Becker C, Bruning R, et al. Computed tomography of the abdomen with multidetector-array CT. Radiology 1999;39:652–661.
28. Foley WD, Mallisee TA, Hohenwalter MD, et al. Multiphase hepatic CT with a multirow detector CT scanner. AJR Am J Roentgenol 2000;175:679–685.
29. Kadota M, Yamashita Y, Nakayama Y, et al. Valuation of small hepatocellular carcinoma with multidetector-row helical CT of the liver: the value of dual phase arterial scanning. Radiology 1999;213(P):124.
30. Murakami T, Kim T, Takahashi S, et al. The usefulness of double arterial phase imaging of multislice helical CT for the detection of hypervascular hepatocellular carcinoma. Radiology 1999;213(P):126.
31. Urban BA, Fishman EK, Kuhlman JE, et al. Detection of focal hepatic lesions with spiral CT: comparison of 4- and 8-mm interscan spacing. AJR Am J Roentgenol 1993;160:783–785.
32. Schwartz LH, Gandras EJ, Colangelo SM, et al. Prevalence and importance of small hepatic lesions found at CT in patients with cancer. Radiology 1999;210:71–74.
33. Van Hoc L, Van Cutsem E, Vergote I, et al. Size quantification of liver metastases in patients undergoing cancer treatment: reproducibility of one-, two-, and three-dimensional measurements determined with spiral CT. Radiology 1997;202:671–675.
34. Brink JA, Wang G, McFarland EG. Optimal section spacing in single-detector helical CT. Radiology 2000;214:575–578.
35. Bluemke DA, Fishman EK. Spiral CT arterial portography of the liver. Radiology 1993;186:576–579.
36. Ichikawa T, Ohtomo K, Takhashi S. Hepatocellular carcinoma: detection with double-phase helical CT during arterial portography. Radiology 1996;198:284–287.
37. Silverman PM, Robert SC, Ducic I, et al. Assessment of a technology that permits individual scan delays on helical hepatic CT: a technique to improve efficiency in use of contrast material. AJR Am J Roentgenol 1996;167:79–84.
38. Fishman EK, Wyatt SH, Ney DR, et al. Spiral CT of the pancreas with multiplanar display. AJR Am J Roentgenol 1992;159:1209–1215.
39. Dupuy DE, Costello P, Ecker CP. Spiral CT of the pancreas. Radiology 1992;183:815–818.
40. Lu DSK, Vedantham S, Krasny RM, et al. Two-phase helical CT for pancreatic tumors: pancreatic versus hepatic phase enhancement of tumor, pancreas, and vascular structures. Radiology 1996;199:697–701.
41. Hollett MD, Jorgensen MJ, Jeffrey RB. Quantitative evaluation of pancreatic enhancement during dual-phase helical CT. Radiology 1995;195:359–361.
42. Bluemke DA, Cameron JL, Hruban RH, et al. Potentially resectable pancreatic adenocarcinoma: spiral CT assessment with surgical and pathologic correlation. Radiology 1995;197:381–385.
43. Foley WD. Helical CT: clinical performance and imaging strategies. Radiographics 1994;14:894–904.
44. Van Hoe L, Gryspeerdt S, Marchal G, et al. Helical CT for the preoperative localization of islet cell tumors of the pancreas: value of arterial and parenchymal phase images. AJR Am J Roentgenol 1995;165:1437–1439.
45. Brink JA, Heiken JP, Balfe DM. Noninvasive cholangiography with spiral CT. Radiology 1992;185:141.
46. Van Beers BE, Lacrosse M, Trigaux JP, et al. Noninvasive imaging of the biliary tree before or after laparoscopic

cholecystectomy: use of three-dimensional spiral CT cholangiography. AJR Am J Roentgenol 1994;162:1331–1335.

47. Fleischmann D, Ringl H, Schoft R, et al. Three-dimensional spiral CT cholangiography in patients with suspected obstructive biliary disease: comparison with endoscopic retrograde cholangiography. Radiology 1996;198:861–868.
48. Klein HM, Wein B, Truong S, et al. Computed tomographic cholangiography using spiral scanning and 3D image processing. Br J Radiol 1993;66:762–767.
49. Stockberger SM, Wass JL, Sherman S, et al. Intravenous cholangiography with helical CT: comparison with endoscopic retrograde cholangiography. Radiology 1994;192:675–680.
50. Caoili EM, Paulson EK, Heyneman LE, et al. Helical CT cholangiography with three-dimensional volume rendering using an oral biliary contrast agent: feasibility of a novel technique. AJR Am J Roentgenol 2000;174:487–492.
51. Soto JA, Velez SM, Guzmán J. Choledocholithiasis: diagnosis with oral-contrast-enhanced CT cholangiography. AJR Am J Roentgenol 1999;172:943–948.
52. Heiken JP, Brink JA, Sagel SS. Helical CT: abdominal applications. Radiographics 1994;14:919–924.
53. Silverman SG, Seltzer SE, Adams DF, et al. Spiral CT of the small indeterminate renal mass: results in 48 patients. Radiology 1991;181:125.
54. Silverman SG, Lee BY, Seltzer SE, et al. Small (≤3 cm) renal masses: correlation of spiral CT features and pathologic findings. AJR Am J Roentgenol 1994;163:597–605.
55. Maki DD, Birnbaum BA, Chakraborty DP, et al. Renal cyst pseudoenhancement: beam-hardening effects on CT numbers. Radiology 1999;213:468–472.
56. Coulam CH, Sheafor DH, Leder RA, et al. Evaluation of pseudoenhancement of renal cysts during contrast-enhanced CT. AJR Am J Roentgenol 2000;174:493–498.
57. Heneghan JP, Spielmann AL, Sheafor DH, et al. Pseudoenhancement of simple renal cysts: a comparison of single and multidetector helical CT. Radiology 2000;217(P):580.
58. Birnbaum BA, Maki DD, Chakraborty DP, et al. Renal cyst pseudoenhancement: evaluation with an anthropomorphic body CT phantom. Radiology 2000;217(P):579.
59. Birnbaum BA, Jacobs JE, Ramchandani P. Multiphasic renal CT: comparison of renal mass enhancement during the corticomedullary and nephrographic phases. Radiology 1996;200:753–758.
60. Cohan RH, Sherman LS, Korobkin M, et al. Renal masses: assessment of corticomedullary-phase and nephrographic-phase CT scans. Radiology 1995;196:445–451.
61. Szolar DH, Kammerhuber F, Altziebler S, et al. Multiphasic helical CT of the kidney: increased conspicuity for detection and characterization of small (<3-cm) renal masses. Radiology 1997;202:211–217.
62. Urban BA. The small renal mass: what is the role of multiplanar helical scanning? Radiology 1997;202:22–23.
63. Chernoff DM, Silverman SG, Kikinis R, et al. Three-dimensional imaging and display of renal tumors using spiral CT: a potential aid to partial nephrectomy. Urology 1994;43:125–129.
64. Quillin SP, Brink JA, Heiken JP, et al. Spiral CT angiography: identification of crossing vessels at the ureteropelvic junction. AJR Am J Roentgenol 1996;166:1125–1130.
65. Platt JR, Ellis JH, Korobkin M, et al. Potential renal donors: comparison of conventional imaging with helical CT. Radiology 1996;198:419–423.
66. Sommer FG, Jeffrey RBJ, Rubin GD, et al. Detection of ureteral calculi in patients with suspected renal colic: value of reformatted noncontrast helical CT. AJR Am J Roentgenol 1995;165:509–513.
67. Smith RC, Verga M, McCarthy S, et al. Diagnosis of acute flank pain: value of unenhanced helical CT. AJR Am J Roentgenol 1996;166:97–101.
68. Katz DS, Lane MJ, Sommer FG. Unenhanced helical CT of ureteral stones: incidence of associated urinary tract findings. AJR Am J Roentgenol 1996;166:1319–1322.
69. Brink JA, Heiken JP, Semenkovich J, et al. Abnormalities of the diaphragm and adjacent structures: findings on multiplanar spiral CT scans. AJR Am J Roentgenol 1994;163:307–310.
70. Rubin GD, Beaulieu CF, Argiro V, et al. Perspective volume rendering of CT and MR images: applications for endoscopic imaging. Radiology 1996;199:321–330.
71. Hara AK, Johnson CD, Reed JE, et al. Colorectal polyp detection with CT colonography: two-versus three-dimensional techniques. Radiology 1996;200:49–54.

Protocol 1:
ABDOMEN SURVEY (Fig. 3)

INDICATION:	*Screening, R/O metastases, evaluate liver*
SCANNER SETTINGS:	kV(p): 120–140 mA: 210–330
ORAL CONTRAST:	600–800 mL, 45–60 min before study initiation. An additional 200 mL given just before scanning.
PHASE OF RESPIRATION:	Suspended inspiration or expiration
ROTATION TIME:	0.5–1.0 sec
ACQUISITION SLICE THICKNESS:	2.5 to 5.0 mm
PITCH:	0.75–1.5 (HQ = 3:1; HS = 6:1)
RECONSTRUCTION SLICE THICKNESS/INTERVAL FOR FILMING:	2.5–5.0 mm/5.0–7.0 mm

ANATOMIC COVERAGE:
  SUPERIOR EXTENT:
  INFERIOR EXTENT:
	
	Dome of the diaphragm
	Iliac crest

IV CONTRAST:

Concentration:	Low osmolar contrast medium (LOCM) 300–370 mg iodine/mL or high osmolar contrast medium (HOCM) 282 mg iodine/mL (60% solution)
Rate:	2–3 mL/sec
Scan Delay:	70 sec
Total Volume:	125–150 mL

COMMENTS:

1. For three-dimensional imaging, save the raw data, retrospectively reconstruct images at 1- to 2-mm intervals depending on acquisition thickness for three dimensional model. Keep the series in exact order by location. Do not alter field of view, matrix size, or center within the series.

2. If there is any question of renal abnormalities, rescan the kidneys after medullary and collecting system opacification. If densely enhancing abnormalities are seen that need to be differentiated from calcifications, perform a few delayed cuts.

3. If available, an automated scan delay using bolus triggering (e.g., CAST or SmartPrep) can be used to scan the liver. A threshold of 50 HU of enhancement over baseline is recommended. Using the full-contrast dose (150 mL), this provides improved contrast enhancement and less interpatient variability. If desired, results equivalent to using 150 mL with a standard fixed scan delay can be achieved with 125 mL and automated triggering.

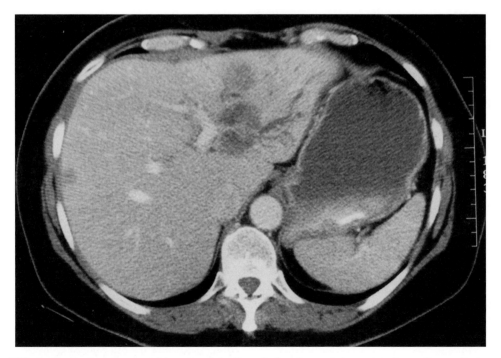

FIG. 3. Computed tomographic scan of the liver during the portal venous phase demonstrates a solid hypoattenuating mass along the medial aspect of the left portal vein. The mass causes biliary obstruction in the lateral segment of the left hepatic lobe. Other hypoattenuating masses are also noted.

Protocol 2:
ABDOMEN AND PELVIS SURVEY (Fig. 4)

INDICATION:	*Tumor staging, abscess*
SCANNER SETTINGS:	kV(p): 120–140 mA: 210–330
ORAL CONTRAST:	600–800 mL, 45–60 min before study initiation. An additional 200 mL given just before scanning.
PHASE OF RESPIRATION:	Suspended inspiration or expiration
ROTATION TIME:	0.5–1.0 sec
ACQUISITION SLICE THICKNESS:	2.5 to 5.0 mm
PITCH:	0.75–1.5 (HQ = 3:1; HS = 6:1)
RECONSTRUCTION SLICE THICKNESS/INTERVAL FOR FILMING:	5.0–7 mm/5.0–7.0 mm

ANATOMIC COVERAGE:
  SUPERIOR EXTENT:
  INFERIOR EXTENT:
	
	Dome of the diaphragm
	Symphysis pubis

IV CONTRAST:

Concentration:	LOCM 300–370 mg iodine/mL or HOCM 282 mg iodine/mL (60% solution)
Scan Delay:	70 sec
Technique:	Uniphasic
Uniphasic:	*Rate:* 2–3 mL/sec *Volume:* 125–150 mL

COMMENTS:

1. A uniphasic injection for helical CT is recommended. In very thin (e.g., less than 120 lb) patients, it may be possible to use lower milliamperes for the helical scan. Frequently, when the pelvis is scanned, the bladder has not opacified with contrast material. If bladder opacification is necessary, additional 5-mm scans through the bladder may be performed after a 5–10 min delay.
2. It is preferable to use 330 mA for patients up to 250 lb; up to 400 mA in patients more than 250 lb.

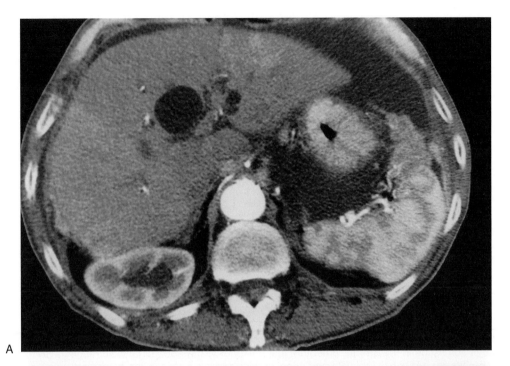

A

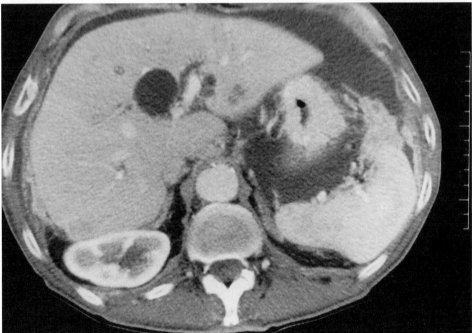

B

FIG. 4. A: Computed tomographic scan of the upper abdomen during the arterial phase demonstrates a hepatic cyst near the liver hilum. A hyperenhancing perfusion abnormality is also identified in the posterior segment of the right hepatic lobe. There is also evidence of ascites and nodular capsular thickening along the right hepatic lobe, posterolaterally. **B:** During the venous phase, there is much more vivid hepatic parenchymal enhancement and more uniform splenic enhancement. During this phase, a nodular soft tissue mass is more apparent along the anterior aspect of the spleen. There are also solid hypoattenuating masses in the liver suggesting parenchymal metastases.

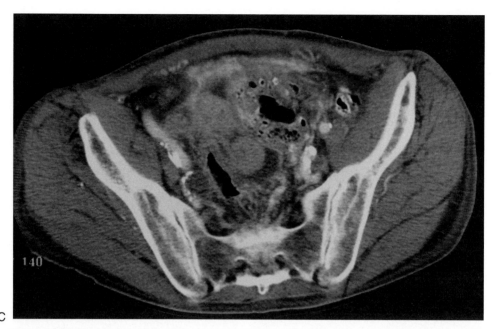

C

FIG. 4. *Continued.* **C:** An image through the midpelvis demonstrates a hyperenhancing mantel of soft tissue in the greater omentum just posterior to the abdominal wall. Findings from all three figures are consistent with peritoneal carcinomatosis from a colon carcinoma.

Protocol 3:
SURVEY FOR ABDOMINAL/PELVIC TRAUMA (Fig. 5)

INDICATION:	*Assess presence and extent of trauma*
SCANNER SETTINGS:	kV(p): 120–140 mA: 210–330
ORAL CONTRAST:	600–800 mL, 45–60 min before study initiation or as soon as possible before the examination. An additional 200 mL given just before scanning.
PHASE OF RESPIRATION:	Suspended inspiration or expiration
ROTATION TIME:	0.5–1.0 sec
ACQUISITION SLICE THICKNESS:	2.5 to 5.0 mm
PITCH:	0.75–1.5 (HQ = 3:1; HS = 6:1)
RECONSTRUCTION SLICE THICKNESS/INTERVAL FOR FILMING:	2.5–5.0 mm/5.0–7.0 mm

ANATOMIC COVERAGE:
  SUPERIOR EXTENT:
  INFERIOR EXTENT:
	
	Dome of the diaphragm
	Symphysis pubis

IV CONTRAST:		
	Concentration:	LOCM 300–370 mg iodine/mL or HOCM 282 mg iodine/mL (60% solution)
	Rate:	2–3 mL/sec
	Scan Delay:	60–70 sec
	Total Volume:	125–150 mL

COMMENTS:

1. This technique is essentially an abdominal/pelvis survey. It also can be used as a protocol for abdominal trauma. A few noncontrast scans through the spleen can be obtained to observe for acute hemorrhage appearing as high density.

2. A 4 × 3.75-mm detector configuration with a pitch of 1.5 mm is an attempt to increase speed without sacrificing image quality.
3. As with conventional CT, it is imperative to scan the pelvis. Some patients may have a significant intra-abdominal bleed with minimal blood in the abdomen but extensive blood in the pelvis.
4. Remove all leads and extraneous devices before scanning.

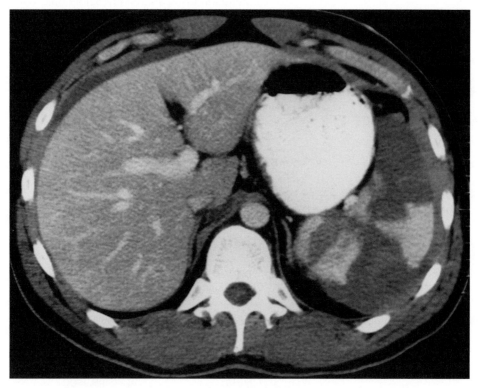

FIG. 5. Computed tomographic scan of the upper abdomen during the venous phase in a patient who sustained blunt trauma. Although the liver appears normal, the spleen demonstrates multiple wedge-shaped hypoenhancing defects consistent with extensive injury. There is also evidence of a small amount of perihepatic and perisplenic blood.

Protocol 4:
THORAX/ABDOMEN (Fig. 6)

INDICATION:	*Combined study, oncologic survey/follow-up*
SCANNER SETTINGS:	kV(p): 120–140 mA: 250–330 (abdomen) 150–250 (thorax)
ORAL CONTRAST:	600–800 mL, 45–60 min befor study initiation. An additional 200 mL given just before scanning.
PHASE OF RESPIRATION:	Suspended inspiration
ROTATION TIME:	0.5–1.0 sec
ACQUISITION SLICE THICKNESS:	2.5 to 5.0 mm
PITCH:	0.75–1.5 (HQ = 3:1; HS = 6:1)
RECONSTRUCTION SLICE THICKNESS/INTERVAL FOR FILMING:	2.5–5.0 mm/5.0–7.0 mm

ANATOMIC COVERAGE:
  SUPERIOR EXTENT:
  INFERIOR EXTENT:
	
	Lung apices
	Iliac crest

IV CONTRAST:

Concentration:	LOCM 300–370 mg iodine/mL or HOCM 282 mg iodine/mL (60% solution)
Technique:	Uniphasic *Rate:* 2–3 mL/sec *Volume:* 150 mL
Scan Delay:	15–30 sec
Total Volume:	150 mL

COMMENTS:

1. It is possible to scan from lung apices to iliac crest in one breath-hold but recommend starting chest after a 20–30-sec delay, then pausing the scanner at the dome of the liver until 60–70 sec, at which time, the entire abdomen is scanned.

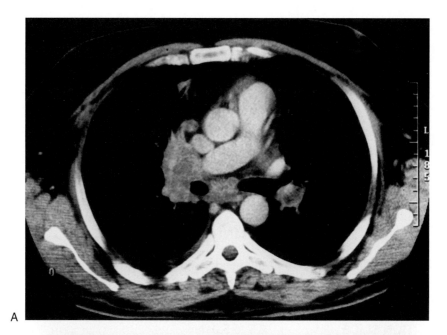

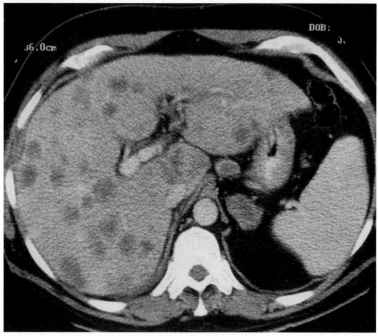

FIG. 6. Computed tomographic scan in a patient with metastatic lung carcinoma. **A:** Image through the midthorax demonstrates a nodular hypoenhancing mass encasing the right mainstem bronchi. There also appears to be left hilar lymphadenopathy. **B:** Scan through the upper abdomen during the venous phase demonstrates numerous hypoenhancing liver metastases, a left adrenal metastasis, and lymphadenopathy along the gastrohepatic ligament. **C:** Scan through the kidneys during the nephrographic phase reveals a subtle, poorly defined hypoenhancing mass in the intrapolar region on the right. **D:** During the excretory phase, the hypoenhancing defect in the right kidney persists. Note the presence of retrocaval lymphadenopathy, as well.

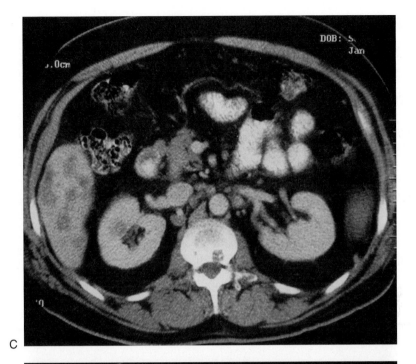

C

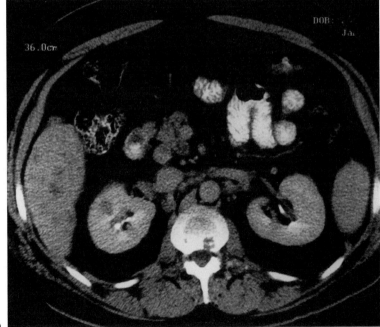

D

FIG. 6. *Continued.*

Protocol 5:
THORAX/ABDOMEN/PELVIS (Fig. 7)

INDICATION:	*Combined study, oncologic screening*
SCANNER SETTINGS:	kV(p): 120–140 mA: 210–330 (abdomen portion) 150–250 (thorax portion)
ORAL CONTRAST:	600–800 mL, 45–60 min before study initiation. An additional 200 mL given just before scanning.
PHASE OF RESPIRATION:	Suspended inspiration
ROTATION TIME:	0.5–1.0 sec
ACQUISITION SLICE THICKNESS:	2.50 to 5.0 mm
PITCH:	0.75–1.5 (HQ = 3:1; HS = 6:1)
RECONSTRUCTION SLICE THICKNESS/INTERVAL FOR FILMING:	2.5–5.0 mm/5.0–7.0 mm

ANATOMIC COVERAGE:
  SUPERIOR EXTENT:
  INFERIOR EXTENT:
	
	Lung apices
	Pubic symphysis

IV CONTRAST:

Concentration:	LOCM 300–370 mg iodine/mL or HOCM 282 mg iodine/mL (60% solution)
Scan Delay:	15–30 sec (chest) 60–70 sec (abdomen/pelvis)
Total Volume:	150 mL
Technique:	Uniphasic *Rate:* 2–3 mL/sec *Volume:* 125–150 mL

COMMENTS:

1. Recommend starting the chest after a 20–30-sec delay, then pausing the scanner at the dome of the liver until 60–70 sec, at which time, the entire abdomen and pelvis is scanned.

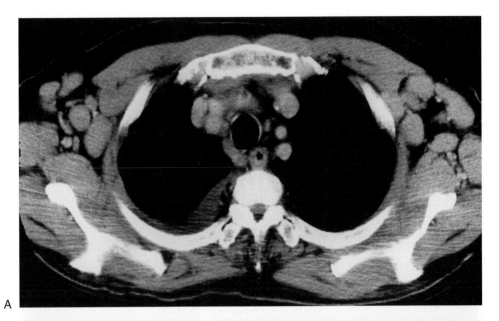

A

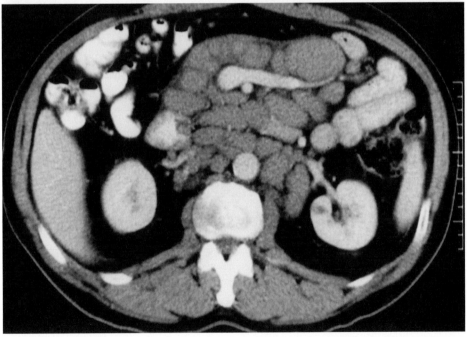

B

FIG. 7. Computed tomographic scan in a patient with non-Hodgkin's lymphoma. **A:** Scan through the upper thorax reveals extensive axillary lymphadenopathy, bilaterally. There is also a small right pleural effusion. **B:** Scan through the midabdomen during the venous phase demonstrates extensive retroperitoneal and mesenteric lymphadenopathy. **C:** Scan through the pelvis reveals external iliac lymphadenopathy, bilaterally. An obturator lymph node is also identified on the left.

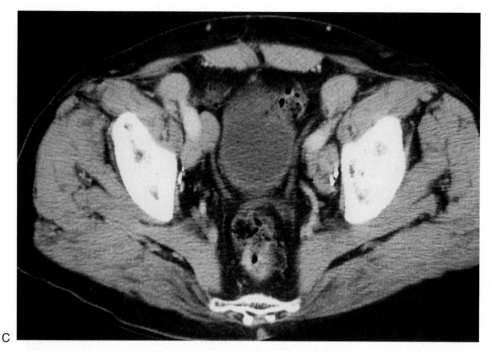

C

FIG. 7. *Continued.*

Protocol 6:
PELVIS (Fig. 8)

INDICATION:	*Oncologic staging of prostate, cervical, endometrial, or ovarian cancer*
SCANNER SETTINGS:	kV(p): 120–140 mA: 165–275
ORAL CONTRAST:	600–800 mL, 45–60 mm before study initiation, rectal contrast media or air is optional
PHASE OF RESPIRATION:	Suspended inspiration or expiration
ROTATION TIME:	0.5–1.0 sec
ACQUISITION SLICE THICKNESS:	2.5–5.0 mm
PITCH:	0.75–1.00 (HQ = 3:1)
RECONSTRUCTION SLICE THICKNESS/INTERVAL FOR FILMING:	5.0 mm/5.0–10.0 mm, 2–3 mm optimal for staging pelvic tumors
ANATOMIC COVERAGE: **SUPERIOR EXTENT:** **INFERIOR EXTENT:**	 Superior iliac crest Inferior portion of symphysis pubis

IV CONTRAST:

Concentration:	LOCM 300–370 mg iodine/mL or HOCM 282 mg iodine/mL (60% solution)
Rate:	2–3 mL/sec
Scan Delay:	70–80 sec
Total Volume:	100–125 mL

COMMENTS:

1. For pelvic malignancies, it may be advantageous to scan the pelvis in a caudal-cranial direction, beginning at the level of the lower symphysis pubis. This technique optimizes visualization of pelvic vasculature.
2. Delayed scans can be performed if bladder opacification is desired.

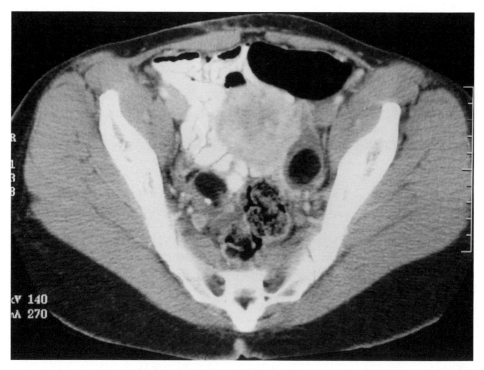

FIG. 8. Computed tomographic scan through the midpelvis reveals bilateral adnexal masses, each having the attenuation characteristics of fat internally. There is also a small calcification on the right side, posteriorly. These masses are consistent with dermoid cysts.

Protocol 7:
DEDICATED LIVER: DUAL PHASE
(Figs. 9 and 10)

INDICATION:	*Primary evaluation of suspected hypervascular hepatic tumors, including focal nodular hyperplasia, hepatic adenoma, hepatocellular carcinoma, hemangioma, and metastases from carcinoid, islet cell carcinoma, thyroid carcinoma, renal cell carcinoma, choriocarcinoma, breast carcinoma, melanoma, and various sarcomas*
SCANNER SETTINGS:	kV(p): 120–140 mA: 210–330
ORAL CONTRAST:	600–800 mL, 45–60 min before study initiation. An additional 200 mL given just before scanning.
PHASE OF RESPIRATION:	Suspended inspiration or expiration
ROTATION TIME:	0.5–1.0 sec
ACQUISITION SLICE THICKNESS:	2.5 to 5.0 mm
PITCH:	0.75–1.5 (HQ = 3:1; HS = 6:1)
RECONSTRUCTION SLICE THICKNESS/INTERVAL FOR FILMING:	2.0–5.0 mm/5.0–7.0 mm

ANATOMIC COVERAGE:
    SUPERIOR EXTENT:
    INFERIOR EXTENT:
	
	Dome of the diaphragm
	Iliac crest

IV CONTRAST:

Concentration:	LOCM 300–370 mg iodine/mL or HOCM 282 mg iodine/mL (60% solution)
Rate:	4–5 mL/sec
Scan Delay:	30–35 sec for arterial phase 60–65 sec for venous phase (or ASAP)
Total Volume:	150 mL

COMMENTS:

1. Unenhanced scans of the liver may be performed before contrast injection.
2. If an intrahepatic cholangiocarcinoma is suspected, rescan the liver 15–30 min after the bolus.
3. If a hemangioma is suspected, it may be helpful to rescan the lesion every 5 min as needed.
4. If the patient's IV access catheter cannot accommodate a high injection flow rate (e.g., hand vein or smaller than 20 G), omit arterial phase and perform only venous phase examination. Modify scan delay according to flow rate (Table 1).
5. Scan delay for the hepatic arterial phase can be automated using bolus triggering. Venous phase initiated about 35 sec after end of arterial phase.

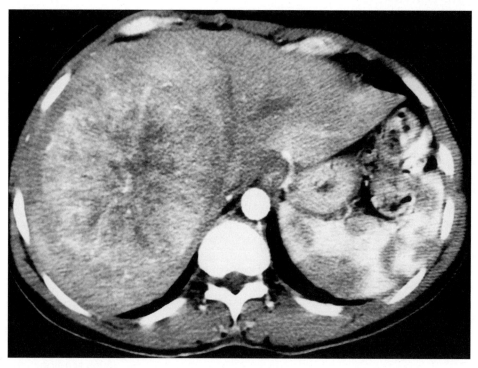

A

FIG. 9. Computed tomographic scan on a patient who is status post–right nephrectomy for renal cell carcinoma. **A:** Scan through the upper abdomen during the arterial phase demonstrates a large hyperenhancing mass occupying most of the right hepatic lobe and extending into the left. **B:** During the venous phase, the mass is hypoenhancing. **C:** Scan through the midabdomen reveals a large lobulated heterogenous soft tissue mass in the mesentery on the right side. Note that the mass contains a ringlike calcification and low-attenuation areas, suggesting necrosis.

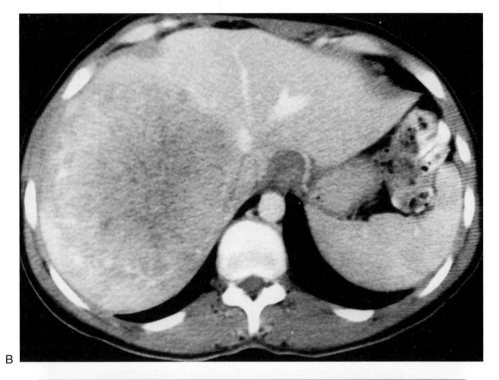

B

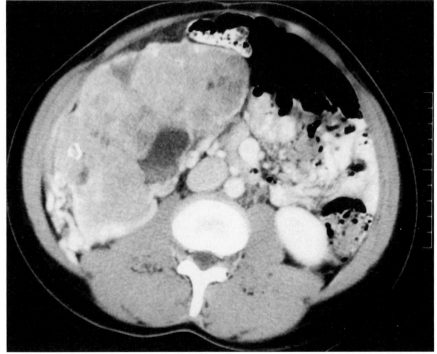

C

FIG. 9. *Continued.*

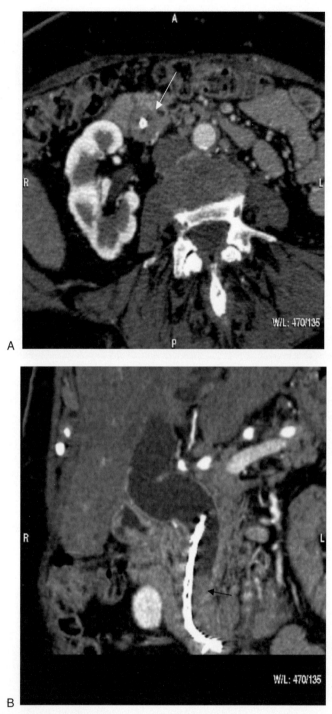

FIG. 10. A 78-year-old female with cholangiocarcinoma arising in the distal common bile duct resulting in marked biliary dilatation. **A:** Transaxial image reveals tumor (*arrow*) filling the distal common bile duct (a biliary stent is in place). **B:** Paracoronal reformation reveals a tumor in the distal bile duct (*arrow*) adjacent to the biliary stent.

Protocol 8:
LIVER: CT ARTERIAL PORTOGRAPHY

INDICATION: *To determine resectability and to plan surgical resection of neoplastic hepatic disease*

SCANNER SETTINGS: kV(p): 120–140
mA: 210–330

ORAL CONTRAST: None

PHASE OF RESPIRATION: Suspended inspiration or expiration

ROTATION TIME: 0.5–10 sec

ACQUISITION SLICE THICKNESS: 2.5 to 5.0 mm

PITCH: 0.75–1.5 (HQ = 3:1; HS = 6:1)

RECONSTRUCTION SLICE THICKNESS/INTERVAL FOR FILMING: 2.5–5.0 mm/5.0 mm

ANATOMIC COVERAGE:
  SUPERIOR EXTENT: Dome of the diaphragm
  INFERIOR EXTENT: Iliac crest

IV CONTRAST:

Concentration:	HOCM 200 mg iodine/mL (or 2:1 dilution of HOCM 282 mg iodine/mL)
Rate:	2–3 mL/sec
Scan Delay:	35 sec
Total Volume:	135 mL

COMMENTS:

1. Contrast material is injected via a small (5-Fr) catheter placed in either the proximal superior mesenteric artery or the splenic artery. If there is a replaced right hepatic artery, the catheter tip must be positioned distal to the origin of this anomalous vessel.

2. Delayed scans at 4 to 6 hr may be obtained. After the CTAP has been completed, administer an additional 50 mL of HOCM (282 mg iodine/mL) before the patient leaves the department. Then schedule a second CT scan (without additional IV contrast medium) to be done 4 to 6 hr after the initial scan.

Protocol 9:
PANCREAS (Fig. 11)

INDICATION:	*Evaluate pancreatitis*
SCANNER SETTINGS:	kV(p): 120–140 mA: 210–330
ORAL CONTRAST:	600–800 mL, 45–60 min before study initiation. An additional 200 mL given just before scanning.
PHASE OF RESPIRATION:	Suspended inspiration or expiration
ROTATION TIME:	0.5–1.0 sec
ACQUISITION SLICE THICKNESS:	2.5 to 5.0 mm
PITCH:	0.75–1.5 (HQ = 3:1; HS = 6:1)
RECONSTRUCTION SLICE THICKNESS/INTERVAL FOR FILMING:	2.5–5.0 mm/5.0–7.0 mm
ANATOMIC COVERAGE: SUPERIOR EXTENT: INFERIOR EXTENT:	Dome of the liver Iliac crest or inferiorly to the pelvis, depending on extent of disease

IV CONTRAST:

Concentration:	LOCM 300–370 mg iodine/mL
Rate:	2–3 mL/sec
Scan Delay:	40–60 sec
Total Volume:	100–150 mL

COMMENTS:

1. This protocol specifies scanning from the diaphragm to the iliac crest. This covers the entire area typically involved in pancreatitis. Occasionally, additional scans may be needed if pseudocysts extend cranially into the mediastinum or caudally into the pelvis.
2. IV contrast media is important to evaluate the viability of the pancreas tissue amidst extensive pancreatic inflammation to assess for glandular necrosis, an important prognostic factor.

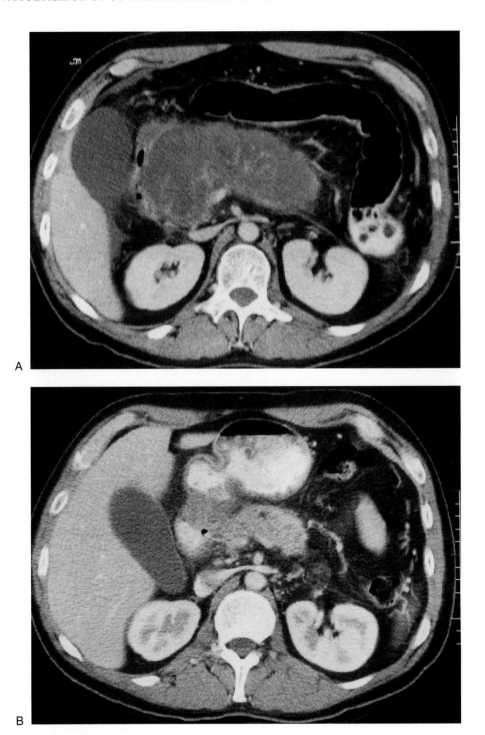

FIG. 11. Computed tomographic scan in a patient with acute pancreatitis. **A:** Scan through the upper abdomen during the venous phase reveals an enlarge hypoenhancing pancreas. Note displacement and narrowing of the duodenal lumen, as well as a dilated loop of transverse colon. **B:** Scan through the upper abdomen several weeks later demonstrates near-complete resolution of the inflammatory process and relatively normal enhancement of the pancreas.

Protocol 10:
DEDICATED PANCREAS: DUAL PHASE
(Figs. 12 through 14)

INDICATION:	*Primary evaluation of known or suspected pancreatic neoplasms; dedicated pancreas study*
SCANNER SETTINGS:	kV(p): 120–140 mA: 210–330
ORAL CONTRAST:	600–800 mL, 45–60 min before study initiation. An additional 200 mL given just before scanning.
PHASE OF RESPIRATION:	Suspended inspiration or expiration
ROTATION TIME:	0.5–1.0 sec
ACQUISITION SLICE THICKNESS:	Arterial/Pancreatic phase: 1.25 to 2.5 mm Venous phase: 2.5 to 5.0 mm
PITCH:	Arterial phase: 1.50 (HS = 6:1) Pancreatic phase/Venous phase: 0.75–1.5 (HQ = 3:1; HS = 6:1)
RECONSTRUCTION SLICE THICKNESS/INTERVAL FOR FILMING:	Arterial/Pancreatic phase: 1.25–2.5 mm/ 2.5–5.0 mm Pancreatic/venous phase: 2.5–5.0 mm/5 mm

ANATOMIC COVERAGE:
  SUPERIOR EXTENT:
  INFERIOR EXTENT:
	Dome of the diaphragm
	Third portion of the duodenum

IV CONTRAST:

Concentration:	LOCM 300–370 mg iodine/mL or HOCM 282 mg iodine/mL (60% solution)
Rate:	4–5 mL/sec
Scan Delay:	30 sec for arterial phase 40 sec for pancreatic phase 60 sec for venous phase (or ASAP)
Total Volume:	150–175 mL

COMMENTS:

1. It may be prudent to perform unenhanced scan to determine the location of the third portion of the duodenum.
2. It may be helpful to perform helical scanning in caudal-cephalad direction beginning at the third portion of the duodenum or inferior tip of liver, whichever is more caudal.
3. For suspected islet cell tumors, the entire liver should be scanned during both postcontrast phases.
4. If the patient's IV access catheter cannot accommodate a high injection flow rate (e.g., hand vein, smaller than 20 G), omit arterial phase and perform only parenchymal/venous phase examination. Modify scan delay according to flow rate (see Table 1).
5. Water can be substituted for oral contrast media.
6. The scan delay for the arterial phase can be automated by bolus triggering.
7. The arterial phase is rendered in three dimensions to evaluate the peripancreatic arteries for tumor encasement. This rendering should include curved MPR images to assess the perivascular soft tissue.

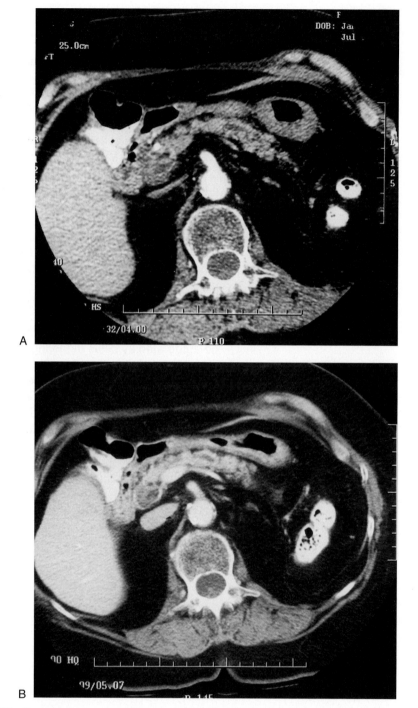

FIG. 12. Computed tomographic scan in a patient with pancreatic adenocarcinoma. **A:** Thin-section, small field-of-view image of the pancreas during the pancreatic phase demonstrates dilatation of the main pancreatic duct. **B:** During the venous phase, a small round heterogenous hypoenhancing mass in the pancreatic head is more apparent. There is no arterial or venous encasement or evidence of peripancreatic lymphadenopathy.

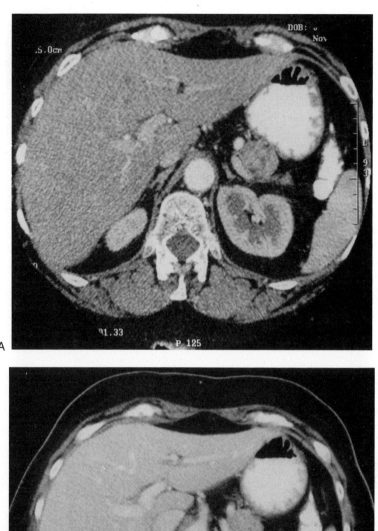

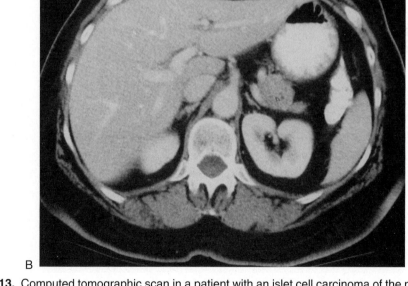

FIG. 13. Computed tomographic scan in a patient with an islet cell carcinoma of the pancreas. **A:** Thin-section, small field-of-view (FOV) scan through the upper abdomen during the pancreatic or parenchymal phase reveals a round enhancing solid mass in the pancreatic tail. **B:** During the venous phase, an image with a thicker section and larger FOV reveals that the mass has similar enhancement characteristics to those of the healthy pancreas. There is no upstream dilation of the main pancreatic duct and no evidence of splenic vein thrombosis.

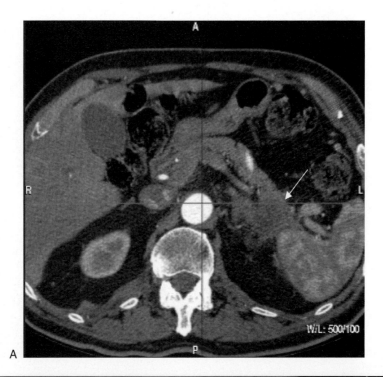

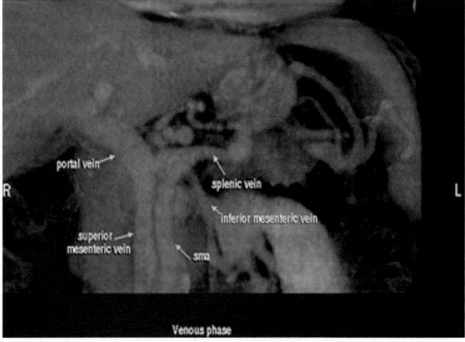

FIG. 14. A 58-year-old man with ductal cell adenocarcinoma in the tail of the pancreas. **A:** Transaxial source image reveals an invasive carcinoma arising from the tail of the pancreas (*arrow*). **B:** Volume-rendered image reveals the mass in the pancreatic tail (*white arrow*) narrowing the splenic vein, resulting in varices in the gastrosplenic ligament.

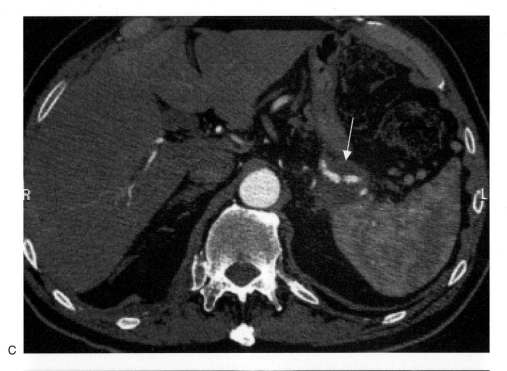

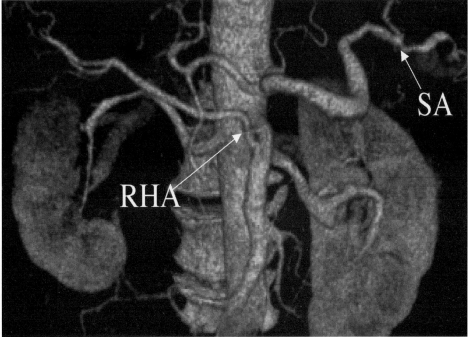

FIG. 14. *Continued.* **C:** Transaxial image reveals narrowing of the splenic artery by the mass (*arrow*). **D:** Volume-rendered coronal image reveals irregular narrowing of the splenic artery *(SA).* A replaced right hepatic artery *(RHA)* is also noted arising from the superior mesenteric artery.

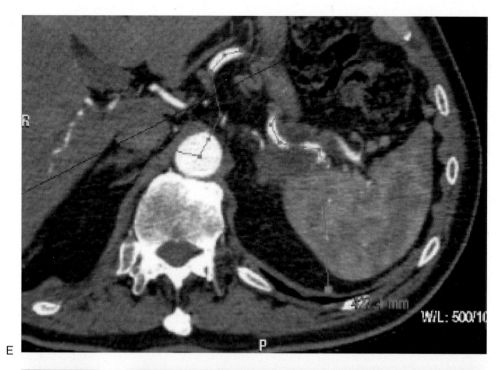

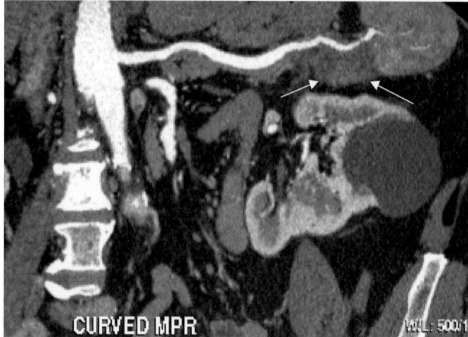

FIG. 14. *Continued.* **E:** A curved planar cut line is deposited in the splenic artery. **F:** Curved planar reformation reveals narrowing of the splenic artery by the pancreatic tumor (*arrows*).

Protocol 11:
SPLEEN SURVEY (Fig. 15)

INDICATION:	*Detecting traumatic injury, infarcts, abscesses, and neoplasms*
SCANNER SETTINGS:	kV(p): 120–140 mA: 210–330
ORAL CONTRAST:	Optional
PHASE OF RESPIRATION:	Suspended inspiration or expiration
ROTATION TIME:	0.5–1.0 sec
ACQUISITION SLICE THICKNESS:	5.0 mm
PITCH:	0.75 (HQ = 3:1)
RECONSTRUCTION SLICE THICKNESS/INTERVAL FOR FILMING:	2.5–5.0 mm/5.0–7.0 mm

ANATOMIC COVERAGE:
  SUPERIOR EXTENT:
  INFERIOR EXTENT:
	
	Dome of the liver
	Superior iliac crest

IV CONTRAST:

Concentration:	LOCM 300–370 mg iodine/mL or HOCM 282 mg iodine/mL (60% solution)
Rate:	2–3 mL/sec
Scan Delay:	60–70 sec
Total Volume:	100– 150 mL

COMMENTS:

1. One of the difficulties in evaluating the spleen is that the spleen normally will have an early rippled, mottled, or striated enhancement pattern when contrast is injected as a bolus and scanned dynamically. Therefore, it is best to delay scanning for about 60 sec after the bolus is initiated. Occasionally, delayed scans will be needed in equivocal cases. Irregular splenic enhancement is most common in patients with decreased cardiac output.
2. On occasion, the early enhancement pattern may reveal curvilinear lucencies that mimic a lesion.

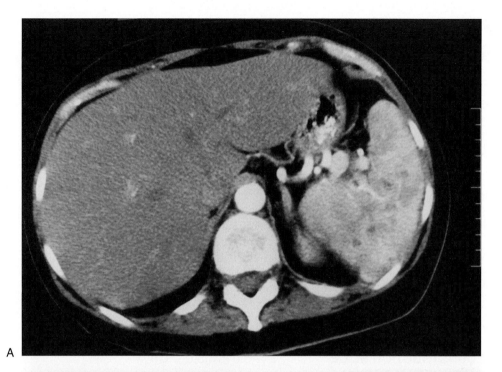

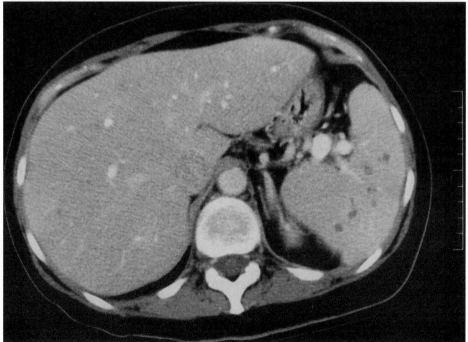

FIG. 15. CT scan in an immunocompromised patient with candidiasis. **A:** Scan of the upper abdomen during the arterial phase reveals mottled enhancement of the spleen. Small hypoattenuation defects are identified. **B:** During the venous phase, the spleen enhances uniformly and the numerous small hypoattenuation defects persist. Note that the arterial phase adds little information to the venous phase.

Protocol 12:
KIDNEYS (Fig. 16)

INDICATION:	*General screening abdomen/kidneys, renal vein thrombosis, or other renal abnormalities*
SCANNER SETTINGS:	kV(p): 120–140 mA: 210–330
ORAL CONTRAST:	600–800 mL, 45–60 min before study initiation. An additional 200 mL given just before scanning.
PHASE OF RESPIRATION:	Suspended inspiration or expiration
ROTATION TIME:	0.5–1.0 sec
ACQUISITION SLICE THICKNESS:	2.5 to 5.0 mm
PITCH:	0.75–1.5 (HQ = 3:1; HS = 6:1)
RECONSTRUCTION SLICE THICKNESS/INTERVAL FOR FILMING:	2.5–5.0 mm/5.0–7.0 mm

ANATOMIC COVERAGE:
  SUPERIOR EXTENT:
  INFERIOR EXTENT:
	
	Above the adrenals
	Below the kidneys

IV CONTRAST:

Concentration:	LOCM 300–320 mg iodine/mL or HOCM 282 mg iodine/mL (60% solution)
Rate:	2–3 mL/sec
Scan Delay:	60–70 sec
Total Volume:	125–150 mL

COMMENTS:

1. Many institutions perform noncontrast scans, followed by contrast-enhanced scans after a 70–80-sec delay. The goal is to obtain images without corticomedullary distinction (low-attenuation medulla, high-attenuation cortex).
2. Preliminary noncontrast images allow for detection of renal calculi and for determining if a mass enhances postcontrast.

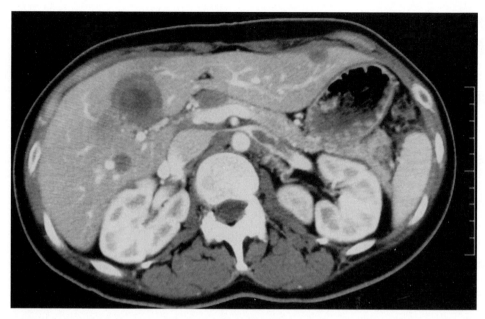

FIG. 16. CT scan of the mid-abdomen during the venous phase in a patient with colon carcinoma. There are several liver metastases and a nonocclusive thrombus in the left renal vein. Note that the kidneys demonstrate corticomedullary differentiation during which phase of enhancement small centrally located renal lesions can be missed.

Protocol 13:
KIDNEYS: DUAL PHASE (Figs. 17 and 18)

INDICATION:	*Primary evaluation of known or suspected renal neoplasms or other noncalculous focal renal lesions, dedicated renal study*
SCANNER SETTINGS:	kV(p): 120–140 mA: 210–330
ORAL CONTRAST:	600–800 mL, 45–60 min before study initiation. An additional 200 mL given just before scanning.
PHASE OF RESPIRATION:	Suspended inspiration or expiration
ROTATION TIME:	0.5 to 1.0 sec
ACQUISITION SLICE THICKNESS:	2.5 to 5.0 mm
PITCH:	0.75–1.5 (HQ = 3:1; HS = 6:1)
RECONSTRUCTION SLICE THICKNESS FOR FILMING:	2.5–5.0 mm/5.0–7.0 mm
ANATOMIC COVERAGE:	
SUPERIOR EXTENT:	Above the adrenals
INFERIOR EXTENT:	Inferior portion of symphysis pubis

IV CONTRAST:

Concentration:	LOCM 300–350 mg iodine/mL or HOCM 282 mg iodine/mL (60% solution)
Rate:	2–3 mL/sec
Scan Delay:	70–80 sec for the nephrographic phase 120–180 sec for the excretory phase
Total Volume:	100–150 mL

COMMENTS:

1. Always perform preliminary noncontrast scan for baseline attenuation measurements and to detect calcifications or calculi.
2. During the nephrographic phase, the entire abdomen should be scanned from the diaphragm to the iliac crests. During the excretory phase, the entire collecting system, including the urinary bladder, should be scanned.

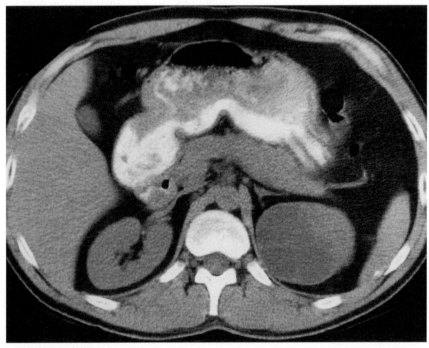

A

FIG. 17. CT scan in a patient with a cystic renal cell carcinoma. **A:** Image through the kidneys before the administration of intravenous contrast material reveals a hypoattenuating mass in the upper pole of the left kidney. There are no obvious calcifications or evidence of intralesional hemorrhage. **B:** During the nephrographic phase, the mass is noted to be complex with a multilocular cystic appearance posteromedially and a solid enhancing appearance anterolaterally. **C:** During the excretory phase, the mass persists. Note that the mass either obliterates or displaces the upper pole calix on the left.

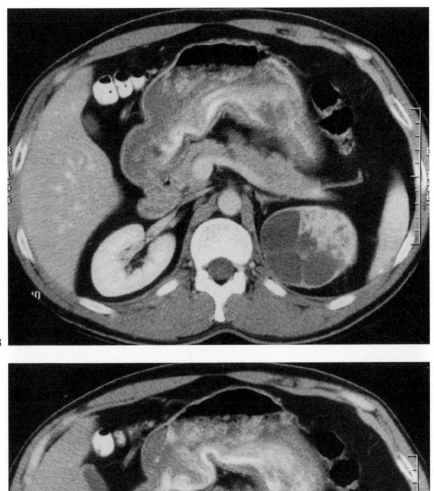

B

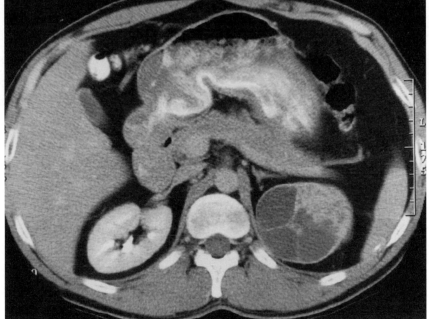

C

FIG. 17. *Continued.*

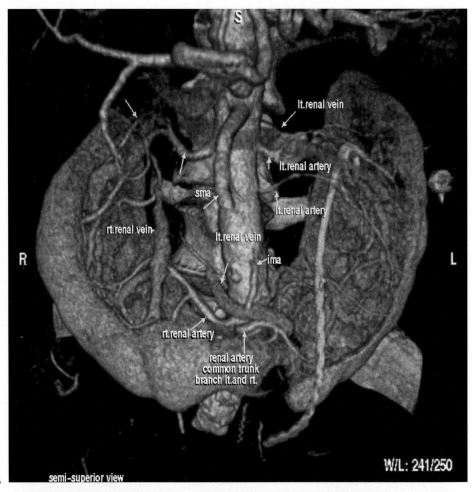

FIG. 18. A 63-year-old man with a horseshoe kidney and a transitional cell carcinoma of the left proximal ureter. Dual-phase imaging with computed tomographic angiography is being done for preoperative assessment before left nephroureterectomy. **A:** Volume-rendered image reveals complex vascular anatomy. **B:** Increased segmentation reveals renal arteries and veins with less overlapping renal parenchyma.

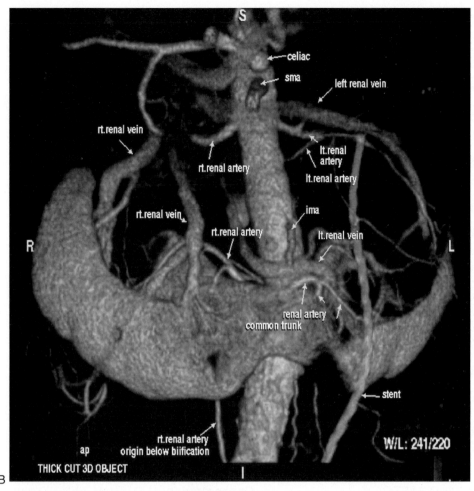

FIG. 18. *Continued.*

Protocol 14:
UPJ OBSTRUCTION (Fig. 19)

INDICATION:	*Evaluation of primary or secondary UPJ obstruction for detection of vessels crossing the UPJ that may be causative or complicate repair*
SCANNER SETTINGS:	kV(p): 120–140 mAs: 210–330
ORAL CONTRAST:	None
PHASE OF RESPIRATION:	Suspended inspiration or expiration
ROTATION TIME:	0.5–1.0 sec
ACQUISITION SLICE THICKNESS:	1.25 to 2.5 mm
PITCH:	1.5 (HS = 6:1)
RECONSTRUCTION SLICE THICKNESS/INTERVAL FOR FILMING:	1.25–2.5 mm/0.5–1.25 mm (targeted to affected kidney)
ANATOMIC COVERAGE:	
SUPERIOR EXTENT:	1 cm superior to main renal arteries
INFERIOR EXTENT:	2 cm below UPJ

IV CONTRAST:

Concentration:	LOCM 300–370 mg iodine/mL or HOCM 282 mg iodine/mL (60% solution)
Rate:	5 mL/sec
Scan Delay:	30 sec for arterial phase 10–15 min for excretory phase
Total Volume:	150 mL

COMMENTS:

1. Clamp nephrostomy tube (if present) when patient arrives to distend the renal pelvis for scanning.
2. Consider administering sterile saline via nephrostomy tube to distend the pelvicalceal system. This may aid in differentiating the ureter from the renal pelvis.
3. Perform interactive interpretation on a workstation using transaxial, three-dimensional and MPR images.

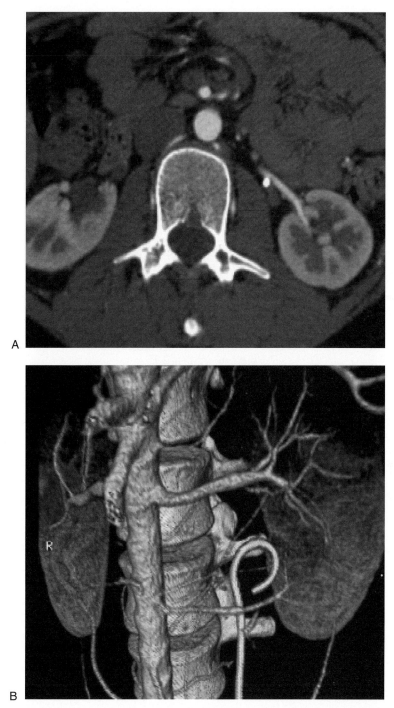

FIG. 19. A 37-year-old woman with congenital ureteropelvic junction (UPJ) obstruction, being evaluated preoperative for endopyelotomy. Computed tomographic angiography is being done to exclude a crossing vessel at the UPJ. **A:** Transaxial image reveals an accessory left renal artery crossing the UPJ anteriorly. Volume-rendered images in the **(B)** right posterior oblique (RPO), and **(C)** craniocaudal projects confirm anatomic relationships.

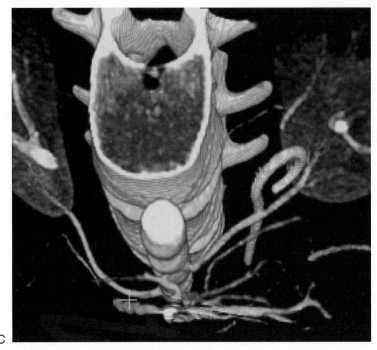

FIG. 19. *Continued.*

Protocol 15:
RENAL COLIC (Fig. 20)

INDICATION:	*Evaluation of patients with known or uspected renal or ureteral calculi as a cause for acute flank pain*
SCANNER SETTINGS:	kV(p): 120–140 mA: 210–330
ORAL CONTRAST:	None
PHASE OF RESPIRATION:	Suspended inspiration or expiration
ROTATION TIME:	0.5–1.0 sec
ACQUISITION SLICE THICKNESS:	2.5 to 5.0 mm
PITCH:	0.75–1.5 (HQ = 3:1; HS = 6:1)
RECONSTRUCTION SLICE THICKNESS /INTERVAL FOR FILMING:	5.0 mm (2.0 mm in regions of concern with FOV targeted to suspicious regions)/5.0 mm

ANATOMIC COVERAGE:
    SUPERIOR EXTENT:
    INFERIOR EXTENT:
	
	Upper pole of kidneys
	Symphysis pubis

IV CONTRAST:	None
COMMENTS:	1. When calcifications are detected at the ureterovesical junction (UVJ), consider rescanning the pelvis in prone position to distinguish a mobile stone in the bladder from stones impacted at the UVJ. Another alternative is to scan patients routinely in the prone position.

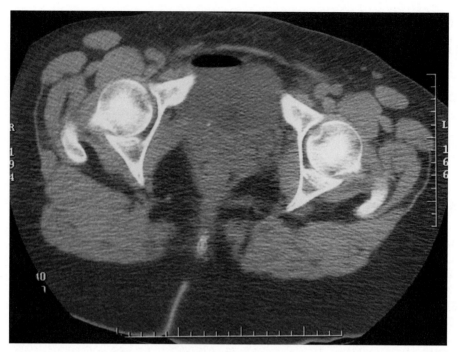

FIG. 20. Computed tomographic scan in a patient with right flank pain. Scan through the pelvis without either intravenous or oral contrast material reveals a 2-mm calcific focus at the level of the right ureterovesical junction. There is also evidence of gas in the urinary bladder from Foley catheter insertion.

Protocol 16:
ADRENAL GLANDS (Fig. 21)

INDICATION:	*Rule out adrenal hemorrhage, mass, or hyperplasia*
SCANNER SETTINGS:	kV(p): 120–140 mA: 250–330
ORAL CONTRAST:	Optional, preferred
PHASE OF RESPIRATION:	Suspended inspiration or expiration
ROTATION TIME:	0.5–1.0 sec
ACQUISITION SLICE THICKNESS:	2.5 mm
PITCH:	0.75 (HQ = 3:1)
RECONSTRUCTION SLICE THICKNESS/INTERVAL FOR FILMING:	2.5–5 mm/5 mm
ANATOMIC COVERAGE: **SUPERIOR EXTENT:**	Localizing scans are obtained to find the area just cephalad to the superior aspect of the adrenal glands
INFERIOR EXTENT:	Caudad to the inferior border of the adrenal glands

IV CONTRAST:	**Concentration:**	LOCM 300–320 mg iodine/mL or HOCM 282 mg iodine/mL (60% solution)
	Rate:	2–3 mL/sec
	Scan Delay:	60–70 sec
	Total Volume:	100–150 mL

COMMENTS:

1. To rule out pheochromocytoma, scans can usually be performed without contrast material at 1-cm intervals. If adrenal glands are normal, scanning through the aortic bifurcation, organs of Zuckerkandl, or even to the bladder should be performed to assess for extraadrenal pheochromocytoma (see Protocol 17).
2. Thinner section scans may be made in patients with MEA syndrome.

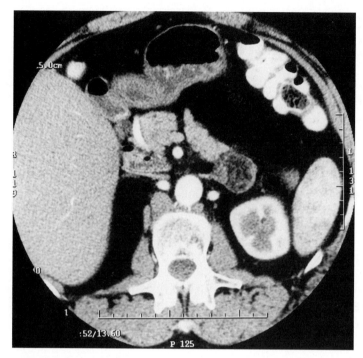

FIG. 21. Thin-section, small field-of-view image through the upper abdomen during the venous phase reveals a solid heterogenous mass in the left adrenal gland. Note that the mass has internal elements of near-fatty attenuation. This is consistent with a choristoma or myelolipoma.

Protocol 17:
ADRENAL GLANDS

INDICATION:	*Suspected pheochromocytoma*
SCANNER SETTINGS:	kV(p): 120 mA: 250–330
ORAL CONTRAST:	600–800 mL oral contrast media given 45 min before the study. An additional 200 mL given just before scanning.
PHASE OF RESPIRATION:	Suspended inspiration or expiration
ROTATION TIME:	0.5–1.0 sec
ACQUISITION SLICE THICKNESS:	2.5 to 5.0 mm
PITCH:	0.75–1.5 (HQ = 3:1; HS = 6:1)
RECONSTRUCTION SLICE THICKNESS/INTERVAL FOR FILMING:	2.5–5.0 mm/5.0 mm depending on the size of the mass
ANATOMIC COVERAGE:	
SUPERIOR EXTENT:	Just cephalad to the upper poles of kidneys or top of adrenal glands, depending on organs of interest
INFERIOR EXTENT:	Aortic bifurcation (may continue to symphysis pubis if biochemical documentation is present but no mass is seen as a small percentage of pheochromocytomas may involve the bladder)
IV CONTRAST:	Use at physician's discretion. Some adverse reactions have been reported.

COMMENTS:

1. IV contrast media may not be necessary for examination of the adrenal glands.
2. The risk of a hypertensive crisis in a patient with a pheochromocytoma after IV administration of iodinated contrast media is not well documented in the literature, but it appears to be extremely low. If the radiologist is using IV contrast media in a patient with biochemical evidence of a pheochromocytoma, he or she should have phentolamine (an α-adrenergic blocker) available in case of a hypertensive reaction.

5

Multislice Computed Tomography In Pediatrics

Sanjeev Bhalla* and Marilyn J. Siegel*

*Mallinckrodt Institute of Radiology, Washington University School of Medicine,
St. Louis, Missouri 63110

Over the past several years, single-slice helical computed tomography (HCT) has been demonstrated to have multiple benefits in pediatric patients (1–4), primarily because high-resolution images can be obtained with shorter examination times. The rapid acquisition times reduce motion artifacts, decrease the need for sedation (5), and enable scanning of a designated area during multiple phases of contrast enhancement. Furthermore, multiplanar reconstructions (MPRs) can be obtained, which can clarify anatomic relationships without increasing radiation exposure.

Multislice CT (MSCT) expands on the advantages of HCT (6–8), by allowing slices to be acquired thinner than the original reconstruction, which reduces partial volume artifacts, leading to a higher spatial resolution in the z-axis. MSCT scanners are up to eight times faster than HCT scanners, resulting in fewer motion artifacts, thereby improving temporal resolution. Moreover, the increase in speed improves contrast enhancement and further decreases the need for sedation.

This chapter addresses current techniques and presents guidelines for the performance of MSCT in pediatric patients. The contemporary applications of this technique and the CT appearances of various common disorders in children are also presented.

TECHNIQUE

Sedation

The increase in speed of MSCT scanners decreases the need for sedation (9), although it may not entirely eliminate it in some infants and young children. The use of sedation requires attention to strict standards of care. These are based on the recommendations of the Joint Commission on Accreditation of Health Care Organizations, the American Academy of Pediatrics (AAP) (10), and the American Society of Anesthesiologists Task Force (11). Aspiration is a major clinical concern in sedated children, and non per os (or "nothing by mouth") guidelines should be as stringent as those used for general anesthesia. Based on guidelines set by the AAP, clear liquids are allowed up to 2 hours before the procedure for patients of any age. Semisolid liquids (including breast milk) and solid foods are allowed up to 4 hours before the procedure for children younger than 6 months; up to 6 hours before the procedure for children age 6 to 36 months; and up to 8 hours before the procedure for older children.

The drugs most frequently used for sedation are oral chloral hydrate and intravenous (IV) pentobarbital sodium. Oral chloral hydrate (50 to 100 mg/kg, with a maximum dose of 2,000 mg) is the drug of choice for children younger than 18 months. IV pentobarbital sodium (6 mg/kg, with a maximum dose of 200 mg) is advocated in children older than 18 months. It is injected slowly in fractions of one-fourth the total dose and is titrated against the patient's response. This is an effective form of sedation, with a failure rate of less than 5%. Regardless of the method of sedation, the child must be closely monitored during and after the CT examination. Proper equipment and personnel trained in pediatric resuscitation and cardiorespiratory support must be present.

Intravenous Contrast Material

If IV contrast material is to be administered, it is helpful to have an IV line in place when the child arrives in the radiology department. This reduces patient agitation that otherwise would be associated with a venipuncture performed just before the administration of contrast material. The largest gauge butterfly needle or plastic cannula that can be placed is recommended.

Contrast may be administered by hand injection or a mechanical injector (12). Hand injections are used when IV access is via a small antecubital catheter (e.g., 24 gauge [G]), a butterfly needle or a central venous catheter (CVC) placed via a peripheral vein. Power injectors may be used when a 22-G or larger cannula can be placed in an antecubital vein. The contrast injection rate is determined by the caliber of the IV catheter (Table 1). A power injection also can be used to administer contrast media via a CVC if the rate of injection is slow (1 mL per second). The site of injection is closely monitored during the initial injection of contrast, to minimize the risk of contrast extravasation. The benefits of power injection are the uniformity and predictability of contrast delivery. This allows for optimal enhancement and the routine use of multiphase imaging of a targeted area (such as arterial, portal venous, and hepatic venous phase imaging of the liver).

Low osmolar (nonionic) contrast material (LOCM) (280 to 320 mg of iodine per milliliter of contrast) is used, usually at a dose of 2 mL/kg (not to exceed 4 mL/kg or 150 mL, whichever is lower). The advantages of low osmolar agents over high osmolar (ionic) agents are a decrease in gastrointestinal side effects, less discomfort at the site of injection, decreased patient motion during IV administration (13), and the decreased risks of cutaneous side effects if extravasation occurs (14).

Because of their varying body sizes, no one scan time will suffice for pediatric patients. The scan delay time will depend on the volume of contrast medium and the rate at which it is administered. In adult patients, the ideal delay time from the start of the injection to scanning is 50 to 70 seconds. In older children and adolescents, who inherently receive larger volumes of contrast medium, the initiation of scanning is often within this time range and usually coincides with the completion of the contrast injection or shortly thereafter. In infants and small children, who will inherently receive smaller volumes of contrast, the administration of contrast may be complete well before 50 seconds. In these patients, the time between the completion of injection and initiation of scanning will need to be delayed. The goal is to scan in

TABLE 5.1. *Rate of Contrast Injection Versus Needle Size*

Needle size (gauge)	Flow rate* (mL/sec)
22	1.5
20	2.0
18	3.0–5.0

*Maximum flow rate

the portal venous phase. The delay time from the completion of the injection to scanning should not exceed 20 seconds (15).

Alternatively, computer-automated scan technology (CAST), also referred to as bolus tracking methods, can be used to optimize contrast enhancement. This technology has proven particularly useful in optional imaging of the liver and in CT angiography (CTA). This method employs a series of low-dose axial images at a predetermined level that is representative of the scan volume. Once a designated threshold has been achieved (in Hounsfield units [HU]), the low-dose scanning terminates and the diagnostic examination begins at the desired range (16). A default delay can be programmed in case the desired threshold is not achieved. This method can be used with both hand and power injectors.

Imaging of the chest and neck begins sooner than a routine abdominal examination. For a mediastinal or hilar survey, scanning should begin 20 to 30 seconds after initiation of the IV contrast administration, regardless of whether hand or power injection is used. A shorter scan initiation time is needed for vascular protocols.

Depending on the clinical indication for the examination, an arterial phase image may add value to the CT examination. This is particularly true in the liver. This technique, also referred to as dual-phase imaging in reference to the imaging of the liver in both arterial and portal venous phases of enhancement, can increase the detection of hypervascular lesions, such as hemangioendotheliomas (17). Dual-phase imaging requires a short scan delay of 10 to 15 seconds. After an interscan delay of another 25 to 30 seconds, the same range is scanned again.

Bowel Contrast Medium

Opacification of the small and large bowel is necessary for most examinations of the abdomen because un-opacified bowel loops can simulate a mass or abnormal fluid collection. The exceptions are patients with depressed mental status who are at risk of aspiration and those with acute blunt abdominal trauma in whom there may be insufficient time for contrast administration. The agent most often used is a dilute mixture of iodinated contrast in water. Lemonade or other fruit flavors can be added to mask the metallic taste. The mixture can be either given orally or via a nasogastric tube.

To achieve optimal bowel opacification, the contrast is given 45 minutes to 1 hour before scanning. This initial volume should approximate an average feeding. The remaining contrast (about one half the additional volume) can be given about 15 minutes before scanning. If distal bowel opacification is inadequate, additional contrast can be given orally, and scanning can be repeated after a delay to allow the contrast medium to pass distally. The volumes of oral contrast material versus patient age are given in Table 2. Rectal contrast material may be administered if necessary to delineate pelvic pathology.

There may be a role for negative bowel contrast agents or those that lower the attenuation of the bowel lumen in the evaluation of intestinal or gastric mucosa (18,19). Tap water is an

TABLE 5.2. *Amount of Oral Contrast Material by Age*

Age	Initial volume (45 min before study)	Additional volume (15 min before study)
<1 mo	2–3 ounces (60–90 mL)	1–1.5 ounces (30–45 mL)
1 mo to 1 yr	4–8 ounces (120–240 mL)	2–4 ounces (60–120 mL)
1–5 yr	8–16 ounces (240–480 mL)	4–8 ounces (120–240 mL)
6–12 yr	16–24 ounces (480–720 mL)	8–12 ounces (240–360 mL)
≥13 yr	24–36 ounces (720–1080 mL)	12–18 ounces (360–540 mL)

excellent negative oral contrast agent. Its role in abdominal imaging continues to evolve, but currently, it is useful in evaluating suspected hypervascular masses in the ampullary or peri-portal region or common duct stones that may be masked by adjacent dense oral contrast. It is also valuable when three-dimensional (3D) imaging or maximum intensity projections (MIPs) are contemplated to reduce artifact from bowel.

TECHNICAL PARAMETERS

MSCT requires the selection of a number of variable parameters (Fig. 1), including detec-tor row thickness, table speed per rotation, slice-reconstruction thickness, and exposure fac-tors (kilovoltage, milliamperes). In MSCT, multiple detector rows are used (as opposed to 1 detector in HCT). The collimation of each detector row or array can be set at 1.25 to 5.0 mm for equal-width detectors and 1.0 to 5.0 mm for unequal-width detector design arrays (6). The collimation determines the nominal or effective section thickness, which can be changed after the patient has left the department, provided that the raw data have been saved.

Pitch, which is defined as the table speed (in millimeters per gantry rotation ÷ individual detector row collimation), is another factor that must be determined before the initiation of scanning. (It should be noted that some authors have defined pitch as table speed (in millime-ters) per gantry rotation ÷ individual detector row collimation × number of detector rows, to allow MSCT pitch values to be comparable to their single-slice counterparts [7].) In conven-tional HCT, pitch can vary between 1 and 2 (as long as a 180-interpolation algorithm is used). In multisection CT, various pitches can be selected. The pitch can vary depending on the ven-dor. Some vendors have a fixed binary pitch (either 3 or 6) (8), whereas other vendors allow for more variability in pitch using a sliding scale (7).

Image reconstruction can be performed at an interval that is equal to or less than that of the nominal section thickness. Thus, a chest CT may be reconstructed as a standard examination and then as a high-resolution examination without rescanning the patient or needing additional radiation. For example, if the chest is scanned with the 4- by 5-mm detector configuration

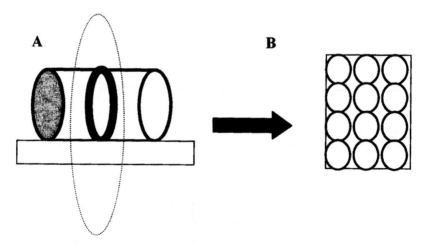

FIG. 1. Schematic of multislice computed tomography terms. The cylinder is representative of the body to be scanned. **A:** The collimation of each detector array (*dark circle*) and the pitch (table speed per rotation/collimation) are entered before scanning. Reconstructions are se-lected once the patient has been scanned. **B:** The collimation determines the nominal or ef-fective slice thickness of each image (*circles*).

(four slices per gantry rotation, each 5 mm thick) and a pitch of 0.75, the minimum slice thickness is 5 mm. If the chest is scanned with the 4- by 2.5-mm detector configuration and a pitch of 1.5, the slices can be reconstructed at 2.5, 3.75, or 5 mm, in the same time as 4 by 5 mm, pitch 0.75. This feature is of great importance in characterizing small lesions in the chest or abdomen in small patients and in acquiring MPRs or 3D images.

In general, the selection of slice thickness and pitch should be individualized on the basis of the area to be covered, contrast resolution of the structures to be imaged, size of the abnormality, and the potential radiation dose. When evaluating the chest or abdomen for gross pathologic processes, such as blood or bulky tumor, thicker slices and larger pitches are used to decrease the acquisition time and the radiation dose. When evaluating small focal lesions, thin slices and smaller pitches are advantageous. A thin slice and a pitch of 1.0 or 1.5 should be used when spatial resolution is very important and the temporal resolution is less important (non-breath-hold or nonangiographic imaging). A thicker slice and a pitch closer to 2 should be used when the temporal resolution is paramount, such as multiphase imaging or CTA (Fig. 1).

Chest and abdominal imaging in older children (older than 5 years) and adolescents should be performed during a single breath-hold. When suspended respiration is not possible, scanning is performed during shallow breathing.

RADIATION DOSE IN PEDIATRIC MULTISLICE COMPUTED TOMOGRAPHY

An important consequence of multislice imaging is the potential for a substantial increase in radiation exposure to the pediatric population (20,21). MSCT actually has increased radiation dose compared with HCT as a function of more widely open collimators. This relative increase is reduced at faster table speeds.

The tube currents listed in Table 3 are recommended for routine chest and abdomen examinations; these are based on patient weight.

Another technique that is useful in reducing radiation dose is to decrease the kilovolts from 120 to 80 kV. This increases contrast resolution, although there may be a reduction in signal-to-noise ratio.

CLINICAL APPLICATIONS

Neck

The main applications of neck CT in children are the differentiation of lymphadenitis from abscess and the evaluation of tumor extent. Typical slice thickness ranges between 3 and 5 mm. (Fig. 2).

TABLE 5.3. *Suggested Tube Current (mA) by Weight and Type of Examination*

Weight (kg)	mA (chest)	mA (abdomen/pelvis)
<10	30	40
10–25	40	60
26–50	65	80
51–70	80	100
>70	>120	>140

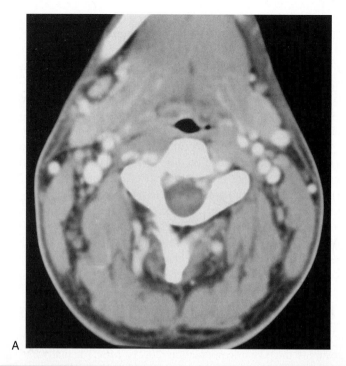

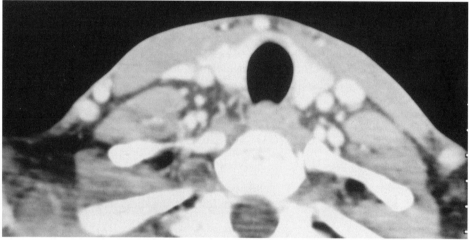

FIG. 2. Contrast-enhanced neck examination. **A, B:** Two computed tomographic (CT) scans from a normal neck examination in a 15-year-old boy. This study was performed simultaneously with chest, abdomen, and pelvis examinations using one injection. Note the uniform enhancement of the neck vessels (scan parameters: thickness, 5 mm; pitch, 0.75; reconstruction slice thickness/interval for filming, 5 mm). **C, D:** Two CT scans in an 11-year-old girl with cat-scratch disease show multiple, low-attenuation lymph nodes (*arrows*). There is no evidence of abscess. (Scan parameters: thickness, 2.5 mm; pitch, 0.75; reconstruction slice thickness/interval for filming, 3 mm.)

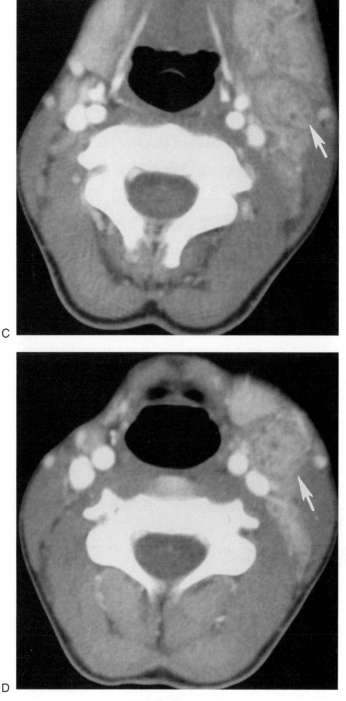

FIG. 2. *Continued.*

Chest

The major applications for helical chest CT include (a) thoracic survey for evaluation of metastatic disease (i.e., pulmonary nodules) in a patient with a known malignancy; (b) characterization of a focal parenchymal mass suspected or detected on chest radiography; (c) characterization of a hilar/mediastinal mass suspected or detected on chest radiography; (d) evaluation of vascular and cardiac anomalies; (e) assessment of congenital or acquired abnormalities of the tracheobronchial tree; and (f) evaluation of lung disease.

Thoracic Survey

HCT has become the established method for the detection and characterization of pulmonary nodules in children with known malignancies that have a high propensity for pulmonary dissemination. The presence of a nodule often changes the treatment plan and may lead to surgery or additional chemotherapy or radiation therapy. HCT is highly sensitive for the detection of pulmonary nodules (22–24), particularly if images can be obtained in one breath-hold. The improved temporal and spatial resolution afforded by multisection CT enhances both the detection and the characterization of pulmonary nodules. Most importantly, the use of thin collimation allows routine retrospective reconstructions without the need to rescan and deliver an additional radiation dose. This allows easy identification of calcification and provides the potential to acquire 3D images through the nodules (Fig. 3).

Thoracic studies obtained to exclude pulmonary nodules are performed with a slice thickness of 2.5 and a pitch of 0.75 (high quality [HQ] = 3:1). Original reconstructions are usually

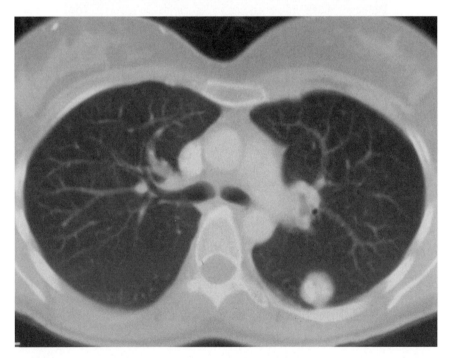

FIG. 3. Pulmonary nodule due to osteosarcoma. Computed tomographic scan shown at lung window setting shows a well-circumscribed nodule containing calcification in the left lower lobe. (Scan parameters: thickness, 2.5 mm; pitch, 0.75; reconstruction slice thickness/interval for filming, 5 mm.)

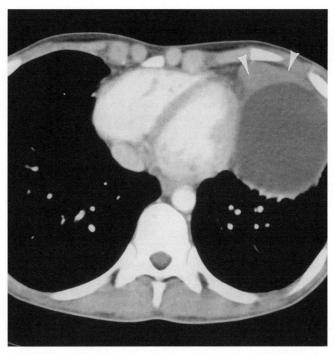

FIG. 4. Focal mass in a 15-year-old girl. Thin-section computed tomographic scans show a low-attenuation mass with a soft tissue rind (*arrowheads*). The appearance mimics that of a cyst, but the attenuation values are equal to those of soft tissue (30 HU). The lesion abuts the chest walls but does not invade it. Final diagnosis was Hodgkin's disease. (Scan parameters: thickness, 2.5 mm; pitch, 0.75; reconstruction slice thickness/interval for filming, 5 mm.)

performed using 5-mm effective slice thickness. If a potential nodule is seen, retrospective reconstructions can be performed using an effective slice thickness as low as the collimation of a single detector (2.5 mm in this case), provided that the raw data are still available. Retrospective reconstructions are advantageous in reducing radiation exposure and allowing the questioned area to be reevaluated confidently, avoiding respiratory misregistration.

Mediastinal/Hilar Survey

An important indication for CT is the evaluation of the character and extent of a mediastinal or hilar mass or mediastinal widening suspected or clearly identified on chest radiography. CT can facilitate identification of mediastinal infiltration, vascular encasement, and hilar lymph nodes (Fig. 5, pg. 240), due to its capability of enabling consistent vascular enhancement and contiguous thin-section reconstructions. These advantages are particularly valuable in the detection of small nodal masses and the identification of calcification. The resultant information can alter the diagnosis, increase the accuracy of tumor staging, and facilitate surgical planning or radiation. MPRs can be used to show encasement or displacement of adjacent vessels or other anatomic structures, which provides valuable information for the surgeon.

Mass Characterization

The volumetric CT images can be useful to characterize complex masses (Fig. 4) and determine their extent. Most focal masses in children are of congenital origin and usually either

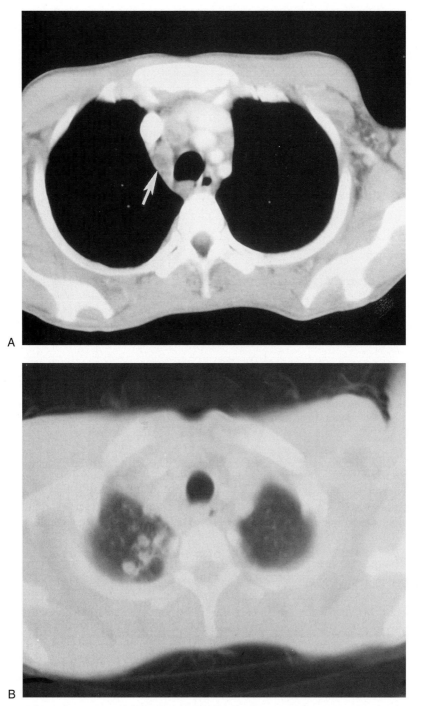

FIG. 5. Adenopathy in an 18-year-old girl with mediastinal enlargement on chest radiography. **A:** Computed tomographic (CT) scan at the level of the great vessels demonstrates paratracheal (*arrow*) lymph node enlargement. **B:** CT scan at a similar level with lung windows shows several small nodular densities in the right upper lobe. Final diagnosis was *Mycobacterium avium-intracellulare* infection. (Scan parameters: thickness, 2.5 mm; pitch, 0.75; reconstruction slice thickness/interval for filming, 5 mm.)

a pulmonary sequestration or a cystic adenomatoid malformation. The most important information derived from CT is the presence of feeding and draining vessels, which allows a diagnosis of sequestration to be established. Even if there are no abnormal vessels, knowledge of lesion extent is important for planning surgery or medical treatment.

Typically, images are acquired with a thin collimation (1.0 or 1.25 mm) and then reconstructed at thin intervals. A targeted field of view is used to increase x–y resolution and allow for maximal mass characterization.

Vascular Imaging

Indications for CTA include evaluation of (a) congenital anomalies of the aorta, great vessels, pulmonary arteries, and superior vena cava, (b) congenital intracardiac or extracardiac shunt lesions, and (c) postoperative vascular shunts (Figs. 6 through 8). The ability to acquire data with improved contrast enhancement increases the conspicuity of arteries, veins, and pathologic conditions. Scanning with thin sections allows the production of high-quality MPRs and detailed 3D images, which are valuable for showing the characteristic diagnostic features of vascular anomalies.

In blunt thoracic trauma, CT has become the method of choice for evaluation of mediastinal widening on chest radiography. The use of MSCT allows excellent vascular enhancement of mediastinal vessels. Improved vascular enhancement allows clearer definition of indirect signs of aortic injury (periaortic hematoma) and direct signs (acute coarctation, flap, pseudoaneurysm) (25). Although not a frequent indication in children, detection of pulmonary embolism can be done with CT scanning. The faster scan times of multisection CT allow the

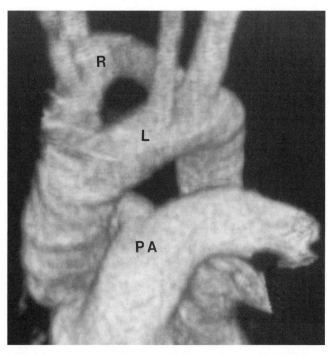

FIG. 6. Mediastinal vascular anomaly. Surface-shaded volumetric reconstruction shows a double aortic arch. (R, right arch; L, left arch; PA, main pulmonary artery.) (Scan parameters: thickness, 3 mm; pitch, 0.75; reconstruction slice thickness/interval for filming, 3 mm.)

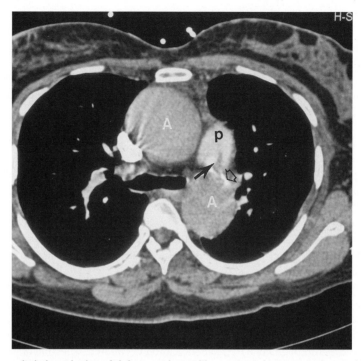

FIG. 7. Congenital shunt lesion. Adolescent boy with a patent ductus arteriosus. Note the flow of un-opacified blood (*arrow*) from the aorta into the pulmonary artery *(p)*. Calcifications of the ductus (*open arrow*) can be seen adjacent to the jet. The aorta *(A)* is enlarged due to the shunting of blood from the pulmonary artery. (Scan parameters: thickness, 3 mm; pitch, 1.5; reconstruction slice thickness/interval for filming, 3 mm.)

study to be completed in a single breath-hold with decreased motion artifact, allowing for improved MPRs. Coronal reconstructions and MIPs can be very helpful in distinguishing potential emboli from adjacent hilar lymphadenopathy.

Tracheobronchial Tree

Because of the ease and quality of MPRs, helical CT is ideal for imaging the tracheobronchial tree (Fig. 9). Indications for a dedicated tracheobronchial CT include evaluation of congenital anomalies, detection of complications after surgery or lung transplantation, and evaluation of abnormal pulmonary function tests. Axial images are useful for lesion identification, and coronal and sagittal MPRs and 3D images ("virtual bronchoscopy") can aid in lesion localization before bronchoscopy or surgery (26,27). Whenever possible, images should be obtained in suspended respiration to minimize misregistration artifacts that will corrupt reconstructions. Increasing pitch often allows the scans to be acquired in one breath-hold. The gain in using a 1.0- to 1.25-mm collimation is negated if the examination needs two breath-holds.

Although endobronchial tumors are uncommon in children, when they are present, CT offers a noninvasive method of assessing their local extent and invasion. Exact delineation of tumor size and length is important when surgical resection is planned. Coronal and/or parasagittal reconstructions are particularly important in demonstrating tumor extent. Multisection CT,

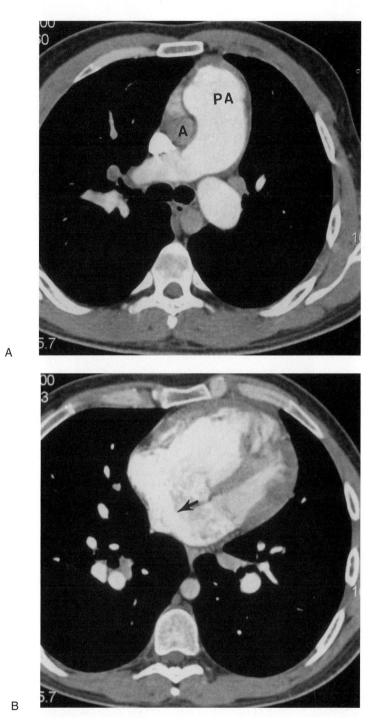

FIG. 8. Atrioseptal defect (ostium secundum). **A:** Axial image shows the large pulmonary artery *(PA)* and un-opacified aorta. **B:** More caudad scan shows un-opacified blood *(arrow)* flowing from the left to the right atrium. (Scan parameters: thickness, 3 mm; pitch, 0.75; reconstruction slice thickness/interval for filming, 3 mm.)

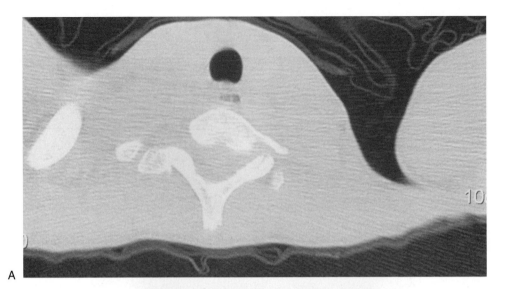

A

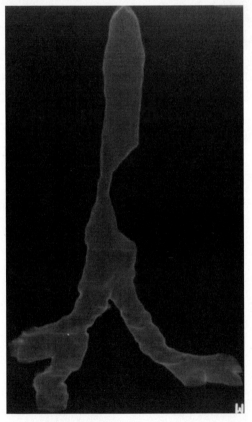

B

FIG. 9. Airway assessment. A 10-year-old boy with dyspnea and stridor on physical exertion. **A:** Inspiration axial image above the thoracic inlet shows a normal trachea. Expiration scan (not shown) was also normal. An area of narrowing was seen on more caudal scans and was further evaluated using volume-rendered techniques. **B:** Edge-enhanced reconstruction in a coronal plane (simulating a bronchogram) clearly shows the area of narrowing. **C:** Surface-rendered image demonstrates an area of soft tissue (*arrow*) along the left tracheal wall, found to represent granulation tissue at surgery. Patient had a remote history of intubation as an infant. (Scan parameters: thickness, 1.25 mm; pitch, 1.5; reconstruction slice thickness/interval for filming, 2.5 mm.)

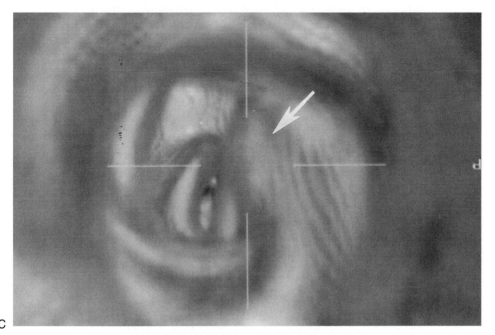

C

FIG. 9. *Continued.*

particularly with its multiplanar capabilities, also may be useful for evaluating the central air-ways for foreign body aspiration. The foreign body can be precisely localized with CT before bronchoscopic removal.

The general coverage for the tracheobronchial tree includes larynx to the main-stem bronchi.

Dynamic high-resolution scans have become important in identifying areas of air trapping associated with small airways disease, such as bronchiolitis obliterans (28–31), or cystic lung disease associated with Langerhans cell histiocytosis and tuberous sclerosis. When CT is used as a screening examination to detect small airways disease, thin sections (1 to 2 mm thickness) are acquired at representative levels (thoracic inlet, aortic arch, carina, and lung bases) during deep inspiration and forced expiration. Lung attenuation is then subjectively or objectively as-sessed in selected areas. In the normal lung, attenuation increases homogeneously during ex-halation. Air trapping is seen as a paradoxical decrease in lung attenuation during expiration.

Interstitial Lung Disease

The indications for CT in the evaluation of interstitial lung disease include (a) detection of subtle lung disease not detected by conventional radiography; (b) characterization of radio-graphically apparent lung disease before transplantation; and (c) detection of complications related to end-stage lung disease. The fast scan times of MSCT allow for the entire chest to be scanned in one breath-hold, decreasing motion-related artifacts (Fig. 10). Some vendors have a combination mode that allows the same raw data to be processed as both a conventional tho-racic–pulmonary survey and a high-resolution thin-section CT. This avoids the added scan times and radiation dose required by a second scan. Occasionally, subtle lung findings can be more apparent on MIPs (Fig. 11).

246

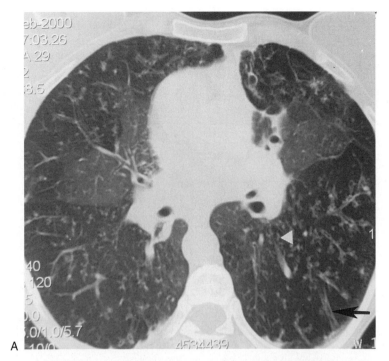

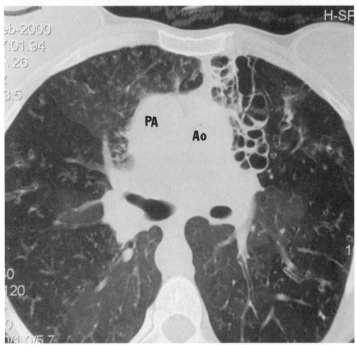

FIG. 10. Interstitial lung disease in an adolescent girl with a history of sinusitis and immotile cilia. **A:** Lung windows show areas of abnormally low-attenuation lung posteriorly, shown to be due to air trapping on expiratory scans. Note the "tree-in-bud" pattern of bronchiolectasis (*white arrowhead*) and bronchiectasis (*black arrow*). **B:** Cystic bronchiectasis is seen adjacent to the left mediastinal border. Both images show the main pulmonary artery *(PA)* anterior and to the right of the aorta *(AO)*. **C:** Image through the upper abdomen shows situs inversus with the liver on the left and the spleen on the right. Given the situs inversus, this patient was diagnosed with Kartagener syndrome. (Scan parameters: thickness, 1 mm; pitch, 1.5; reconstruction slice thickness/interval for filming, 5 mm.)

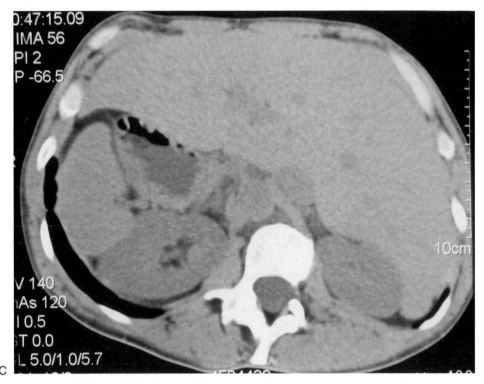

FIG. 10. *Continued.*

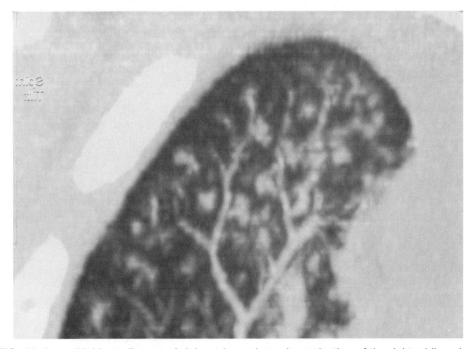

FIG. 11. Interstitial lung disease. Axial maximum intensity projection of the right midlung in a patient with a lung allograft demonstrating bronchiolectasis ("tree in bud"). In this patient, the bronchiolectasis was secondary to *Mycobacterium avium-intracellulare.* (Scan parameters: thickness, 1.25 mm; pitch, 1.5; reconstruction slice thickness/interval for filming, 5 mm.)

Abdomen/Pelvis

The frequent indications for CT of the abdomen and pelvis in children are as follows: (a) evaluation of the character and extent of neoplastic and inflammatory processes of the kidneys, adrenal glands, liver, pancreas, and presacral space; (b) detection of abscess; (c) evaluation of the extent of abdominal trauma; and (d) evaluation of causes of acute abdominal pain, such as appendicitis and ureteral calculi. Less often, CT is used to evaluate vascular abnormalities of solid organs or the great vessels.

Kidney And Adrenal Glands

The most common indications for CT of the pediatric retroperitoneum are suspected tumors of the kidneys or adrenal glands. Wilms' tumor is the most common primary renal neoplasm in children. Typically, it is quite large, and the goal of imaging is not detection, but staging and operative planning (Fig. 12). The rapid scanning afforded by multisection CT improves vascular enhancement, which can improve the conspicuity of vascular pathology. For renal tumors, the most important information derived from CT is the presence of renal vein, caval, or right atrial tumor extension. Even when vessels are not invaded, knowledge of displacement or effacement is important for surgical planning. Valuable information about the presence or absence of small contralateral lesions and tumor thrombus can be obtained by scanning the kidney during both arterial and nephrogenic phases of enhancement. MPRs may be useful to display the full longitudinal extent of the mass or the tumor thrombus.

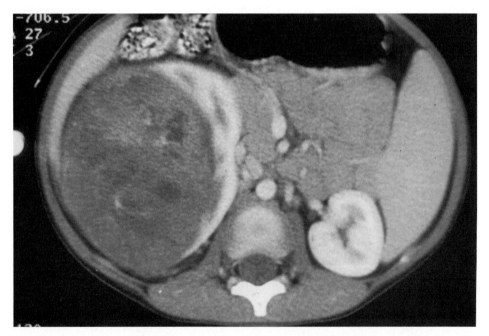

FIG. 12. Renal mass. Wilms tumor in a 5-year-old boy. Axial computed tomography shows a large mass with areas of central necrosis arising within the right kidney. A rim of normal enhancing parenchyma surrounds the tumor. The soft tissue density in the left abdomen represents un-opacified bowel loops. (Scan parameters: thickness, 2.5 mm; pitch, 0.75; reconstruction slice thickness/interval for filming, 3 mm.)

Inflammatory disease, particularly pyelonephritis, and renovascular disease, such as renal artery stenosis, are less common indications for multisection CT in children.

Neuroblastoma is the most common extrarenal retroperitoneal neoplasm in children (Fig. 13). Approximately two thirds of retroperitoneal neuroblastoma arise from the adrenal glands. Less common retroperitoneal lesions include adrenal carcinomas, pheochromocytomas (Fig. 14), and retroperitoneal sarcomas or germ cell tumors. In neuroblastoma, the most important information for treatment planning is the presence of midline extension of tumor, vessel encasement, contralateral lymph nodes, and hepatic metastases. MPRs may help in determining the effect of the tumor on adjacent organs or vessels (Fig. 13).

Liver

Approximately two thirds of hepatic neoplasms in children are malignant and usually hepatoblastomas. The remainder are benign and most often hemangioendotheliomas. Because the liver has blood supply from the hepatic artery and the portal vein, there are several phases of enhancement that occur after the IV administration of contrast material. These include the hepatic arterial, the portal venous, and the equilibrium phases. Scanning during the arterial and portal venous phases can be particularly helpful in characterizing vascular hepatic neoplasms. The arterial phase is usually initiated 10 to 15 seconds after the start of the contrast injection.

The principal contribution of helical CT in imaging hepatic malignancy is the determination of the intrahepatic extent of tumor (segmental or multisegmental involvement) and vascular invasion. MPRs and 3D displays of the data set can be useful in precisely localizing and defining the extent of tumor for surgical planning. A less common application of multisection hepatic CT is the assessment of acquired vascular abnormalities, such as portal or hepatic venous thrombosis.

Pancreas

Most pancreatic diseases in children are inflammatory. Pancreatic tumors in children are extremely rare. CT is most often used to evaluate the extent of pancreatitis and the presence of complications, such as pseudocyst formation, pseudoaneurysm, or abscess. The use of multisection CT allows excellent vascular enhancement, which improves definition of peripancreatic tissue planes, particularly given the paucity of fat in children, as well as vascular abnormalities.

Pelvis

Ultrasonography is the initial study of choice for evaluating suspected pelvic lesions. However, CT is used as an adjunctive study for determining the extent of tumors arising in the reproductive organs (e.g., ovary, uterus, and prostate); bladder; and lymph nodes. Magnetic resonance imaging (MRI) is the preferred adjunctive study for assessing the character and extent of presacral tumors and congenital anomalies of the female genital tract. Axial CT facilitates identification of tumor margins and pelvic infiltration, vessel encasement, and lymph node enlargement by tumor as a result of its capability to allow high levels of vascular enhancement. MPRs also can provide additional information about the relationship between large tumors and adjacent structures (Fig. 15).

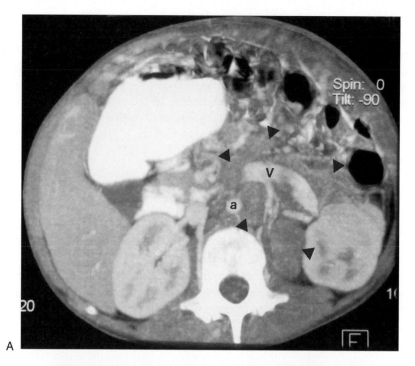

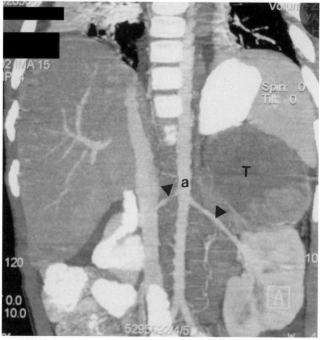

FIG. 13. Adrenal neoplasm. Neuroblastoma. **A:** Contrast-enhanced axial computed tomographic scan in a 2-year-old girl shows a left retroperitoneal mass (*arrows*) extending across the midline in the retroperitoneum and encasing the aorta *(a)* and left renal vein *(V)*. **B:** Coronal reconstruction demonstrates the tumor *(T)* arising in the left adrenal gland and extending inferiorly and across the midline. The tumor encases the aorta *(a)* and surrounds both renal arteries (*arrowheads*). (Scan parameters: thickness, 2.5 mm; pitch, 0.75; reconstruction slice thickness/interval for filming, 2.5 mm.)

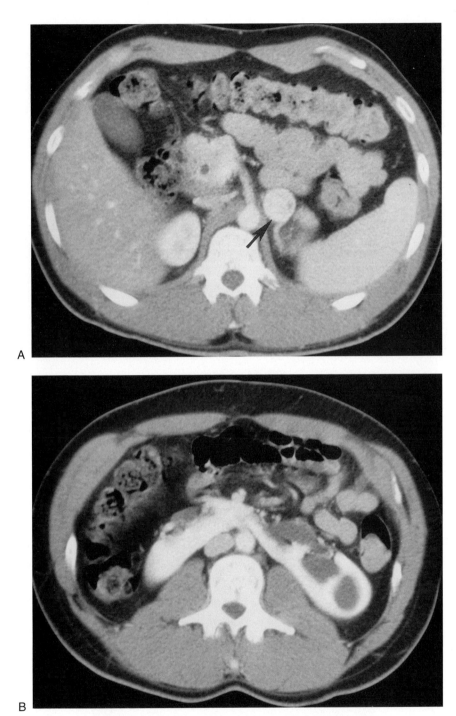

FIG. 14. Adrenal neoplasm. A 10-year-old boy with a history of hypertension. **A:** Axial image shows a hyperenhancing mass in the left adrenal gland (*arrow*) found to be pheochromocytoma at surgery. **B:** Caudally, a horseshoe kidney was incidentally discovered. **C:** Volume-rendered coronal reconstruction shows the single renal arteries to each moiety (*arrows*) and the left pheochromocytoma (*arrowhead*). The inferior paired arteries (*open arrows*) represent lumbar arteries. (Scan parameters: thickness, 2.5 mm; pitch, 0.75; reconstruction slice thickness/interval for filming, 2.5 mm.)

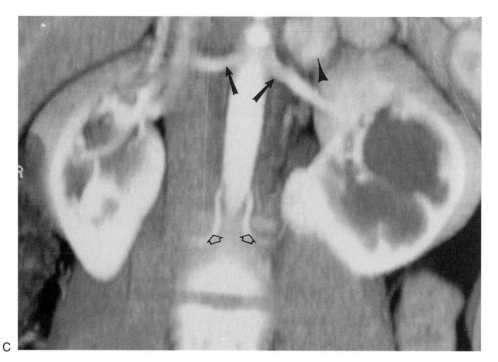

FIG. 14. *Continued.*

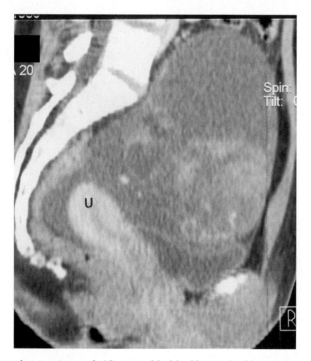

FIG. 15. Cystic ovarian teratoma. A 13-year-old girl with a palpable pelvic mass. Sagittal multiplanar reconstruction shows a large, predominantly low-density (near water attenuation) mass with scattered areas of soft tissue and calcifications anterior and superior to the uterus *(U)*. The extent of the mass and its relationships to adjacent structures are easily seen on the sagittal reconstruction. (Scan parameters: thickness, 2.5 mm; pitch, 0.75; reconstruction slice thickness/interval for filming, 3 mm.)

Abdominal Abscess

CT is the method of choice for the evaluation of an abdominal and/or pelvic abscess suspected on clinical or other imaging examinations. Abdominal and pelvic abscesses in children are usually a complication of perforated appendicitis or inflammatory bowel disease, or they may be a postoperative complication. The ability of multisection CT to provide high-quality MPRs and thinner images can increase confidence that a fluid-filled structure is an abscess and not a loop of bowel.

Abdominal Trauma

CT is the screening tool of choice for the evaluation of blunt abdominal trauma (Fig. 16). The rapid acquisition allows for one bolus to be used for both the chest and the abdomen and/or pelvis. Imaging during peak enhancement improves sensitivity for small visceral injuries. Thinner collimation reconstructions may improve confidence in the detection of a small amount of fluid (versus volume averaging) and reduce the number of motion artifacts simulating free fluid.

Acute Abdominal Pain

Multisection CT is increasingly being used for the evaluation of appendicitis in children (Fig. 17). Various techniques have been advocated in the performance of appendiceal CT.

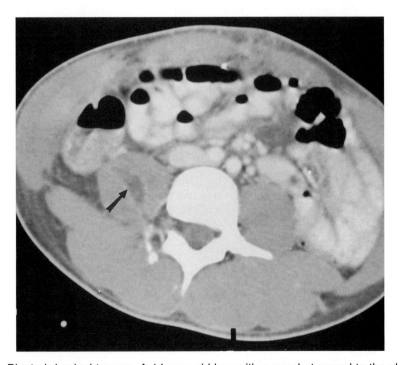

FIG. 16. Blunt abdominal trauma. A 14-year-old boy with a gunshot wound to the abdomen. Axial image shows the bullet tract through the right psoas (*arrow*) and the fracture of the transverse process of L3. (Scan parameters: thickness, 2.5 mm; pitch, 1.5; reconstruction slice thickness/interval for filming, 5 mm.)

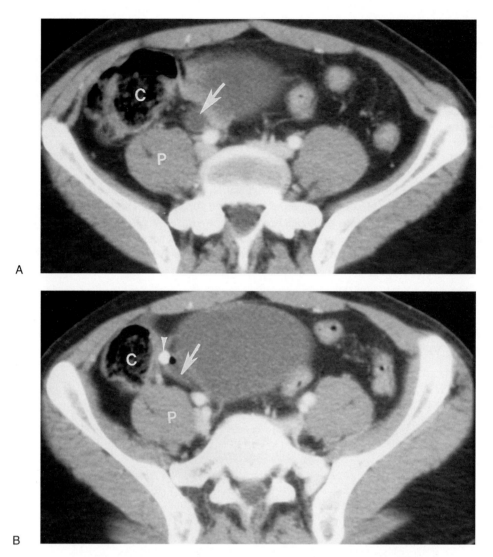

FIG. 17. Acute appendicitis. **A, B:** Two axial computed tomographic images through the pelvis show a fluid-filled appendix (*arrows*) anterior to the psoas *(P)* muscle and adjacent to the cecum *(C).* The increased focus of attenuation represents an appendicolith (*arrowhead*). (Scan parameters: thickness, 2.5 mm; pitch, 0.75; reconstruction slice thickness, 3 mm.)

These include (a) full abdominopelvic scanning after IV and oral contrast administration, (b) imaging limited to the lower abdomen and pelvis without any contrast material (32), (c) imaging limited to the lower abdomen and pelvis with the use of oral and rectal contrast material, and (d) imaging of the lower abdomen and pelvis with the use of only rectal contrast material (33).

The use of helical CT to detect acutely obstructing renal or ureteral calculi producing renal colic is also increasing. The ability to acquire multiple thin sections improves the detection of small stones not recognized on abdominal radiography.

Pitfalls

The increasing speed of MSCT can lead to a number of potential pitfalls in diagnosis (34,35). In the spleen, early sinusoidal enhancement produces a heterogeneous appearance that may be misinterpreted as splenic pathology. In the kidney, the renal cortex enhances before the medulla, which can make the diagnosis of medullary and collecting system lesions, such as obstruction, small tumors, and traumatic disruption, difficult. Flow artifacts caused by mixing of contrast material and un-opacified blood, usually at the junction of the inferior vena cava with the renal veins, may mimic thrombus formation. In the liver, the hepatic veins may not enhance and may conceivably be misinterpreted as low-attenuation lesions. Finally, in the pelvis, early scanning can result in poor bladder opacification, which can preclude a diagnosis of laceration or disruption. Obtaining delayed images can help minimize most of these potential problems.

Musculoskeletal System

CT is a useful adjunct to conventional radiography and skeletal scintigraphy, which remain the conventional imaging studies for evaluating suspected skeletal abnormalities in children. The advantages of MSCT in bone and joint imaging are related to the speed of acquisition and the ability to acquire MPRs (36). Given the ability of MRI to image the soft tissues and bone marrow, CT is usually reserved to clarify complex osseous anatomy, define the full extent of fractures, and determine the origin and location of a nidus in osteoid osteoma. The nominal slice thickness, pitch, and reconstruction intervals depend on the length of the bone or joint to be imaged. Narrower parameters are used for growth-plate injuries and small lesions, particularly in the wrist, ankle, and foot. For the pelvis, hips, and spine, wider parameters may be used. The volumetric imaging of MSCT allows for excellent reconstructions. Developmental hip dysplasia is a common indication for musculoskeletal CT in children. In neonates, sonography is the first imaging test used. Post–closed reduction and CAST immobilization CT play an important role in assessing the amount of acetabular coverage and the morphology of the femoral head, even when the femoral head is unossified (Fig. 18).

Tarsal coalition is a common cause of rigid flatfoot and perineal spasm in pediatrics. Calcaneonavicular coalitions are best seen on a plane paralleling that of the long axis of the foot, and talocalcaneal coalitions are best visualized on scans perpendicular to the long axis of the foot (Fig. 19). Imaging both feet is essential because many coalitions are bilateral (as much as 50%). Fibrous and cartilaginous coalitions may be more easily detected when a comparison foot is available. Multisection CT further increases the ability of CT to define and characterize fractures (Fig. 20). Multiplanar images can allow a fracture to be visualized in any plane and can improve visualization of the relationship of the fracture to the articular surfaces and physeal plates.

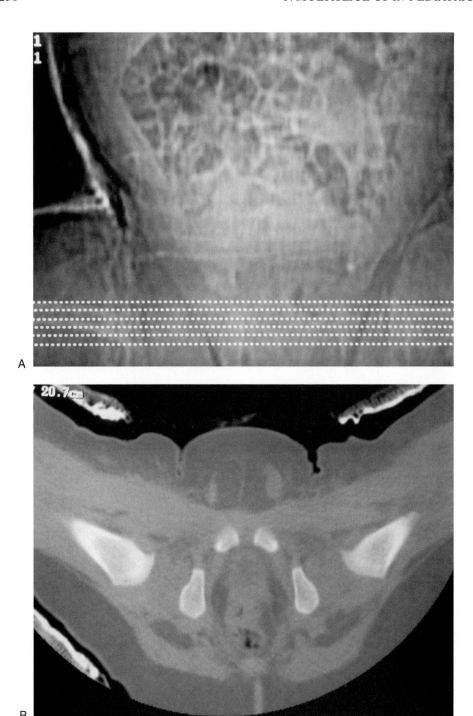

FIG. 18. Developmental hip dysplasia in a 4-month-old boy. Computed tomographic scan performed to evaluate acetabular coverage after closed hip reduction. **A:** Scout image shows the levels of the scan. **B:** Axial image shows the femoral metaphyses directed toward the acetabulum. The femoral heads are unossified. (Scan parameters: thickness, 2.5 mm; pitch, 0.75; reconstruction slice thickness/interval for filming, 3 mm.)

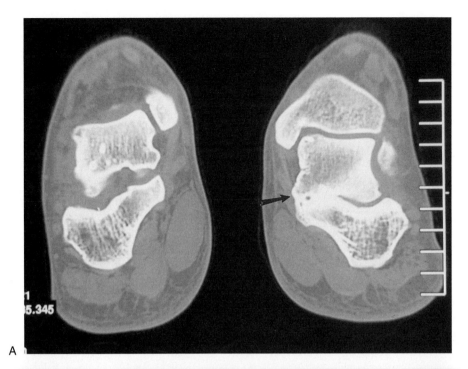

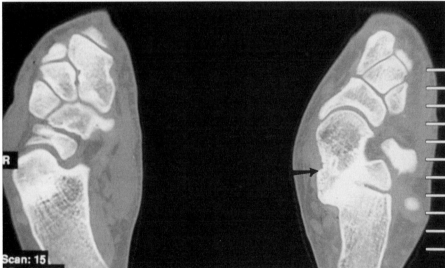

FIG. 19. Talocalcaneal tarsal coalition. **A:** Because a talocalcaneal coalition was suspected, images were obtained supine with knees bent, so that the acquisition would be perpendicular to the long axis of the foot (better delineating the talocalcaneal joint). **B:** Reconstructions were then made parallel to the long axis of the foot. (Coalition is indicated by an arrow.) (Scan parameters: thickness, 1 mm; pitch, 0.75; reconstruction slice thickness/interval for filming, 2 mm.)

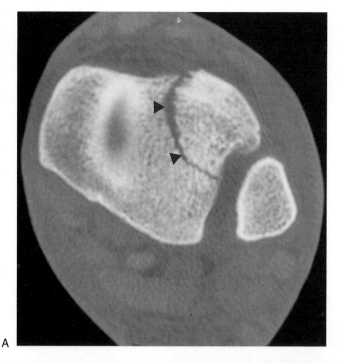

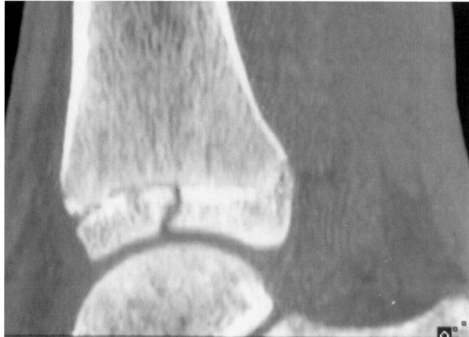

FIG. 20. Complex fractures. **A:** Direct axial images in computer-automated scan technology show a distracted tibial fracture (*arrowheads*). **B:** Sagittal and **(C)** coronal reconstructions confirm the triplanar configuration of this fracture. (Scan parameters: thickness, 1 mm; pitch, 0.75; reconstruction slice thickness/interval for filming, 2 mm.)

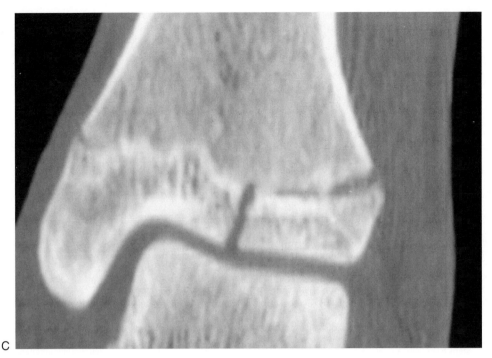

C

FIG. 20. *Continued.*

REFERENCES

1. Siegel MJ. Techniques. In: Siegel MJ, ed. Pediatr Body CT. Philadelphia: Lippincott Williams & Wilkins, 1999.
2. Siegel MJ, Luker GD. Pediatric applications of helical (spiral) CT. Radiol Clin North Am 1995;33:997–1022.
3. White KS. Invited article: helical/spiral CT scanning: a pediatric radiology perspective. Pediatr Radiol 1996;26:5–14.
4. Frush DP, Siegel MJ, Bisset GS. From the RSNA refresher courses: challenges of pediatric spiral CT. Radio-Graphics 1997;17:939–959.
5. Kaste SC, Young CW, Holmes TP, et al. Effect of helical CT on the frequency of sedation in pediatric patients. AJR Am J Roentgenol 1997;168:1001–1003.
6. Hu H, He HD, Foley WD, et al. Four multidetector-row helical CT: image quality and volume coverage speed. Radiology 2000;215:55–62.
7. Rydberg J, Buckwalter KA, Caldemeyer KS, et al. Multisection CT: scanning techniques and clinical applications. RadioGraphics 2000;20:1787–1806.
8. Klingenbeck-Regn K, Schaller S, Flohr T, et al. Subsecond multislice computed tomography: basics and applications. Eur J Radiol 1999;31:110–124.
9. Pappas JN, Donnelly LF, Frush DP. Reduced frequency of sedation of young children using new multislice helical CT [Abstract]. Radiology 1999;213:418.
10. American Academy of Pediatrics, Committee on Drugs. Guidelines for monitoring and management of pediatric patients during and after sedation for diagnostic and therapeutic procedures. Pediatrics 1992;89:1110–1115.
11. American Society of Anesthesiologists Task Force. Practice guidelines for sedation and analgesia by non-anesthesiologist: a report by the American Society of Anesthesiologists Task Force on sedation and analgesia by non-anesthesiologists. Anesthesiology 1996;84:459–471.
12. Kaste SC, Young CW. Safe use of power injectors with central and peripheral venous access devices for pediatric CT. Pediatr Radiol 1995;26:499–501.
13. Stockberger SM, Hickling JA, Liang Y, et al. Spiral CT with ionic and nonionic contrast material: evaluation of patient motion and scan quality. Radiology 1998;206:631–636.
14. Cohan RH, Ellis JH, Garner WL. Extravasation of radiographic contrast material: recognition, prevention and treatment. Radiology 1996;200:593–604.
15. Frush DP, Donnelly LF, Bisset GS. Effect of scan delay on hepatic enhancement for pediatric abdominal multislice helical CT. AJR Am J Roentgenol 2001;176:1559–1561.

16. Silverman PM, Roberts S, Tefft MC, et al. Helical CT of the liver: clinical application of an automated computer technique, SmartPrep, for obtaining images with optimal contrast enhancement. AJR Am J Roentgenol 1995;165:73–78.
17. Bonaldi VM, Bret PM, Reinhold C, et al. Helical CT of the liver: value of an early arterial phase. Radiology 1995;197:357–363.
18. Winter TC, Ager JD, Nghiem HV, et al. Upper gastrointestinal tract and abdomen: water as an orally administered contrast agent for helical CT. Radiology 1996;201:365–370.
19. Walker D, Blaquiere RM. Technical note: low density contrast in upper abdominal computed tomography. Br J Radiol 1995;68:80–81.
20. Brenner DJ, Elliston CD, Hall EJ, et al. Estimated risks of radiation-induced fatal cancer from pediatric CT. AJR Am J Roentgenol 2001;176:3289–3296.
21. Donnelly LF, Emery KH, Brody AS, et al. Minimizing radiation dose for pediatric body applications for single-detector helical CT: strategies at a large children's hospital. AJR Am J Roentgenol 2001;176:303–306.
22. Costello P, Anderson W, Blume D. Pulmonary nodule: evaluation with spiral volumetric CT. Radiology 1991;179:875–876.
23. Remy-Jardin, Remy J, Giraud F, et al. Pulmonary nodules: detection with thick-section spiral CT versus conventional CT. Radiology 1993;187:513–520.
24. Wright AR, Collie DA, Williams JR, et al. Pulmonary nodules: effect on detection of spiral CT pitch. Radiology 1996;199:837–841.
25. Fishman JE. Imaging of blunt aortic and great vessel trauma. J Thorac Imaging 2000;15:97–103.
26. Rapp-Bernhardt U, Welte T, Doehring W, et al. Diagnostic potential of virtual bronchoscopy: advantages in comparison with axial CT slices, MPR and MIP? Eur Radiol 2000;10:981–988.
27. Zeiberg AS, Silverman PM, Sessions RB, et al. Helical (spiral) CT of the upper airway with three-dimensional imaging: technique and clinical assessment. AJR Am J Roentgenol 1996;166:292–299.
28. Gilkeson.RC, Ciancibello LM, Hejal RB, et al. Tracheobronchomalacia: dynamic airway evaluation with multi-detector CT. AJR Am J Roentgenol 2001;176:205–210.
29. Siegel MJ, Bhalla S, Gutierrez FR, et al. Post–lung transplantation bronchiolitis obliterans syndrome: usefulness of expiratory thin-section CT for diagnosis. Radiology 2001;220:455–462.
30. Stern EJ, Webb WR, Golden JA, et al. Cystic lung disease associated with eosinophilic granuloma and tuberous sclerosis: air trapping at dynamic ultra-fast-high-resolution CT. Radiology 1992;182:325–329.
31. Stern EJ, Frank MS. Small airway disease of the lungs: findings at expiratory CT. AJR Am J Roentgenol 1994;163:37–41.
32. Lane MJ, Katz DS, Ross BA, et al. Unenhanced helical CT for suspected appendicitis. AJR Am J Roentgenol 1997;168:465–469.
33. Rao PM, Rhea JT, Novelline RA, et al. Helical CT combined with contrast material administered only through the colon for imaging suspected appendicitis. AJR Am J Roentgenol 1997;169:1275–1280.
34. Herts BR, Einstein DM, Paushter DM. Spiral CT of the abdomen: artifacts and potential pitfalls. AJR Am J Roentgenol 1993;161:1185–1190.
35. Silverman PM, Cooper CJ, Weltman DI, et al. Helical CT: practical considerations and potential pitfalls. Radio-Graphics 1995;15:225–236.
36. Buckwalter KA, Rydberg J, Kopecky KK, et al. Musculoskeletal imaging with multislice CT. AJR Am J Roentgenol 2001;176:979–986.

Protocol 1:
NECK (Fig. 2)

INDICATION: *Abscess, adenopathy, mass*

SCANNER SETTINGS: kV(p): 120
mA: Based on weight

Weight (kg)	mA
<10	30
10–25	40
26–50	65
51–70	80
>70	>120

ORAL CONTRAST: None

PHASE OF RESPIRATION: Suspended inspiration

ROTATION TIME: 0.5 to 1.0 sec

ACQUISITION SLICE   2.5–3 mm
  THICKNESS:

PITCH: 0.75, 1.5 (HQ = 3:1; HS = 6:1)

RECONSTRUCTION SLICE   2.5–3.0 mm/2.5–3.0 mm
  THICKNESS/INTERVAL
  FOR FILMING:

ANATOMIC COVERAGE:
  SUPERIOR EXTENT: Angle of mandible
  INFERIOR EXTENT: Sternal notch

IV CONTRAST:

Concentration:	Low osmolar contrast medium (LOCM) 280–320 mg iodine/mL

Rate and Scan Delay:
Hand injection:
  Rate: Rapid push bolus
  Scan Delay: 20–30 sec
Power injection:
  Rate: Dependent on needle size

Needle size	**Flow rate**
22 gauge	1.5 mL/sec
20 gauge	2.0 mL/sec
18 gauge	3.0 mL/sec

  Scan Delay: 20–30 sec

Total volume: 2 mL/kg (maximum 4 mL/kg or 150 mL, whichever is less)

COMMENTS:

1. If patient is sedated, scans are obtained at shallow breathing. In cooperative patients, scanning is performed during a single breath-hold.
2. If mass is large, a larger nominal slice thickness (5 mm) may be used.
3. Pitch varies with patient size. In larger patients, the pitch can be increased to 1.5.

Protocol 2:
THORACIC SURVEY (Fig. 3)

INDICATION: *Oncologic staging, pulmonary metastases*

SCANNER SETTINGS: kV(p): 120
mA: Based on weight

Weight (kg)	mA
<10	30
10–25	40
26–50	65
51–70	80
>70	>120

ORAL CONTRAST: None

PHASE OF RESPIRATION: Suspended inspiration

ROTATION TIME: 0.5 to 1.0 sec

ACQUISITION SLICE THICKNESS: 2.5–3.75 mm

PITCH: 0.75 (HQ = 3:1)

RECONSTRUCTION SLICE THICKNESS/INTERVAL FOR FILMING: 5.0 mm/5.0 mm

ANATOMIC COVERAGE:
   SUPERIOR EXTENT: Superior margins of clavicles (above lung apices)
   INFERIOR EXTENT: Adrenal glands or posterior sulci (whichever is lower)

IV CONTRAST: None

COMMENTS:
1. If patient is sedated or uncooperative, CT scans are obtained at quiet breathing.
2. Collimation and pitch are based on length of the patient. The goal is to image the chest in one breath-hold. In larger patients, the pitch can be increased to 6 (6:1) by increasing table speed, but leaving collimation at 2.5.

3. In smaller patients, nominal slice thickness can be reduced to 2.5 mm.
4. When parenchymal lung metastases are the main concern, IV contrast medium is not needed.

Protocol 3:
FOCAL PULMONARY MASS (Fig. 4)

INDICATION:	*Congenital mass (cystic adenomatoid malformation, sequestration, vascular malformations) abscess, tumor*

SCANNER SETTINGS:

kV(p): 120
mA: Based on weight

Weight (kg)	mA
<10	30
10–25	40
26–50	65
51–70	80
>70	>120

ORAL CONTRAST: None

PHASE OF RESPIRATION: Suspended inspiration

ROTATION TIME: 0.5 to 1.0 sec

ACQUISITION SLICE THICKNESS: 2.5–3.0 mm

PITCH: 0.75 (HQ = 3:1)

RECONSTRUCTION SLICE THICKNESS/INTERVAL FOR FILMING: 3.0–5.0 mm/3.0–5.0 mm

ANATOMIC COVERAGE:
SUPERIOR EXTENT: Just above top of mass
INFERIOR EXTENT: Just below bottom of mass

IV CONTRAST:

Concentration:	LOCM 280–320 mg iodine/mL

Rate and Scan Delay:
Hand injection:
  Rate: Rapid push bolus
  Scan Delay: 20–30 sec after start of injection
Power injection:
  Rate: Dependent on needle size

Needle size	Flow rate
22 gauge	1.5 mL/sec
20 gauge	2.0 mL/sec
18 gauge	3.0 mL/sec

  Scan Delay: 20–30 sec after start of injection
Total Volume: 2 mL/kg (maximum
                                     5 mL/kg or 150
                                     mL, whichever is
                                     lower)

COMMENTS:

1. If tumor is suspected, additional sections should be obtained through the entire chest to detect metastases.
2. MPR can be useful when an abnormal vessel is suspected or if the relationship with the diaphragm needs to be clarified.
3. For smaller masses or vasculare anomalies, such as sequestration, 1.0 mm (1.25 mm) slice thickness should be used.

Protocol 4:
MEDIASTINAL/HILAR SURVEY (Fig. 5)

INDICATION: *Mass lesion*

SCANNER SETTINGS: kV(p): 120
                               mA: Based on weight

Weight (kg)	mA
<10	30
10–25	40
26–50	65
51–70	80
>70	>120

ORAL CONTRAST: None

PHASE OF RESPIRATION: Suspended inspiration

ROTATION TIME: 0.5 to 1.0 sec

ACQUISITION SLICE   2.5–3.75 mm
   THICKNESS:

PITCH: 0.75 (HQ = 3:1)

RECONSTRUCTION SLICE   3.75–5.0 mm/3.75–5.0 mm
   THICKNESS/INTERVAL
   FOR FILMING:

ANATOMIC COVERAGE:
   SUPERIOR EXTENT: Lung apices
   INFERIOR EXTENT: Adrenal glands or posterior sulci (whichever is
                                  lower)

IV CONTRAST:

Concentration:	LOCM 280–320 mg iodine mL

Rate and Scan Delay:
Hand injection:
   Rate: Rapid push bolus
   Scan Delay: 20–30 sec after start of injection
Power injection:
   Rate: Dependent on needle size

Needle size	**Flow rate**
22 gauge	1.5 mL/sec
20 gauge	2.0 mL/sec
18 gauge	3.0 mL/sec

   Scan Delay: 20–30 sec after start of injection

Total Volume:	2 mL/kg (maximum 4 mL/kg or 150 mL, whichever is lower)

COMMENTS:

1. If child is sedated or uncooperative, CT scans are obtained in quiet respiration.
2. Acquisition slice thickness should be based on length of coverage.

Protocol 5:
VASCULAR DISEASE (Figs. 6 through 8)

INDICATION: *Congenital anomalies, intracardiac and extracardiac shunts*

SCANNER SETTINGS: kV(p): 120
mA: based on weight

Weight (kg)	mA
<10	30
10–25	40
26–50	65
51–70	80
>70	>120

ORAL CONTRAST: None

PHASE OF RESPIRATION: Suspended inspiration

ROTATION TIME: 0.5 to 1.0 sec

ACQUISITION SLICE THICKNESS: 2.5–3.75 mm

PITCH: 0.75, 1.5 (HQ = 3:1; HS = 6.1)

RECONSTRUCTION SLICE THICKNESS/INTERVAL FOR FILMING: 2.5–3.75 mm/2.5–3.75 mm

ANATOMIC COVERAGE:
SUPERIOR EXTENT: Lung apices
INFERIOR EXTENT: Diaphragm

IV CONTRAST:

Concentration:	LOCM 280–320 mg iodine/mL

Rate and Scan Delay:
Hand injection:
  Rate: Rapid push bolus
  Scan Delay: 10–20 sec after start of injection
Power injection:
  Rate: Dependent on needle size

Needle size	*Flow rate*
22 gauge	1.5 mL/sec
20 gauge	2.0 mL/sec
18 gauge	3.0 mL/sec

  Scan Delay: 10–20 sec after start of injection

Total Volume: 2 mL/kg (maximum 4 mL/kg or 150 mL, whichever is lower)

COMMENTS:

1. If child is sedated or uncooperative, CT scans are obtained in quiet respiration.
2. MPR and 3D reconstructions are routinely obtained to provide an overview of anatomy.
3. Shorter scan times (10 seconds) are needed in neonates and small infants.
4. Pitch is selected to maximize coverage in a given scan time. Larger pitch used in larger (taller) patients.

Protocol 6:
TRACHEOBRONCHIAL TREE (Fig. 9)

INDICATION:	*Congenital anomalies, tracheal stenosis, postoperative complications*

SCANNER SETTINGS:

kV(p): 120
mA: Based on weight

Weight (kg)	mA
<10	30
10–25	40
26–50	65
51–70	80
>70	>120

ORAL CONTRAST:	None
PHASE OF RESPIRATION:	Suspended inspiration
ROTATION TIME:	0.5 to 1.0 sec
ACQUISITION SLICE THICKNESS:	1.0–1.25 mm
PITCH:	1.5 (HS = 6:1)
RECONSTRUCTION SLICE THICKNESS/INTERVAL FOR FILMING:	2.5 mm/2.5 mm for filming (1 mm thickness for 3D)
ANATOMIC COVERAGE: SUPERIOR EXTENT: INFERIOR EXTENT:	Just above vocal cords Main-stem bronchi (below carina)
IV CONTRAST:	None

COMMENTS:

1. Aim for single breath-hold. The pitch should be changed to scan the area of interest in a single breath-hold in cooperative patients.
2. If tracheomalacia is suspected, scans can be obtained in expiration.
3. MPRs and 3D reconstructions are useful to provide an overview of anatomy for surgical planning.

Protocol 7:
DIFFUSE LUNG DISEASE (Figs. 10 and 11)

INDICATION: *Extent and characteristics of diffuse
                                          interstitial disease*

SCANNER SETTINGS: kV(p): 120
                                          mA: Based on weight

Weight (kg)	mA
<10	30
10–25	40
26–50	65
51–70	80
>70	>120

ORAL CONTRAST: ·   None

PHASE OF RESPIRATION: Suspended inspiration and occasionally
                                          suspended expiration

ROTATION TIME: 0.5 to 1.0 sec

**ACQUISITION SLICE
  THICKNESS:**   1.0–1.25 mm

PITCH: 1.5 (HS = 6:1)

**RECONSTRUCTION SLICE
  THICKNESS/INTERVAL
  FOR FILMING:**   5 mm/5 mm

ANATOMIC COVERAGE:
  SUPERIOR EXTENT: Clavicles
  INFERIOR EXTENT: Adrenal glands

IV CONTRAST: None

COMMENTS: 1. Expiration imaging can be useful to
                                             evaluate suspected areas of air
                                             trapping.
                                          2. Subtle lung findings may be more
                                             apparent on MIPs.

Protocol 8:
ABDOMINAL/PELVIC SURVEY
(Figs. 12 through 15)

INDICATION:

Tumor staging, abscess, parenchymal inflammation (pancreatitis, pyelonephritis)

SCANNER SETTINGS:

kV(p): 120
mA: Based on weight

Weight (kg)	mA
<10	40
10–25	60
26–50	80
51–70	100
>70	>140

ORAL CONTRAST:

Oral contrast (water soluble) given 45 min to 1 hr before scan. Additional dose given 15 min before scanning.
Dose: Depends on age

Age	Initial volume (45 min before study)	Additional volume (15 min before study)
<1 month	2–3 ounces (60–90 mL)	1–1.5 ounces (30–45 mL)
1 mo to 1 yr	4–8 ounces (120–240 mL)	2–4 ounces (60–120 mL)
1–5 yr	8–16 ounces (240–480 mL)	4–8 ounces (120–240 mL)
6–12 yr	16–24 ounces (480–720 mL)	8–12 ounces (240–360 mL)
≥13 yr	24–36 ounces (720–1080 mL)	12–18 ounces (360–540 mL)

PHASE OF RESPIRATION:

Suspended inspiration

ROTATION TIME:

0.5 to 1.0 sec

ACQUISITION SLICE THICKNESS (COLLIMATION):

2.5–3.0 mm

PITCH:

0.75, 1.5 (HQ = 3:1; HS = 6.1)

RECONSTRUCTION SLICE THICKNESS/INTERVAL FOR FILMING:

2.5–3.0 mm/2.5–3.0 mm

ANATOMIC COVERAGE:
  SUPERIOR EXTENT: Diaphragm
  INFERIOR EXTENT: Pubic symphysis

IV CONTRAST:

Concentration:	LOCM 280–320 mg iodine/mL
Rate and Scan Delay:	
Hand injection:	
Rate: Rapid push bolus	
Scan Delay: 40–60 sec from start of injection	
Power injection:	
Rate: Dependent on needle size	
Needle size	***Flow rate***
22 gauge	1.5 mL/sec
20 gauge	2.0 mL/sec
18 gauge	3 mL/sec
Scan Delay: 40–60 sec from start of injection	
Total Volume:	2 mL/kg (maximum 4 mL/kg or 150 mL, whichever is lower)

COMMENTS:

1. In infants and small children, who will inherently receive smaller volumes of contrast medium, it may be necessary to use a shorter scan delay time. However, the delay time should not exceed 20 sec from the completion of the injection to initiation of scanning.
2. In sedated patients, scans are obtained at quiet breathing.
3. If contrast has not reached the colon, delayed images can be obtained or rectal contrast can be administered.
4. Delayed images may be helpful if an abnormality of the bladder or renal collecting system is suspected.
5. Arterial phase images are of value in characterization of hepatic masses.
6. MPRs or 3D reconstructions can help define the full longitudinal extent of a tumor.
7. Pitch will vary with patient size. Larger pitch used in larger (taller) patients to maximize coverage in a shorter scan time.

Protocol 9:
ABDOMINAL/PELVIC TRAUMA SURVEY
(Fig. 16)

INDICATION:	*Trauma*

SCANNER SETTINGS: kV(p): 120
mA: Based on weight

Weight (kg)	mA
<10	40
10–25	60
26–50	80
51–70	100
>70	>140

ORAL CONTRAST: Oral contrast (water soluble) given 45–60 min
before scan. Additional dose given 15 min before
scanning.
Oral contrast should be used with caution if patient
has a depressed level of consciousness.
Dose: Depends on age

Age	Initial volume (45 min before study)	Additional volume (15 min before study)
<1 mo	2–3 ounces (60–90 mL)	1–1.5 ounces (30–45 mL)
1 mo to 1 yr	4–8 ounces (120–240 mL)	2–4 ounces (60–120 mL)
1–5 yr	8–16 ounces (240–480 mL)	4–8 ounces (120–240 mL)
6–12 yr	16–24 ounces (480–720 mL)	8–12 ounces (240–360 mL)
≥13	24–36 ounces (720–1080 mL)	12–18 ounces (360–540 mL)
	See adult protocols	See adult protocols

PHASE OF RESPIRATION: Suspended inspiration

ROTATION TIME: 0.5 to 1.0 sec

ACQUISITION SLICE THICKNESS: 2.5 mm

PITCH: 1.5 (HS = 6:1)

RECONSTRUCTION SLICE THICKNESS/INTERVAL FOR FILMING: 5.0 mm/5.0 mm

ANATOMIC COVERAGE:
   SUPERIOR EXTENT: Diaphragm
   INFERIOR EXTENT: Pubic symphysis

IV CONTRAST:

Concentration:	LOCM 280–320 mg iodine/mL
Rate and Scan Delay:	
Hand injection:	
Rate: Rapid push bolus	
Scan Delay: 40–60 sec from start of injection	
Power injection:	
Rate: Dependent on needle size	
Needle size	***Flow rate***
22 gauge	1.5 mL/sec
20 gauge	2.0 mL/sec
18 gauge	3.0 mL/sec
Scan Delay: 40–60 sec from start of injection	
Total Volume:	2 mL/kg (maximum 4 mL/kg or 150 mL, whichever is smaller)

COMMENTS:

1. In infants and small children, who will inherently receive smaller volumes of contrast medium, it may be necessary to use a shorter scan delay. However, the delay time should not exceed 20 sec from the completion of the injection to initiation of scanning.
2. If patient is obtunded or sedated, scans are obtained at quiet breathing.
3. Delayed images may be helpful if bladder or renal injury is suspected.
4. Images of upper abdomen should be reviewed at lung windows to detect small amounts of free intraperitoneal air.
5. If pancreatic injury is a question, thin reconstructions can be obtained though the area of interest.

Protocol 10:
SUSPECTED APPENDICITIS (Fig. 17)

INDICATION: *Suspected appendicitis*

SCANNER SETTINGS: kV(p): 120
                                    mA: Based on weight

Weight (kg)	mA
<10	40
10–25	60
26–50	80
51–70	100
>70	>140

ORAL CONTRAST: Oral contrast (water soluble) given 45–60 min
                                    before scan. Additional dose given 15 min
                                    before scanning.
                                    Dose: Depends on age

Age	Initial volume (45 min before study)	Additional volume (15 min before study)
<1 mo	2–3 ounces (60–90 mL)	1–1.5 ounces (30–45 mL)
1 mo to 1 yr	4–8 ounces (120–240 mL)	2–4 ounces (60–120 mL)
1–5 yr	8–16 ounces (240–480 mL)	4–8 ounces (120–240 mL)
6–12 yr	16–24 ounces (480–720 mL)	8–12 ounces (240–360 mL)
>13	24–36 ounces (720–1080 mL)	12–18 ounces (360–540 mL)

PHASE OF RESPIRATION: Suspended inspiration

ROTATION TIME: 0.5 to 1.0 sec

**ACQUISITION SLICE   2.5–3.0 mm
   THICKNESS:**

PITCH: 0.75 (HQ = 3:1)

**RECONSTRUCTION SLICE   2.5–3.0 mm/2.5–3.0 mm
   THICKNESS/INTERVAL
   FOR FILMING:**

ANATOMIC COVERAGE:
   SUPERIOR EXTENT: Diaphragm
   INFERIOR EXTENT: Pubic symphysis

IV CONTRAST:

Concentration:	LOCM 280– 320 mg iodine/mL

Rate and Scan Delay:
Hand injection:
  Rate: Rapid push bolus
  Scan Delay: 40 to 60 sec from start of injection
Power injection:
  Rate: Dependent on needle size

Needle size	**Flow rate**
22 gauge	1.5 mL/sec
20 gauge	2.0 mL/sec
18 gauge	3.0 mL/sec

  Scan Delay: 40 to 60 sec from start of injection

Total Volume:	2 mL/kg (maximum 4 mL/kg or 150 mL, whichever is smaller)

COMMENTS:

1. Other techniques for performing appendiceal CT include (a) imaging limited to the lower abdomen and pelvis without any contrast material, (b) imaging limited to the lower abdomen and pelvis with the use of oral and rectal contrast material, and (c) imaging of the lower abdomen and pelvis with the use of only rectal contrast material.
2. Rectal contrast is administered through a rectal catheter. The amount of contrast material varies with patient size and the degree of fullness and discomfort that the patient can tolerate when the fluid is instilled. The administered volume of fluid varies with patient size.

Protocol 11:
RENAL COLIC

INDICATION:	*Suspected renal or ureteral calculi*

SCANNER SETTINGS: kV(p): 120
mA: Based on weight

Weight (kg)	mA
<10	40
10–25	60
26–50	80
51–70	100
>70	>140

ORAL CONTRAST: None

PHASE OF RESPIRATION: Suspended inspiration

ROTATION TIME: 0.5 to 1.0 sec

ACQUISITION SLICE THICKNESS: 2.5 mm

PITCH: 0.75–1.5 (HQ = 3:1; HS = 6:1)

RECONSTRUCTION SLICE THICKNESS/INTERVAL FOR FILMING: 5.0 mm/5.0 mm

ANATOMIC COVERAGE:
  SUPERIOR EXTENT: Upper pole of kidney
  INFERIOR EXTENT: Pubic symphysis

IV CONTRAST: None

Protocol 12:
Neontal HIPS (Fig. 18)

INDICATION: *Evaluate acetabular/femoral contiguity after*
                                          closed reduction for dysplasia

SCANNER SETTINGS: kV(p): 120
                                          mA: Based on weight

Weight (kg)	mA
<15	20

ORAL CONTRAST: None

PHASE OF RESPIRATION: Quiet breathing

ROTATION TIME: 0.5 to 1.0 sec

ACQUISITION SLICE   2.5–3.0 mm
** THICKNESS:**

PITCH: 0.75 (HQ = 3:1)

RECONSTRUCTION SLICE
** THICKNESS/INTERVAL**   2.5–3.0 mm/2.5–3.0 mm
** FOR FILMING:**

ANATOMIC COVERAGE:
** SUPERIOR EXTENT:**   Acetabular roof
** INFERIOR EXTENT:**   Femoral necks

IV CONTRAST: None

Protocol 13:
TARSAL COALITION (Fig. 19)

INDICATION:	*Congenital coalitions*
SCANNER SETTINGS:	kV(p): 120 mA: Based on weight

Weight (kg)	mA
5–14	20
15–34	40
35–54	70
>55	100

ORAL CONTRAST:	None
PHASE OF RESPIRATION:	Quiet breathing
ROTATION TIME:	Varies with patient size
ACQUISITION SLICE THICKNESS:	1.0–1.25 mm
PITCH:	0.75 (HQ = 3:1)
RECONSTRUCTION SLICE THICKNESS/INTERVAL FOR FILMING:	2.0–2.5 mm/2.0–2.5 mm (reconstruct 1.0–1.25 mm for MPRs)

ANATOMIC COVERAGE:
    SUPERIOR EXTENT:
    INFERIOR EXTENT:
	
	Anterior to talus
	Through midcalcaneus past talocalcaneal joint

IV CONTRAST:	None
COMMENTS:	1. Bone algorithm should be used. 2. For talocalcaneal coalition, patient is supine with knees bent and feet flat on the gantry table. Tape feet to prevent motion. 3. For calcaneonavicular coalitions, the patient is supine with legs extended and feet perpendicular to the table. 4. Both feet should be imaged. 5. MPRs and 3D reconstructions are routinely obtained.

Protocol 14:
LOCALIZED BONE LESION (Fig. 20)

INDICATION: *Osteoid osteoma, complex fractures*

SCANNER SETTINGS: kV(p): 120
                                  mA: Based on weight

Weight (kg)	mA
5–14	20
15–34	40
35–54	70
>55	100

ORAL CONTRAST: None

PHASE OF RESPIRATION: Quiet breathing

ROTATION TIME: 0.5 to 1.0 sec

**ACQUISITION SLICE
  THICKNESS:**   1.0–1.25 mm

PITCH: 0.75 (HQ = 3:1)

**RECONSTRUCTION SLICE
  THICKNESS/INTERVAL
  FOR FILMING:**   2.0–2.5 mm/2.0–2.5 mm (1 mm thickness
                                     for MPRs)

ANATOMIC COVERAGE:
** SUPERIOR EXTENT:**   Superior to abnormality on plain film
** INFERIOR EXTENT:**   Inferior to abnormality on plain film

IV CONTRAST: None

COMMENTS: 1. Thicker collimation (2.5 mm) can be
                                      used for larger lesions.
                                   2. Use bone algorithm
                                   3. MPRs are routinely obtained.

6

Multislice Imaging of the Musculoskeletal System

Elliot K. Fishman

*Department of Radiology and Oncology, Johns Hopkins Hospital,
Baltimore, Maryland 21287*

Computed tomography (CT) has always played a prominent role in the evaluation of musculoskeletal pathology (1–5, 9, 12–13). With the advent of spiral CT and most recently multidetector-multirow CT (MSCT), the quality of the data sets available for image analysis and for postprocessing and display has unprecedented resolution and detail (12). Concurrent with this advance in image quality has been the continued development of postprocessing techniques, particularly three-dimensional (3D) volume rendering (9, 13). This chapter reviews the current state of musculoskeletal imaging, focusing on MSCT and 3D rendering and its role in clinical practice today. The chapter by its nature focuses on the principles and techniques of MSCT imaging, rather than attempting to be comprehensive in its review of specific pathologies.

STUDY DESIGN AND PROTOCOL SELECTION

The newest scanners provide increased options for protocol design and optimization of both initial data-reconstruction techniques (for the raw data coming from the scanner) and postprocessing tools. The use of spiral CT and more recently MSCT or multislice CT provides increased capabilities in many of the key aspects of musculoskeletal imaging. The quality of a CT data set depends on many factors, ranging from milliamperes to kilovolt(peak) (kV[p]) to slice thickness. Routine CT imaging of bone has classically required thin-section imaging (3 mm or less) and close interscan reconstruction intervals (3 mm or less), particularly when multiplanar reconstruction (MPR) or 3D imaging is needed. With MSCT, the user has increased flexibility, because instead of selecting the slice thickness before the study, the user chooses the scan collimation. On our Siemens Somatom Volume Zoom scanner, we currently use four detectors for data acquisition from each 500-millisecond scan rotation. The typical detectors chosen are either 1 or 2.5 mm, with 1 mm now clearly the selection of choice in small-part imaging (i.e., wrist or hand). With the 1-mm detector, a range of slice thickness can be obtained. For example, we can reconstruct data at slice thickness ranging from 1 to 8 mm. For the best detail and the best 3D reconstruction, we select 1- to 1.25-mm slice thickness and reconstruct the data at 1-mm intervals. The scan protocol typically includes 120 kV(p), 150 mA, and a pitch of 6 to 8. On our scanner, pitch is defined as distance traveled per scan rotation divided by the nominal slice thickness (e.g., 15-mm-per-second travel with 2.5-mm collimators is a pitch of 6). For smaller volumes, we are able to obtain a 0.5-mm slice thickness, although pitch is limited to 2.0, which results in longer scan times for the volume scanned. However, the advantage of a 0.5-mm slice thickness is that the volume becomes an isotropic data set, with the x-, y-, and z-axes being equal in size, as opposed to routine CT data sets, which are anisotropic. The advantage of an isotropic data set is that regardless of the plane in which the patient is scanned, reconstructed data in any plane are of equal resolution. Although currently we are limited by scan speed, the newest scanners (delivered in late 2001 and in 2002) will provide isotropic data sets as routine scanning protocols. With 8-detector scanners now being introduced and 16-detector scanners to soon follow, the use of 0.5-mm section thickness will become more of a standard for small-part imaging.

One of the concerns in the past with spiral CT for skeletal imaging was that the image quality suffered on both the axial and the 3D display because higher pitches were used. This was due not only to the less than optimal scan-reconstruction algorithms available but also to how the single spiral scans were obtained. With higher pitches, the slice profile might increase up to 27% (e.g., a scan with a 5-mm collimation might actually be 6.5 mm) and the milliamperes would actually decrease on the higher pitches, resulting in poorer image quality. With MSCT, the slice thickness selected is the slice thickness achieved without any blooming artifacts. Also, the milliamperes are constant across the scan volume regardless of the pitch selected. One should caution that these assumptions vary between individual scanners, depending on the manufacturer and the system model. It is, therefore, important to be aware of the capabilities, to optimize protocol design.

There are several other key decisions that are routinely made in musculoskeletal CT imaging. These include the following:

- Is intravenous (IV) contrast needed for the study? In cases of pelvic trauma, a noncontrast study is often satisfactory if the question is simply to detect or define a pelvic fracture. In other cases in which a potential vascular injury is suspected, a CT angiogram (CTA) may be done concurrently with the musculoskeletal imaging examination. Numerous articles have shown that CTA has a high accuracy in this situation. In addition, the presence of muscle pathology is best seen after infusion of IV contrast, regardless of whether one is looking at an abscess, tumor, or myositis. Protocol design of CTAs varies but typically includes rapid injection of iodinated contrast material (3 mL per second of 120-mL of Omnipaque-350), a 30-second delay from contrast injection to initiation of data acquisition, and the use of narrow collimation and close interscan spacing (1.25-mm slice thickness reconstructed at 1-mm intervals). In most cases, only an arterial phase is required, although in other cases, two phases (arterial and venous) may be needed.
- Will 3D imaging or MPRs be needed? The need for MPR or 3D imaging demands the use of thin collimation and close interscan spacing. We feel that image postprocessing is a routine part of skeletal imaging, particularly in the setting of trauma and in congenital deformities. The postprocessing of data can be done on scanner-based software or on an independent workstation. Although a freestanding workstation usually has several advantages (e.g., better interface, more functionality, and better reconstruction algorithms), it is not mandatory for some basic 3D mapping.
- What anatomic area needs to be scanned? Scan protocols are defined based also on the volume to be scanned (e.g., tibial plateau vs. the entire tibia). When a large volume is to be scanned, a slice collimation of 3 mm is usually chosen to limit the scan time needed. With MSCT, data can be reconstructed at 1-mm intervals even with 3-mm collimation.
- The reconstruction algorithm must be selected based on the clinical application. In cases in which soft tissue or muscle imaging is the primary process, a standard soft tissue algorithm is used. If bone detail is needed, a high-resolution algorithm is needed. The specific algorithms vary between the various scanner manufacturers, so you must know the individual selections available on your scanner. Please note that the ideal reconstruction algorithm also depends on whether 3D rendering needs to be done. Some high-resolution algorithms cre-

ate images with too much noise and result in 3D images of suboptimal quality. Trial and error may be needed to optimize your scanning protocol and your 3D reconstruction algorithms. In select cases, the data may need to be reconstructed with two algorithms. This should be fairly easy with the flexibility of the current scanners.

- The use of 3D imaging requires a basic understanding of the available rendering techniques and their implementation. In our practice, we routinely use only the volume rendering technique (VRT) for our bone and soft tissue reconstruction protocols. Volume rendering has been shown to be the most flexible technique as well as the most accurate technique. Through the use of a trapezoid-based rendering system, you can easily and accurately display both bone and soft tissue in a range of presentations by changing factors including opacity and brightness. Shaded surface rendering technique can also be used to display bone in 3D, but the imaging quality suffers due to the use of a binary classification technique that uses less than 10% of the data set in creating the image. Volume rendering of bone can be presented in several different presentations, which can vary opacity of bone (or transparency) depending on clinical application or individual physician preference. We routinely review these images in real time to optimize selection of the ideal image display and to be able to view the images in stereo mode. We have found that using preset 3D imaging protocols may not be as valuable as the radiologist or referring physician reviewing the images on a real-time display.

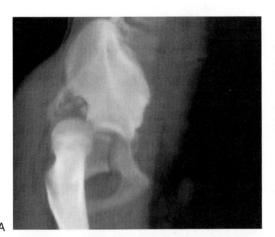

A

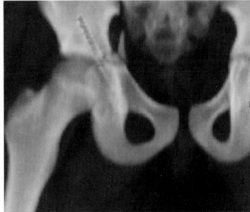

B

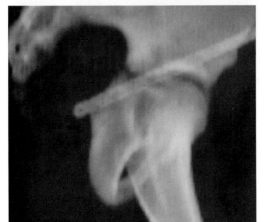

C

FIG. 1. Acetabular fracture with posteriorly dislocated femur with an acetabular fracture in an 11-year-old girl. Postoperative three-dimensional (3D) renderings show the use of 3D in patient management.

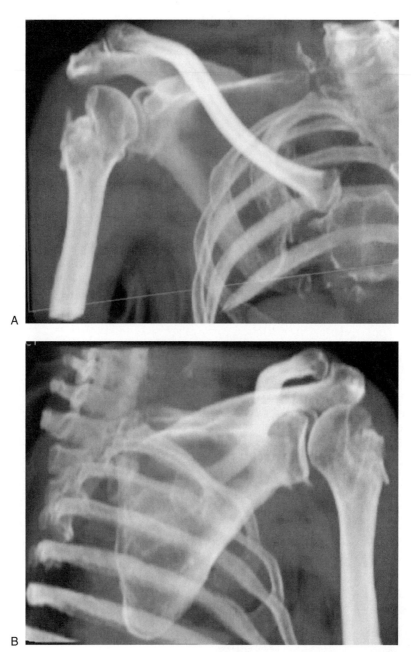

FIG. 2. Impacted fracture of the right humeral head. The three-dimensional rendering defines the impaction of bone and injury to the humerus. Displacement of bone is critical to surgical planning.

CLINICAL APPLICATIONS

Trauma

One of the most classic applications for CT and 3D imaging is the evaluation of musculoskeletal trauma. Even in the earliest days of CT, scanning numerous articles touted the advantages of CT and 3D imaging as both a diagnostic and a patient clinical management tool. Patients commonly referred to CT were either sent as a result of plain films that were indeterminate for fracture or cases of extensive fracture in which the goal was to define the true extent of injury to allow for surgical or nonsurgical planning (Figs. 1 through 3). The addition of 3D imaging in these cases changed the patient management in up to 30% of cases. In many regards, little has changed over the past two decades in terms of referral patterns for many trauma applications.

What has changed, however, is the increased availability and speed of the CT scanners, the placement of CT scanners in or near the emergency room, the need for rapid triage of the patient in the emergency room, and the increased use of CT across all emergency room applications. In the current environment, it is very clear that in many applications, the increased use of CT early in the evaluation of patients provides both a more rapid diagnosis and a more rapid patient triage, which is important particularly with the increased volume of many emergency rooms. For example, new imaging algorithms for spinal trauma using CT as the initial study are becoming more common in centers with a CT scanner in the emergency room (Figs. 4 and 5).

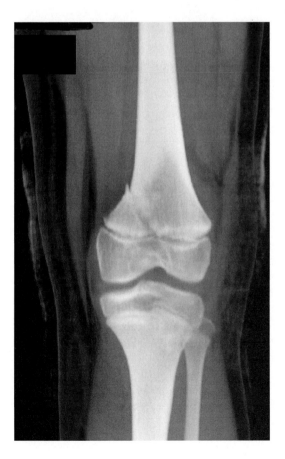

FIG. 3. Fracture of femur with fracture line extending through the metaphysis into the epiphyseal plate.

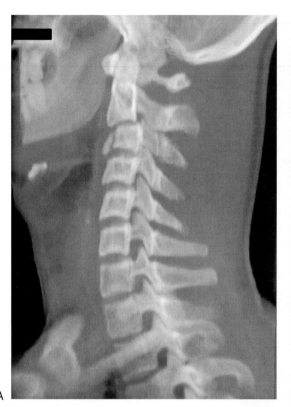
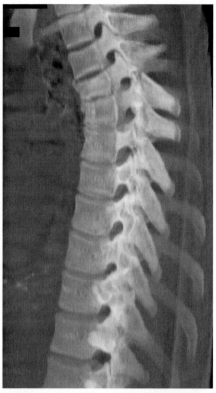

A   B

FIG. 4. Cervical and thoracic spine fractures in patient who had a motor-vehicle accident. **A:** Three-dimensional (3D) computed tomographic (CT) scan of multislice CT (MSCT) data set demonstrates the fracture of the body of C3 with the step off in alignment at C3–4. **B:** 3D MSCT demonstrates fracture of several upper thoracic vertebral bodies, with involvement of the posterior element also seen.

The use of MSCT is ideal in all trauma applications. CT can limit the need for sedation and provide a single comprehensive examination that can combine imaging of the solid organs and the skeletal structures. This is particularly true in pediatric patients in whom the need for sedation is nearly eliminated with the use of MSCT.

The importance of high-quality data sets generated by MSCT is particularly important in small-part imaging such as the wrist (Figs. 6 and 7). In their state-of-the-art review, Goldfarb et al. (5) state, "We prefer not to use reconstructed images for a second plane, unless prior use of a scanner shows that the machine can produce excellent quality reconstructed images that equal the quality of directly acquired images. The use of 0.5-mm slice thickness and isotropic data sets is ideal for this application. Supplemented by 3D renderings, they can produce all of the necessary views for surgical decision making. Isotropic data sets eliminate the need for two views and thereby speed up the examination without compromising quality."

In the evaluation of pelvic trauma, MSCT is ideal for combining skeletal imaging with more complicated studies including CTA to look for vascular injury, as well as CT cystograms to exclude bladder injury in patients with pelvic trauma (Fig. 8). CT cystograms are as accurate as classic cystograms for detecting bladder injury.

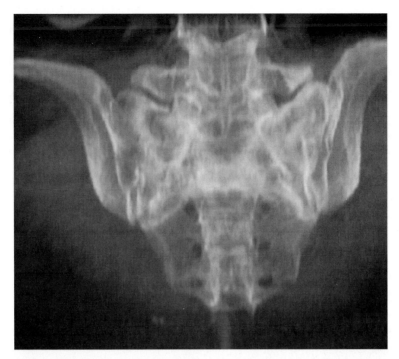

FIG. 5. Elderly woman with back pain has evidence of bilateral sacral stress fractures. Sacral stress fractures are common in elderly women and can be confused with bone metastases or missed on plain radiographs.

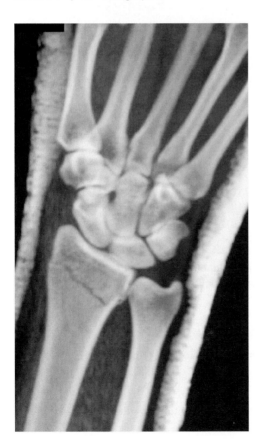

FIG. 6. A 41-year-old woman after a fall. **A:** 0.5-mm thick sections are a key in the detail of this three-dimensional multislice computed tomographic volume-rendered image. Note the detail of the minimally displaced fracture line in the radius.

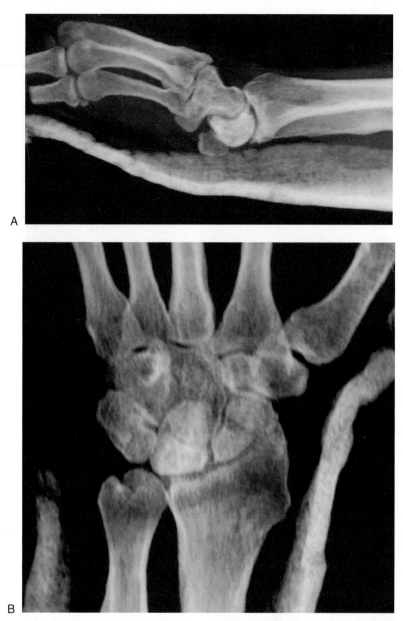

FIG. 7. A 69-year-old man with fracture dislocation of the wrist. **A, B:** Three-dimensional volume renderings define the lunate dislocation and the subtle scaphoid fracture.

Oncologic Applications

The role of CT scanning for oncologic imaging has continued to remain strong even with the continuing evolution of MRI. CT is used in a number of clinical scenarios, which include the following:

- Cases in which there are inconsistencies between interpretation of either plain radiographs or patient symptoms or between bone scans and plain films

- Cases in which there is a need to determine extent of tumor before determining therapy including surgery, chemotherapy, or radiation therapy. Tumor volumes can be accurately calculated using volumes determined from MSCT data sets.
- Cases in which one needs the ability to define the optimal site of a lesion for biopsy. Biopsy can be done with CT guidance and if necessary using CT fluoroscopy. CT fluoroscopy allows biopsy of smaller lesions in more difficult locations. CT fluoroscopy can also be used to guide radiofrequency ablation of osteoid osteoma. Newer MSCT scanners are continuing to focus on the interventional use of real-time CT fluoroscopy.
- Cases in which one must define the presence and extent of disease that may be detected with bone scanning or positron emission tomographic (PET) scanning. CT can help determine whether increased uptake in a bone scan is Paget's disease or metastases in indeterminate cases. CT combined with PET scanning can be used to more precisely define the site of increased tracer uptake on a PET study. Several manufacturers are taking this one step further by combining CT and PET scanning into a single scanner. This appears to be more accurate than trying to merge images retrospectively from two different data sets acquired at separate times on two different imaging devices.

The use of MSCT with optimal scan protocols is routinely supplemented by 3D reconstructions in many of these patients (Figs. 9 and 10). We routinely combine volumetric 3D reconstruction with multiplanar coronal and sagittal reconstruction. The use of MSCT data as a volume display, rather than as a slice-based display, is critical particularly when looking at joint surfaces and articular zones. With ever larger data sets being generated, we feel that the 3D display will become the dominant display.

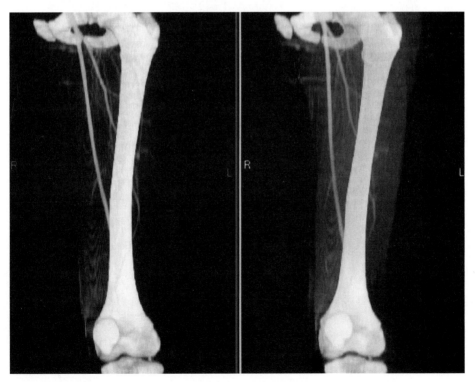

FIG. 8. Computed tomographic angiogram in a patient with pelvic trauma demonstrates no evidence of arterial vascular injury.

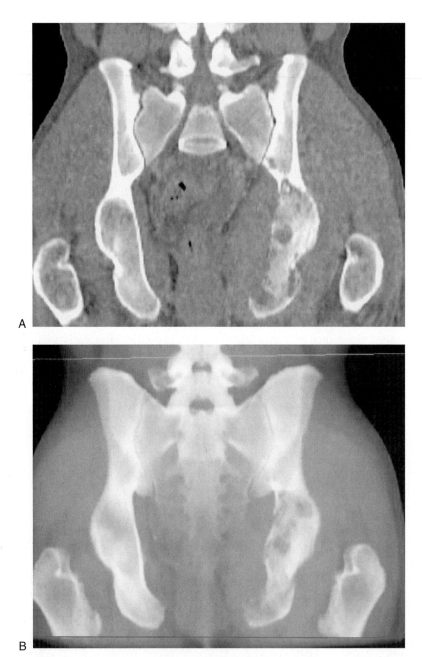

FIG. 9. Infiltration of the left hemipelvis by lymphoma. **A, B:** Coronal multiplanar reconstruction and three-dimensional multislice computed tomographic images define the extent of the bony infiltration and associated soft tissue mass.

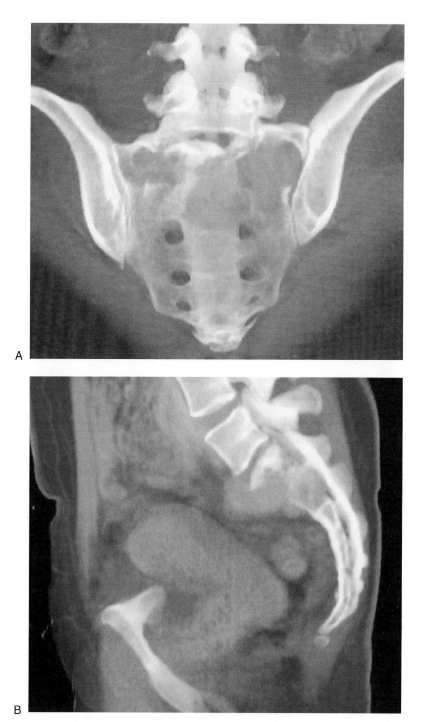

FIG. 10. Three-dimensional computed tomography (CT) of multislice CT data set demonstrates destructive tumor of the sacrum, which was a biopsy proven chordoma. **A, B:** Use of rendering techniques defines both bone and soft tissue component of the tumor.

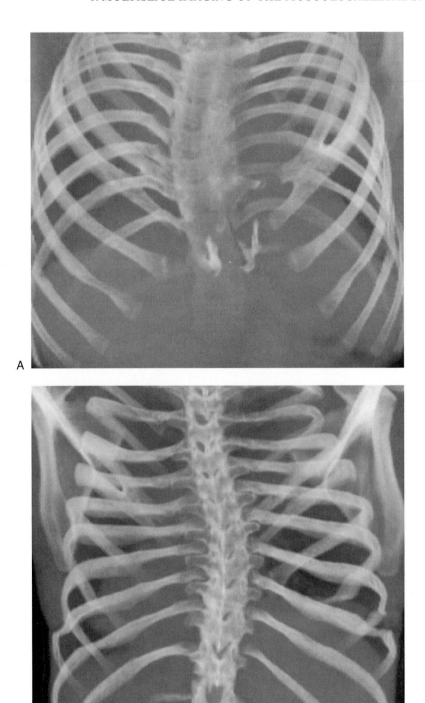

FIG. 11. Preoperative pectus repair. **A, B:** Three-dimensional (3D) multislice computed tomographic data sets are presented as 3D volume renderings and demonstrate the fused ribs anteriorly, as well as scoliosis of the spine.

Congenital Deformities

CT has always been used for the evaluation of a wide range of congenital hip diseases. In a recent review on the radiologic imaging and treatment of developmental dysplasias of the hip, Murray and Crim (9) recommended the use of multidetector CT with thin-section imaging. In addition to the virtual elimination of the need for sedation, the use of MSCT provides ideal data sets for 3D reconstruction. Numerous authors have documented that CT and 3D imaging are invaluable in both preoperative planning and postoperative follow up in patients with developmental dysplasias of the hip. The more severe the deformity, the more valuable the reformation of the data set becomes. In younger patients, it is important to select the lowest scan parameters possible, to minimize the radiation dose to the patient.

Similarly, in other areas such as the chest wall, imaging can be valuable in detecting benign anatomic variations that can simulate disease. We have also found CT to be helpful in the evaluation of patients pre–pectus excavatum repair, as well as inpatients with failed pectus repairs (Fig. 11). In the latter group of patients, Pretorius et al. (11) previously showed how the use of 3D CT has had an impact on management.

The use of isotropic data sets with 0.5-mm collimation is ideal for the evaluation of the painful foot where a tarsal coalition is one of the more common diagnoses. Scans through the hind foot are done in a 15-second period and are ideal for making the dignosis of bony or fibrous unions. The ability to reconstruct data in any plane eliminates the need for a second set of scans while providing a volume display that can help detect and define bony or fibrous unions. It is not surprising that in cases in which tarsal coalition is suspected, other diagnoses are made based on the CT scan to explain the patient's symptoms (Fig. 12).

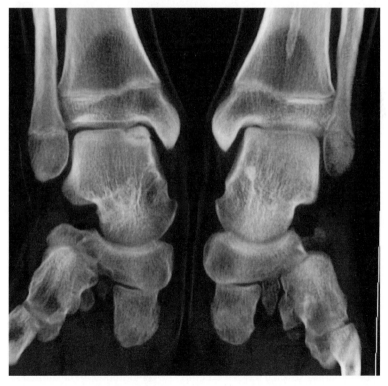

FIG. 12. Isotropic data set imaging of a teenager with right ankle pain. **A:** Three-dimensional multislice computed tomographic display defines avascular necrosis of the right medial dome of the talus. Note old infarct in left tibia.

Postoperative Orthopedic Imaging

One of the most challenging clinical scenarios is in the patient who has had prior orthopedic surgery with the insertion of pins, plates, screws, or joint replacement. Classic axial CT imaging may be limited due to artifacts generated on axial CT scans due to the metal implants. However, image postprocessing can solve this problem. Some CT scanners provide postprocessing software that can reduce artifacts or extend the CT scale to try and minimize the artifacts generated due to beam hardening.

A technique that we find particularly valuable is the generation of MPRs and/or 3D volume renderings using thin collimation and narrow interscan spacing. Because artifacts typically are random on each individual CT slice, the reconstruction of overlapping CT scans limits the artifacts and results in diagnostic quality CT images. Specific applications in which we have found this valuable include looking at fracture healing or suspected postoperative infection, evaluation of suspected failure of orthopedic hardware, or in patients with persistent pain with hardware in place (Figs. 13 and 14). Please note that when using 3D, we have found that using color for metal (blue works best) against the classic opacification usually selected for bone is ideal. Our experience with MDCT is that a slice thickness ranging from 0.5 to 1.25 mm is ideal with a 0.5 to 1.0 mm reconstruction interval (Fig. 12). In these cases, we usually use a standard algorithm to help minimize the artifacts.

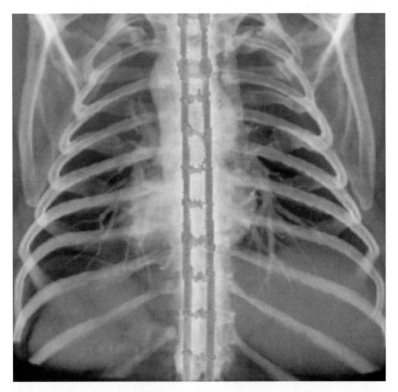

FIG. 13. Three-dimensional (3D) multislice computed tomography demonstration of metal artifact reduction by 3D display. **A:** Color-coded image defines the detail of the spinal rods without any significant artifact.

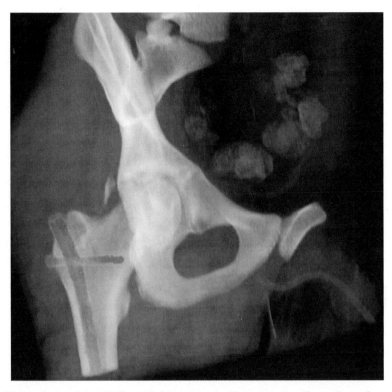

FIG. 14. Three-dimensional (3D) multislice computed tomography of a patient after repair of a femur fracture with an intramedullary rod and pin. Note the fracture of the posterior acetabulum, which is well defined on this 3D map.

Soft Tissue And Muscle Imaging

One of the applications of CT scanning that is continuing to grow, particularly in the emergency room setting, is the evaluation of known or suspected musculoskeletal infection. With the ever-increasing numbers of immunosuppressed patients, be it due to bone marrow transplant, high-dose steroid renal failure, or acquired immunodeficiency syndrome, we are seeing an increasing number of patients with the potential for musculoskeletal infection. Our experience has been that spiral CT is a rapid and accurate technique for evaluating suspected or known musculoskeletal infection. The key advantage parameters in these cases relate to the ability to scan the patient quickly while IV iodinated contrast is accentuating the difference between normal and abnormal structures such as in muscle.

In cases in which IV contrast is not used, but in which there is substantial inflammation present, we can still usually detect the pathologic process. However, information regarding extent of inflammation and level of involvement is substantially inferior. Our protocols for contrast-enhancement techniques are described in the specific protocols, but nevertheless a few comments are in order. The use of IV contrast is typically noted to accentuate the difference between normal and abnormal tissue. When muscle becomes edematous or ischemic, it commonly enlarges and has fewer sharp edges due to edema. With IV contrast, we find that the normal musculature enhances even up to 50 to 70 Hounsfield units (HU), whereas abnormal muscle enhances to a lesser degree.

With MSCT, we typically scan around 30 to 40 seconds after we begin the injection of contrast (100 to 120 mL of Omnipaque-350 injected at 2 to 3 mL per second). We have found this to be an ideal time to be able to optimize differentiation between normal and abnormal muscle. One of the potential limitations, at least from a theoretical perspective, is that enhancing muscle abscesses can look very similar to tumors. However, in most cases, the clinical history is obviously different, and the radiologic interpretation is not typically problematic.

When evaluating muscle inflammation, one must review bone windows through the appropriate scan levels. Often bony involvement is a primary source of the inflammatory process, or it may become secondarily involved. This is particularly true in infections in the chest wall, the sternoclavicular joint, the sacroiliac joints, and the sacrum.

In the evaluation of musculoskeletal infection, we will typically image the patient with a standard algorithm. The high-resolution algorithm or bone algorithms create substantial noise, which makes the images suboptimal for viewing the soft tissues. In cases in which high-resolution images of bone are desired, reconstruction with both algorithms is ideal.

In most cases of musculoskeletal inflammation, 3D or multiplanar imaging is not needed for the detection of the primary disease process. However, it may be very valuable in determining the extent of inflammation, which may be helpful to the surgeon in preoperative planning. This is particularly true in imaging spinal infection, in which it is easier to define disc space involvement on sagittal MPR or 3D sagittal reconstruction formats (Figs. 13 and 14). With MSCT data sets, we are finding that routine use of 3D volume displays is becoming more of a primary display mode due to a number of factors including the number of axial images that may be generated with current and future scanners (Figs. 15 and 16).

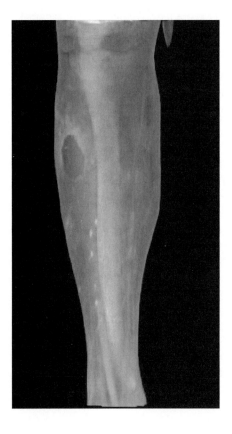

FIG. 15. Soft tissue display defines an ulceration in the soft tissue of the calf. Patient also had venous insufficiency.

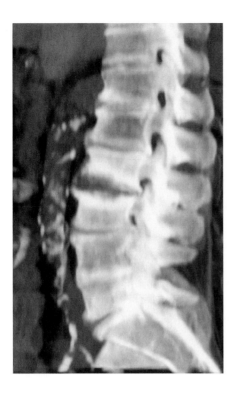

FIG. 16. Osteomyelitis of the L2–3 disc space, with destruction of the endplates of both vertebral bodies. The etiologic agent was *Staphylococcus.*

CONCLUSION

The role of CT in the evaluation of musculoskeletal pathology will continue to grow and evolve with the diffusion of MDCT and its continued evolution. New patient protocols will be developed, particularly in the emergency room setting, in which CT in many cases will be the initial and only study performed in patients with trauma. The use of CT in a volume display mode will also be ideal for the rapid screening of the patient with multisite trauma and will potentially become a cost-effective, time-effective study technique. The next generation of MDCT scanners will also allow routine use of isotropic data sets of 0.5-mm thickness, which will be ideal for high-resolution imaging, which will be particularly valuable in musculoskeletal imaging especially for small-part CT scanning. Whether for trauma, infection, or oncologic applications, we believe the critical role of CT is only now being truly understood.

REFERENCES

1. Beauchamp NJ Jr, Scott WW Jr, Gottlieb LM, et al. CT evaluation of soft tissue and muscle infection and inflammation: a systematic compartmental approach. Skeletal Radiol 1995;24(5):317–324.
2. Daffner R. Cervical radiography for trauma patients: a time effective technique? AJR Am J Roentgenol 2000; 175:1309–1311.
3. Donnelly LF. Use of three-dimensional reconstructed helical CT images in recognition and communication of chest wall anomalies in children. AJR Am J Roentgenol 2001;177:441–445.
4. Fishman EK, Magid D, Robertson DD, et al. Metallic hip implants: CT with multiplanar reconstruction. Radiology 1986:160:675–681.
5. Goldfarb CA, Yin Y, Gilula LA, et al. Wrist fractures: what the clinician wants to know. Radiology 2001;219:11–28.
6. Kuszyk BS, Ney DR, Fishman EK. The current state of the art in 3D oncologic imaging: an overview. Int J Radiat Oncol Biol Phys 1995;33:1029–1039.

7. Kuszyk BS, Heath DG, Bliss DF, et al. Skeletal 3-D CT: advantages of volume rendering over surface rendering. Skeletal Radiol 1996;25:207–214.
8. Link TM, Berning W, Scherf S, et al. CT of metal implants: reduction of artifacts using an extended CT scale technique. J Comput Assisted Tomogr 2000;24(1):165–172.
9. Murray KA, Crim JR. Radiographic imaging for treatment and follow-up of developmental dysplasia of the hip. Semin Ultrasound Comput Tomogr Magn Reson Imaging 2001;22(4):306–340.
10. Ney DR, Drebin RA, Fishman EK, et al. Volumetric rendering of computed tomographic data: principles and techniques. IEEE Comput Graphic Appl 1990;10:24–32.
11. Pretorius ES, Haller JA, Fishman EK. Spiral CT with 3D reconstruction in children requiring reoperation for failure of chest wall growth after pectus excavatum surgery: preliminary observations. Clin Imaging 1998;22:108–116.
12. Pretorius ES, Fishman EK. Volume-rendered three-dimensional spiral CT: musculoskeletal applications. Radio-Graphics 1999;19:1143–1160.
13. Pretorius ES, Fishman EK. Spiral CT and three-dimensional CT of musculoskeletal pathology—emergency room applications. Radiol Clin North Am 1999;37(5):953–974.

Protocol 1:
SUSPECTED METASTASES
(FOCUSED STUDY)

INDICATION:	*Suspected bone metastases*
SCANNER SETTINGS:	kV(p): 120–140 mA: 130
ORAL CONTRAST:	None
PHASE OF RESPIRATION:	Inspiration
ROTATION TIME:	15–30 sec
ACQUISITION SLICE THICKNESS:	2.5 or 1.0 mm
PITCH:	1.5 (HS = 6:1)
RECONSTRUCTION SLICE THICKNESS/INTERVAL FOR FILMING:	1.25–3.0 mm/1.25–3.0 mm
ANATOMIC COVERAGE:	
SUPERIOR EXTENT:	Several cm above and below the area in question
INFERIOR EXTENT:	Several cm above and below the area in question
IV CONTRAST:	None
COMMENTS:	1. This is a specific study to exclude bone metastases. Use dedicated above algorithm for reconstruction bone detail. 2. In select areas when 3D imaging is used the thinnest collimation is most valuable for quality 3D images. 3. IV contrast is used if an associated soft tissue abnormality requires evaluation of soft tissue. If so, 2–3 mL/sec injection of 120 mL of nonionic contrast is used.

Protocol 2:
SUSPECTED OSTEOID OSTEOMA

INDICATION: *Suspected osteoid osteoma*

SCANNER SETTINGS: kV(p): 120
                                         mA:90

ORAL CONTRAST: None

PHASE OF RESPIRATION: Quiet respiration or at full inspiration
                                            depending on the area to be scanned.

ROTATION TIME: 15–30 sec

ACQUISITION SLICE   1.0–1.25 mm
   THICKNESS:

PITCH: 1.5 (HS = 6.1)

RECONSTRUCTION SLICE   1.0 mm/1.0 mm
   THICKNESS/INTERVAL
   FOR FILMING:

ANATOMIC COVERAGE:
   SUPERIOR EXTENT: Region of lesion
   INFERIOR EXTENT: Region of lesion

IV CONTRAST: None

COMMENTS: 1. This is called ultra high-resolution spiral
                                            and is used typically for "small-part
                                            scanning" such as the wrist. It can also
                                            be used for focused examinations such
                                            as osteoid osteoma. If 0.5 mm slice
                                            thickness is available it would be helpful
                                            in defining the nidus in select cases.

Protocol 3:
POSSIBLE MUSCLE ABSCESS

INDICATION:	*R/O muscle abscess*
SCANNER SETTINGS:	kV(p): 120 mA: 165
ORAL CONTRAST:	None
PHASE OF RESPIRATION:	Suspended respiration
ROTATION TIME:	15–30 sec
ACQUISITION SLICE THICKNESS:	2.5 mm
PITCH:	1.5 (HS = 6:1)
RECONSTRUCTION SLICE THICKNESS/INTERVAL FOR FILMING:	2.5–5.0 mm/3.0–5.0 mm

ANATOMIC COVERAGE:
  SUPERIOR EXTENT:
  INFERIOR EXTENT:
	
	Above to below abnormalities
	Above to below abnormalities

IV CONTRAST:

Concentration:	100–150 mL of Omnipaque 350
Injection Rate:	2–3 mL/sec
Scan Delay (sec):	40 sec
3D Technology Used:	typically not needed

COMMENTS:

1. The key parameter is the differential enhancement of healthy muscle and abscess. Without IV contrast, many abscesses would be missed.
2. Bone windows should be reviewed to exclude associated bowel involvement or osteomyelitis.

Protocol 4:
POSSIBLE MUSCLE ABSCESS

INDICATION:	*Muscle, R/O or evaluate suspected tumor*
SCANNER SETTINGS:	kV(p): 120 mA: 165
ORAL CONTRAST:	None needed
PHASE OF RESPIRATION:	N/A
ROTATION TIME:	15–30 sec
ACQUISITION SLICE THICKNESS:	3.0 or 5.0 mm
PITCH:	1.5 (HS = 6.1)
RECONSTRUCTION SLICE THICKNESS/INTERVAL FOR FILMING:	3.0 mm/3.0 mm or 5.0 mm/5.0 mm
ANATOMIC COVERAGE:	
SUPERIOR EXTENT:	Several cm above and below the area in question
INFERIOR EXTENT:	Several cm above and below the area in question

IV CONTRAST:

Volume/Type:	100–150
Rate:	2.5–3 mL/sec
Scan Delay:	40–50 sec
Total Value:	100–150 mL

COMMENTS:

1. A second reconstruction of the data can be done with a bone algorithm for better bone detail. You can film the muscle/soft tissue with the reconstructions from the standard acquisition of soft tissues and bone with the bone algorithm.
2. Narrow window may be helpful to define subtle infiltration.

Protocol 5:
STERNOCLAVICULAR JOINT:
R/O INFECTION, OSTEOMYELITIS

INDICATION:	*Sternoclavicular joint: R/O infection or osteomyelitis*
SCANNER SETTINGS:	kV: 120 mA: 120
ORAL CONTRAST:	None
PHASE OF RESPIRATION:	Suspended respiration and end of inspiration
ROTATION TIME:	15–30 sec
ACQUISITION SLICE THICKNESS:	1.0–1.25 mm
PITCH:	1.5 (HS = 6:1)
RECONSTRUCTION SLICE THICKNESS/INTERVAL FOR FILMING:	1.0–1.25 mm/2.0–3.0 mm

ANATOMIC COVERAGE:
  SUPERIOR EXTENT:
  INFERIOR EXTENT:
	
	Above and below joint space
	Above and below joint space

IV CONTRAST:

Volume/Type:	100–150 mL
Injection **Rate:**	2–3 mL/sec
Scan Delay (sec):	100–150 mL
3D Technique Used:	Volume rendering

COMMENTS:

1. This protocol is found in the ultrahigh resolution in the extremity protocol. Reconstruct the data also with soft tissue algorithm, for an optimal study.
2. Oblique MPRs are often useful in these cases.

Protocol 6:
TRAUMA TO SHOULDER JOINT

INDICATION:	*Shoulder, including humerus and sternoclavicular and acromioclavicular joints*
SCANNER SETTINGS:	kV(p): 120–140 mA: 120
ORAL CONTRAST:	None
PHASE OF RESPIRATION:	Suspended inspiration
ROTATION TIME:	15–30 sec
ACQUISITION SLICE THICKNESS:	1. 25–2.5 mm
PITCH:	1.5 (HS = 6:1)
RECONSTRUCTION SLICE THICKNESS/INTERVAL FOR FILMING:	1.25–2.5 mm/1.25–2.5 mm
ANATOMIC COVERAGE:	
SUPERIOR EXTENT:	Several cm above to several cm below the shoulder joint
INFERIOR EXTENT:	Several cm above to several cm below the shoulder joint
IV CONTRAST:	N/A
COMMENTS:	1. Volume rendering is used for 3D display. 2. 3-mm thick sections reconstructed by 1 or 2 mm is also satisfactory in less cooperative patients.

Protocol 7:
WRIST/HAND

INDICATION:	*Wrist: R/O fracture, R/O fracture/dislocation*
SCANNER SETTINGS:	kV(p): 120 mA: 100–160 mm
ORAL CONTRAST:	None
PHASE OF RESPIRATION:	N/A
ROTATION TIME:	15–30 sec
ACQUISITION SLICE THICKNESS:	0.5–1.0 mm
PITCH:	1.5 (HS = 6:1)
RECONSTRUCTION SLICE THICKNESS/INTERVAL FOR FILMING:	1.0–1.25 mm/1.0–1.25 mm
ANATOMIC COVERAGE:	
SUPERIOR EXTENT:	Entire wrist including proximal radius/ulna as necessary
INFERIOR EXTENT:	Entire wrist including proximal radius/ulna as necessary
IV CONTRAST:	N/A
COMMENTS:	1. This uses the bone algorithm, which is critical for small-part anatomy. 2. Positioning of wrist is less critical when 0.5 mm (isotropic) slides are used.

Protocol 8:
LUMBAR SPINE

INDICATION:	*Evaluate suspected fracture*
SCANNER SETTINGS:	kV(p) 120–140 mA: 200–300
ORAL CONTRAST:	None
PHASE OF RESPIRATION:	Suspended respiration
ROTATION TIME:	15–30 sec
ACQUISITION SLICE THICKNESS:	1.0 or 2.5 cm
PITCH:	1.5 (HS = 6.1)
RECONSTRUCTION SLICE THICKNESS/INTERVAL FOR FILMING:	1.0–3.0 mm/1.0–3.0 mm

ANATOMIC COVERAGE:
  SUPERIOR EXTENT:
  INFERIOR EXTENT:
	
	Several cm above and below area of interest
	Several cm above and below area of interest

IV CONTRAST:	Use will vary on case by case basis

Concentration:	LOCM 300–250 mg iodine/mL or HOCM 282 mg iodine/mL (60% solution)
Rate:	2–3 mL/sec
Scan Delay:	60–70 sec
Total Volume:	100–150 mL

COMMENTS:

1. This provides high spatial resolution at the cost of increased dose. For 3D rendering, reconstruction at a standard abdomen soft tissue algorithm and at a bone algorithm may both be needed.

Protocol 9:
LUMBAR SPINE

INDICATION:	*Detailed spine examinaton/myelographic study*
SCANNER SETTINGS:	kV(p): 140 mA: 300–350
ORAL CONTRAST:	None
PHASE OF RESPIRATION:	Suspended respiration
ROTATION TIME:	15–30 sec
ACQUISITION SLICE THICKNESS:	1.0–1.25 mm
PITCH:	1.5 (HS = 6:1)
RECONSTRUCTION SLICE THICKNESS/INTERVAL FOR FILMING:	1.25 mm/1.25 mm

ANATOMIC COVERAGE:
  SUPERIOR EXTENT:
  INFERIOR EXTENT:
	
	Area of Interest
	Area of Interest

IV CONTRAST:

Concentration:	LOCM 250–300 mg iodine/mL or HOCM 282 mg iodine/mL (60% solution)
Rate:	2–3 mL/sec
Scan Delay:	60–70 sec
Total Volume:	100 mL–150 mL

COMMENTS:

1. Volume rendering reconstruction.
2. This is a good protocol to use, without having to scan with a gantry tilt. MPR with curved sagittals or 3D imaging provides all the information necessary. This is also a good postmyelogram protocol.

Protocol 10:
ACETABULUM/PELVIS

INDICATION:	*Evaluate suspected fracture*
SCANNER SETTINGS:	kV(p): 120–140 mA: 200–250
ORAL CONTRAST:	None
PHASE OF RESPIRATION:	Suspended respiration
ROTATION TIME:	15–30 sec
ACQUISITION SLICE THICKNESS:	1.25 mm
PITCH:	1.5 (HS = 6:1)
RECONSTRUCTION SLICE THICKNESS/INTERVAL FOR FILMING:	1.0 mm–1.25 mm/1.0–1.25 mm

ANATOMIC COVERAGE:
    SUPERIOR EXTENT:
    INFERIOR EXTENT:
	
	Area of Interest
	Area of Interest

IV CONTRAST:	May be used for CT angiogram
COMMENTS:	1. In many cases of isolated pelvic injury, a noncontrast study is satisfactory. If, however, the possibility of vascular or bladder injury is suspected, then the protocol should be done with IV contrast, and a CT angiogram can also be done (see Chapter 7). 2. CT angiogram can be done at the same time if needed.

Protocol 11:
KNEE

INDICATION:	*Trauma*
SCANNER SETTINGS:	kV(p): 120–140
ORAL CONTRAST:	None
PHASE OF RESPIRATION:	None
ROTATION TIME:	15–30 sec
ACQUISITION SLICE THICKNESS:	1.0–1.25 mm
PITCH:	0.75 (HQ = 3:1) or 1.5 (HS = 6.1)
RECONSTRUCTION SLICE THICKNESS/INTERVAL FOR FILMING:	1.0–1.25 mm/1.0–1.25 mm
ANATOMIC COVERAGE:	
SUPERIOR EXTENT:	Above and below area
INFERIOR EXTENT:	Above and below area
IV CONTRAST:	N/A
COMMENTS:	1. Overscanning with 0.75 (HQ = 3.1) improves volumetric data set but at increased radiation dose.

Protocol 12:
FOOT

INDICATION:	*Pain/coalition*
SCANNER SETTINGS:	kV(p): 120–140 mA: 90–110
ORAL CONTRAST:	None
PHASE OF RESPIRATION:	N/A
ROTATION TIME:	15–30 sec
ACQUISITION SLICE THICKNESS:	1.0–1.25 mm
PITCH:	1.5 (HS = 6:1)
RECONSTRUCTION SLICE THICKNESS/INTERVAL FOR FILMING:	1.0–1.25 mm/1.0–1.25 mm
ANATOMIC COVERAGE: **SUPERIOR EXTENT:** **INFERIOR EXTENT:**	 Anatomic area Anatomic area
IV CONTRAST:	N/A
COMMENTS:	1. This protocol also uses the high-resolution algorithm designed for better bone detail. 2. MPR and/or volume rendering 3D are useful in these cases. 3. Two different positions may be needed unless isotrophic data sets are acquired.

Protocol 13:
CERVICAL SPINE

INDICATION:	*Trauma screening*
SCANNER SETTINGS:	kV(p): 120–140 mA: 200–250
ORAL CONTRAST:	None
PHASE OF RESPIRATION:	Suspended respiration
ROTATION TIME:	15–30 sec
ACQUISITION SLICE THICKNESS:	1.25–3.0 mm
PITCH:	1.5 (HS = 6:1)
RECONSTRUCTION SLICE THICKNESS/INTERVAL FOR FILMING:	1.25–3.0 mm/1.25–3.0 mm

ANATOMIC COVERAGE:
   SUPERIOR EXTENT:
   INFERIOR EXTENT:
	
	Area of clinical interest
	Area of clinical interest

IV CONTRAST:	N/A
COMMENTS:	1. Use the bone filter and the soft tissue filter for ideal studies. 2. CT can replace a plain film series.

Protocol 14:
CERVICAL SPINE

INDICATION:	*Trauma extent of injury*
SCANNER SETTINGS:	kV(p): 120–140
ORAL CONTRAST:	mA: 200
PHASE OF RESPIRATION:	N/A
ROTATION TIME:	15–30 sec
ACQUISITION SLICE THICKNESS:	1.0–1.25 mm
PITCH:	1.5 (HS = 6:1)
RECONSTRUCTION SLICE THICKNESS/INTERVAL FOR FILMING:	1.0–1.25 mm/1.0–1.25 mm
ANATOMIC COVERAGE: SUPERIOR EXTENT: INFERIOR EXTENT:	Above area of abnormality Below area of abnormality
IV CONTRAST:	N/A
COMMENTS:	1. Detailed examination is not a screening study to replace plain x-rays. 2. Some suggest 0.5 mm slice thickness. 3. MPR and 3D are valuable in these patients.

Protocol 15:
ORBIT

INDICATION:	*Trauma*
SCANNER SETTINGS:	kV(p): 120 mA:
ORAL CONTRAST:	None
PHASE OF RESPIRATION:	N/A
ROTATION TIME:	15–30 sec
ACQUISITION SLICE THICKNESS:	1.0–1.25 mm
PITCH:	1.5 (HS = 6.1)
RECONSTRUCTION SLICE THICKNESS/INTERVAL FOR FILMING:	1.0–1.25 mm/1.0–1.25 mm

ANATOMIC COVERAGE:
  SUPERIOR EXTENT:
  INFERIOR EXTENT:
	
	Anatomic orbit
	Anatomic orbit

IV CONTRAST:	N/A
COMMENTS:	1. 3D imaging can be very helpful in these cases. 2. Preventing patient motion is key.

Protocol 16:
FACIAL BONES

INDICATION:	*Trauma*
SCANNER SETTINGS:	kV(p): 120–140 mA: 140–160
ORAL CONTRAST:	None
PHASE OF RESPIRATION:	N/A
ROTATION TIME:	15–30 sec
ACQUISITION SLICE THICKNESS:	1.0–1.25 mm
PITCH:	1.5 (HS = 6:1)
RECONSTRUCTION SLICE THICKNESS/INTERVAL FOR FILMING:	1.0–1.25 mm/1.0–1.25 mm

ANATOMIC COVERAGE:
    SUPERIOR EXTENT:
    INFERIOR EXTENT:
	
	Coverage as determined by injury.
	Coverage as determined by injury.

IV CONTRAST:	N/A
COMMENTS:	1. Value data set is ideal for coronal and sagittal reformations, MPR. 2. Sections at 0.5 mm may be useful.

7

Multislice Imaging for Three-dimensional Examinations

Geoffrey D. Rubin

*Department of Radiology, Stanford University School of Medicine,
Stanford, California 94305*

Because helical computed tomographic (CT) data are volumetric, they are well suited to three-dimensional (3D) visualization (1). However, the quality of 3D images is highly dependent on the quality of the acquired CT data. The use of 3D rendering must be anticipated before image acquisition, to optimize the data available for rendering. This chapter first reviews relevant acquisition, contrast administration, and reconstruction issues for optimizing 3D visualization of the blood vessels, airways, and colon, and then the most commonly available rendering techniques and tools for prerendering data preparation (editing) are discussed.

ACQUISITION OPTIMIZATION

The use of multidetector-multirow CT (multislice CT [MSCT]) substantially diminishes the constraints on image acquisition imposed by single-detector–single-row CT (single-slice CT [SSCT]). With prior SSCT, maximum breath-hold duration and contrast medium dose dictated the scan duration, which in turn presented a challenge to balance anatomic coverage with section thickness within the constraints of a maximum pitch of 2.0 with SSCT. Fortunately, the competing ideal of maximized anatomic coverage and narrowest section thickness have virtually disappeared with MSCT using four or more detector rows because most clinically relevant anatomic territories can be acquired within substantially less than a typical 30-second breath-hold, even when using a section thickness of less than 1.5 mm (2).

In general, the highest quality visualization using 3D rendering techniques or multiplanar visualization techniques is going to result from voxel dimensions that are isotropic or the same size in all three dimensions. When recognizing that transverse voxel dimensions are typically between 0.5 and 0.8 mm on CT sections, it should become apparent that true isotropic spatial resolution is still beyond the reach of most standard CT applications. Instead, longitudinal voxel dimensions (effective section thickness) of 1.3 to 3 mm are the norm with MSCT. These represent a substantial improvement over SSCT scanning, and in particular when 1.3—mm effective section thickness data are acquired, longitudinal spatial resolution is virtually indistinguishable from transverse spatial resolution in the clinical setting.

One important strategy that should be used to maximize the opportunity to achieve near-isotropic voxel dimensions, particularly when anatomic territories greater than 15 to 20 cm long are needed, is to maximize pitch. Maximization of the pitch of the scan within the manufacturer's recommendations (typically between 6.0 and 8.0) ensures the fastest table feed for a given nominal section thickness. Although maximization of pitch results in the greatest table feed to effective section thickness ratio, there is one minor limitation associated with higher pitch values: an increase in the helical artifacts. Although this rarely presents significant limitations to CT data interpretation, it is important to be cognizant of this phenomenon. Readers particularly interested in this are referred to reference 3.

CONTRAST ADMINISTRATION

A critical factor that determines the quality of 3D renderings is the contrast to noise ratio. Therefore, for any CT application in which 3D visualization is desired, the contrast differential between the structures of interest and the background tissues should be maximized. Although this does not present difficulties for airway or colonic visualization, in which air provides naturally high contrast, in the blood vessels, contrast opacification must be maximized with intravascular contrast medium. Iodinated contrast medium is administered through an antecubital vein. To ensure maximal vascular opacification, a tight bolus is delivered, so the bolus duration is equivalent to the scan duration; for example, a 40-second helical scan requires a 40-second long bolus. As a result, the contrast dose and flow rate are related as follows:

contrast medium volume (mL) = contrast medium flow rate (mL/sec) × scan duration (sec)

or

contrast medium flow rate (mL/sec) = contrast medium volume (mL) ÷ scan duration (sec)

One exception to this rule applies to the assessment of the lower extremity inflow and runoff, where we have found that a 50-second long injection (180 mL at 3.5 mL per second) suffices for a 60- to 70-second scan (4).

In general, contrast medium with at least 300 mg of iodine per milliliter injected at a flow rate of 4 mL per second is required to achieve consistent opacification within the adult arterial system for high-quality 3D visualization. This value can be reduced to 3 to 3.5 mL per second in patients weighing less than 60 kg. For patients weighing more than 120 kg, higher flow rates may be required. Unless a compelling reason exists to limit the iodinated contrast dose, such as azotemia, the volume of contrast that allows contrast delivery at the appropriate flow rate for a period equivalent to the scan duration should be administered. If contrast dose must be limited, the maximum tolerable volume of contrast should be established, and the flow rate and/or scan duration modified accordingly.

Before initiating the computed tomographic angiogram (CTA), one additional variable must be measured for optimizing the contrast delivery—the scan delay time. Because the bolus duration is equivalent to the scan duration, the enhancement plateau in the arteries of interest must coincide perfectly with the helical CT acquisition. To achieve this, the circulation time for contrast to travel from the site of injection to the target anatomy must be determined individually. Although a delay time of 16 to 24 seconds before scan initiation will likely work in 75% of adults and 95% of adults younger than 50 years, most CTAs are performed in patients older than 50 years who have coexistent vascular disease, frequently involving the heart. As a result, it can be impossible to predict the appropriate scan delay time without a preliminary test injection of contrast material. This is performed with 10 to 15 mL of contrast medium, injected at a rate of 4 mL per second. After an 8-second delay, 5- to 10-mm transverse sections are acquired every 2 to 3 seconds at the anticipated initiation site of the CTA until 40 to 45 seconds have elapsed since the bolus began. A time–density curve is created by positioning a region of interest (ROI) within the center of the vessel. The *peak of the curve* is selected as the delay time between bolus initiation and scan initiation (5).

Most CT scanners offer an algorithm that will allow a contrast injection to be monitored in near real time and then initiate a spiral CT acquisition. Although these bolus tracking (computer-automated scan technology [CAST]) algorithms, previously discussed in Chapter 4, can be very useful in patients with delayed circulation or in patients in whom early arterial opacification is not critical, the latency from the point of contrast arrival to the triggering of the CT acquisition may be too great to be used for CTA of the arterial system (6,7). This latency varies among CT manufacturers and should be considered before incorporating automated bolus tracking CAST into CTA routines.

RECONSTRUCTION

As already mentioned, the quality of 3D renderings is dependent on the contrast to noise ratio of the cross sections. Therefore, a low noise-reconstruction kernel should be used, that is, "soft" or "standard," not "sharp" or "bone." Additionally, the field of view (FOV) should be limited to include the anatomy of interest, rather than subcutaneous tissues. This approach improves the in-plane resolution substantially. Typical in-plane FOVs should be 18 to 25 cm, rather than 36 to 40 cm as is the case for many routine adult chest, abdomen, or pelvic scans. One cautionary note, however, is that many workstations will only render a longitudinal dimension that is less than or equal to the transverse FOV. Therefore, if the table travel distance (anatomic coverage) is greater than the reconstructed FOV, portions of the data will be "cut off" from a 3D view oriented to visualize the longitudinal axis. If a single 3D view that displays all of the imaged anatomy is desired, a practical rule is to reconstruct the data with an FOV that is equivalent to the table travel distance. When large distances (more than 36 cm) are to be covered, the 3D-rendered volume should be subdivided to avoid over-minification and loss of spatial resolution.

One additional critical element for reconstructing the data is that overlapping cross sections should always be generated at a frequency that is at least 50% of the effective section thickness. This improves the longitudinal spatial resolution of the scan and substantially improves the quality of 3D renderings (6–8).

RENDERING

Four main visualization techniques are used on clinical 3D workstations: multiplanar reconstruction (MPR), maximum intensity projection (MIP), shaded surface display (SSD), and volumetric rendering (VR). The first two techniques are limited to external visualization while the latter can be used for either external or immersive visualization for simulating endoscopy.

MPR is a very convenient and available technique for displaying the data. One substantial limitation of traditional MPR is that visualized structures must lie in a plane. Because almost all structures for which 3D visualization is desired do not lie within a single plane, an MPR cannot be created that demonstrates the entirety of a structure. As structures course in and out of the MPR, pseudostenoses are created. The solution to this problem is to use curved planar reformations (CPRs). Similar to MPR, CPR is a single-voxel thick tomogram, but it is capable of demonstrating an uninterrupted longitudinal cross section because the display plane curves along the structure of interest. CPRs are created from points that are manually positioned over a structure of interest as viewed on transverse sections, MPRs, MIPs, SSDs, or VRs. The points are connected to form a 3D curve that is then extruded through the volume perpendicular to the desired view to create the CPR. CPRs are very useful for displaying the interior of tubular structures such as blood vessels, airways, and bowel. They are also useful for visualizing structures immediately adjacent to these lumina, such as mural thrombus and extrinsic or exophytic neoplasia, without any editing of the data. An important limitation of CPRs is that they are highly dependent on the accuracy of the curve. Inaccurately positioned or insufficient numbers of points can result in the curve "slipping off" the structure of interest, creating pseudostenoses. Further, a single curve cannot adequately display eccentric lesions; therefore, at least two curves that are orthogonal to each other should always be created, to provide a more complete depiction of eccentric lesions, particularly stenoses.

MIPs are created when a specific projection is selected (e.g., anteroposterior), and then rays are cast perpendicular to the view through the volume data, with the maximum value encountered by each ray encoded on a two-dimensional (2D) output image (9,10). As a result, the entire volume is "collapsed" with only the brightest structures being visible. Variations of this approach include the minimum intensity projection (minIP), which can be useful for visualizing airways (11), and the ray-sum or average projection (12), which sums all pixel values encountered by each ray to provide an image similar to a radiograph.

An advantage of MIPs over MPRs is that structures that do not lie in a single plane are visible in their entirety. A limitation of MIPs, however, is that bones or other structures that are more attenuative than contrast-enhanced blood vessels, for example, will obscure the blood vessels. Similarly when creating minIPs, air external to the patient will obscure the airways and surrounding lung. There are two approaches to addressing these limitations: slab-MIP and prerendering editing. Slab-MIPs are created when a plane through the data is defined and then "thickened" perpendicular to the plane (13). The process with which the plane is thickened can be MIP, minIP, ray-sum, or VR. By selecting a slab orientation that does not result in overlapped extremely high-attenuation structures (bones or metal) and structures of interest (blood vessels), the structures of interest can be clearly visualized without the need for time-consuming and operator-dependent editing. This approach, however, is generally limited to allowing visualization through slabs that are 5 to 30 mm thick. If an MIP of a larger subvolume of the scan data is desired, the data typically must be edited to remove obscuring structures. The techniques for editing are discussed in the subsequent section. Even after the issues of obscuration are addressed, MIPs have a couple of lingering limitations. They do not provide for an appreciation of depth relationships, and in regions of complex anatomy, such as at the neck of an aortic aneurysm, it can be difficult to be confident when the true origin of a branch is visualized versus a foreshortened branch due to overlap of its proximal extent with the aorta itself.

SSDs provide exquisite 3D representations of anatomy, relying on grayscale to encode surface reflections from an imaginary source of illumination (14,15). Most SSDs created on clinical workstations display a single surface that is the interface between user-selected thresholds. As a result, the 12-bit CT data are reduced to binary data, with each pixel being either within or outside of the threshold range. Some workstations allow several threshold ranges to be defined and displayed with different colored surfaces. In this setting, different tissue types or structures are coded as different colors, to facilitate their visualization relative to adjacent structures. For each classification, data segmentation is required, typically by both thresholding and editing, which increases the required processing time arithmetically. Regardless of the number of tissue groups or classes assigned, the selection of the threshold range that defines each class is typically arbitrary and can substantially limit the accuracy of data interpretation, particularly when attempting to grade stenoses. This is particularly true when calcified plaque accompanies regions of arterial stenosis. The plaque typically falls within the same threshold range as blood vessel lumen, resulting in the spurious appearance of a local dilatation, rather than a stenosis (16).

The final and most complex rendering technique is VR (17–21). There are many different versions and interfaces for VR, but the general approach is that all voxel values are assigned an opacity level that varies from complete transparency to complete opacity. This opacity function can be applied to the histogram of voxel values as a whole or to regions of the histogram that are classified as specific tissue types. With the latter approach, trapezoidal regions are selected that correspond to the range of attenuation values for a structure (22,23). The "walls" of the trapezoid slope from an opacity plateau to the baseline of complete transparency in an attempt to account for partial volume effects at the edges of structures. Regions at the walls of the trapezoidal regions or in positions where the opacity curve has a steep slope are referred to as transition zones in the ensuing protocols and are analogous to threshold levels with SSDs. Lighting effects may be simulated in a similar fashion as with SSD. Because there is no surface definition with VR, lighting effects are applied based on the spatial gradient (i.e., variability of attenuation within a local neighborhood of voxels). Near the edges of structures, the spatial variation in attenuation changes more rapidly (a high gradient) than in the center of structures (a low gradient). Lighting effects are most pronounced in regions of high spatial gradients. Because lighting effects and variations in transparency are simultaneously displayed, it is frequently useful to view VRs in color. The color is applied to the attenuation histogram, to allow differentiation of pixel values and to avoid ambiguity with lighting effects, which are encoded in grayscale. Other variables such as specular reflectivity, which models the "shininess" of a surface, may be available but should be used with caution to avoid confounding the visualization.

EDITING

The challenge of performing efficient and accurate 3D visualization of clinical CT data is to balance the use of visualization techniques that require editing versus those that do not. Editing can span from very quick and simple interactive cut-plane selection to meticulous 2D ROI selection, with intermediate steps being provided by 3D ROI editing, region-growing or connectivity, and slab editing.

When viewing SSDs or VRs, the use of cut-planes can be very helpful to remove obscuring structures that lie between our viewpoint and the anatomy of interest. Cut-planes can usually be oriented arbitrarily, but for the same reasons that MPRs are limited for visualizing curved structures, cut-planes are limited for removing curved structures.

A 3D ROI edit is performed when an ROI is selected by drawing a rectangle or more complex shape and extruding this shape through the volume along an appropriate linear path. The selected region is either removed or exclusively retained for rendering. This is a very quick technique that requires the drawing of a single ROI that can then be applied to many cross sections. It can be useful for eliminating the air around the chest when creating minIPs or for removing the spine from data sets containing only the cervical or lumbar regions of the spine. The easiest way to implement this type of edit is to create an MIP from above or below that allows a cleavage plane to be identified between the spine and the aorta, for example. This usually requires a 10- to 20-degree anterior rotation of the superior aspect of the volume to correct for lumbar lordosis. Unfortunately, this type of editing is not sufficient for removing the pelvis, skull, or large portions of the rib cage, particularly near the thoracic inlet, where a cleavage plane between anatomy of interest and obscuring structures cannot be identified.

There are two main approaches for dealing with this problem: region-growing/connectivity and slab editing. Both can be very effective, but in general, region growing is the most flexible and efficient when combined with boolean operations, such as subtraction. Region growing or connectivity is a threshold-based process, in which a seed point is selected in the structure of interest and allowed to "grow" into contiguous voxels that are within a defined threshold range. Region growing is rarely adequate as the sole editing tool, because there are typically regions of "leakage" where the seed may grow into undesirable structures. To combat this problem, limited cut-planes or "scalpel cuts" can be applied over a variable number of sections to disconnect the structures. A typical application of this technique is the disconnection of the superior gluteal arteries from the sacrum as they exit the pelvis. These predictable sites of leakage between the arteries and bones can be disconnected in seconds. A quick search of the remainder of the cross sections may reveal problematic osteophytes contacting the aorta, which must be similarly disconnected, then the region growing is applied and the aorta and its branches can be selected. There are two approaches to using region growing for editing CT data. The first and most intuitive is the selection of the structure of interest and deletion of all unselected pixels from the data. This approach has several limitations. First, the structure of interest may not be identifiable with a single region-growing step, such as both sides of an occluded blood vessel reconstituted distally by collateral flow or a highly stenotic vessel that becomes discontinuous with thresholding. Second, the edges of structures will be arbitrarily truncated at the threshold selected for the region growing. Therefore, the edge pixels that represent a partial volume effect–mediated transition between the structure of interest and the background are excluded. Although SSDs will look fine, MIPs will appear as though they have been cut from the data with a scissors. This latter limitation can be combated with a simple dilation step, in which the editing is allowed to "grow" by one to four pixels to include these edges; however, the former problem cannot be addressed by dilation. As a result, the preferred approach is to use region growing to identify the bones, dilate them three to four pixels to include the edges, and subtract them from the original data. An MIP of 200 abdomen and pelvis transverse sections can be edited in less than 5 minutes using this approach to display the aortoiliac system free of overlapping bones. The edited data can also be used to create SSDs free of bones, providing a posterior view of the aorta and its branches.

Slab editors can also be efficient means of editing the data. Slab editors work by allowing the user to preselect variable-thickness slabs of data. The slabs are displayed as slab-MIPs and an ROI is drawn on each slab. Fewer slabs require less ROI drawing, but more slabs may be required to remove complex structures. For many applications, 5 to 10 transverse sections are used per slab, improving the efficiency over 2D ROI editing by a factor of 5 to 10. This technique can be limited in regions such as the pelvis, where the iliac arteries lie close to the pelvic sidewall and the pelvis has a sloping contour or at the skull base adjacent to the circle of Willis.

The most time-consuming editing technique is section-by-section 2D ROI editing, in which an ROI is drawn individually on each cross section. This provides the most control but is extremely time consuming and should be reserved only for situations in which none of the above approaches suffices.

ENDOLUMINAL VISUALIZATION

The ability of helical CT to image the inner surfaces of tubular lumina has lead to proposed clinical applications of "virtual endoscopy" to examine the bowel (21,24,25), airways (21,26–28), blood vessels (21,29), and urinary tract (30,31). Although the term virtual endoscopy is catchy, it is vague and loosely applies to any technique that displays the interior of tubular lumina.

The interior surface of tubular lumina can be visualized with SSD or VR. The basic approach is to identify threshold levels for SSD that exclude pixels of similar attenuation to the lumen (−900 to −1,000 HU for air-filled lumina and 150 to 400 HU for contrast-enhanced blood vessels) or an opacity curve for VR that results in complete transparency of the lumen. It is important to recognize that these renderings allow visualization of the interface between luminal contrast and extraluminal attenuation, not the mucosal or intimal surface. Once the intraluminal pixels have been eliminated or rendered transparent, a view must be created that allows unobstructed intraluminal visualization. To that end, there are two main strategies that can be employed: orthographic external rendering with cut-planes and immersive perspective rendering.

Orthographic renderings are the most common type of rendering, particularly for external visualization, and are based on the assumption that light rays reaching our eyes are parallel, as if structures were viewed with a high-powered telescope from far away. As a result, the proximity of structures to the viewpoint does not influence the size with which they are rendered. This approach is contrasted to perspective rendering in the subsequent paragraph. Although orthographic rendering is exclusively used for visualization from a viewpoint that is external to the data, it can be used for internal visualization when combined with cut-planes that are positioned within the lumen of the structure of interest. This is analogous to cutting a window into a piece of pipe, to visualize its interior. This technique is mostly useful for providing regional snapshots but currently cannot provide a continuous display of all interior surfaces within a tubular lumen. Greater inner surface visualization is available with immersive rendering.

Immersive rendering implies that the viewpoint is within the data set. To understand depth relationships from close range, structures must be viewed with perspective, which is an approach that demonstrates spatial relationships similar to the human visual system, where light rays are focused to converge on the retina. The phenomenon of perspective helps us recognize the distance of structures based on their size; for example, a structure close to the eye appears larger than a structure farther away. The extent to which this effect is observed is determined by the FOV of our "virtual lens," which is typically defined as the size of the angle at the apex of a cone of visualization emanating from our viewpoint. A larger angle indicates greater perspective and thus greater disparity in the size–distance relationships. Most perspective renderings of CT data are created with a 20- to 60-degree FOV. Greater viewing angles typically result in substantial peripheral distortion.

Both SSDs and VRs can be rendered with perspective and can be used to create endoluminal views that mimic fiberoptic endoscopy without the mechanical limitations of access to the lumen and view direction. One of the greatest challenges of immersive visualization is navigation. Flying a virtual endoscope is akin to flying a helicopter. There are three spatial degrees of freedom for position and three spatial degrees of freedom for view direction. When considered with the challenge of appropriate threshold (SSD) or opacity table (VR) selection and color, the complexity of creating these visualizations can be daunting. Further, without some external indication of the view position, either on a 3D model or on MPRs, it is easy to lose track of one's location within the lumen. Techniques that automatically create a flight path through the center of a lumen have shown promising results (32). There are likely to be many variations on the performance of virtual endoscopy, aimed at improving efficiency and ease that will be developed in the future (33).

REFERENCES

1. Rubin GD, Napel S, Leung A. Volumetric analysis of volume data: achieving a paradigm shift. Radiology 1996; 200:312–317.
2. Rubin GD, Shiau MC, Leung AN, et al. Aorta and iliac arteries: single versus multiple detector-row helical CT angiography. Radiology 2000;215:670–676.
3. Fleischmann D, Rubin GD, Paik DS, et al. Stair-step artifacts with single versus multiple detector-row helical CT. Radiology 2000;216:185–196.
4. Rubin GD, Schmidt AJ, Logan LJ, et al. Multi-detector row CT angiography of lower extremity arterial inflow and runoff: initial experience. Radiology 2001;221.
5. Rubin GD. Spiral (helical) CT of the renal vasculature. Semin Ultrasound Comput Tomogr Magn Reson Imaging 1996; 17:374–397.

6. Silverman PM, Roberts S, Tefft MC, et al. Helical CT of the liver: clinical application of an automated computer technique, SmartPrep, for obtaining images with optimal contrast enhancement.
7. Silverman PM, Brown B, Wray LT, et al. Optimal contrast enhancement of the liver using helical (spiral) CT: value of SmartPrep. AJR Am J Roentgenol 1995;164:1169–1171.
8. Kalender WA, Polacin A, Süss C. A comparison of conventional and spiral CT: an experimental study on the detection of spherical lesions. J Comput Assisted Tomogr 1994;18:167–176.
9. Keller PJ, Drayer BP, Fram EK, et al. MR angiography with two-dimensional acquisition and three-dimensional display. Radiology 1989;173:527–532.
10. Napel S, Bergin CJ, Paranjpe DV, et al. Maximum and minimum intensity projection of spiral CT data for simultaneous 3-D imaging of the pulmonary vasculature and airways [Abstract]. Radiology 1992;185(P):126.
11. Rubin GD. Techniques of reconstruction. In: Rémy-Jardin M, Rémy J, eds. Spiral CT of the chest. Berlin: Springer-Verlag, 1996:101–128.
12. Zeman RK, Berman PM, Silverman PM, et al. Diagnosis of aortic dissection: value of helical CT with multiplanar reformation and three-dimensional rendering. AJR Am J Roentgenol 1995;164:1375–1380.
13. Napel S, Rubin GD, Jeffrey RB Jr. STS-MIP: a new reconstruction technique for CT of the chest. J Comput Assisted Tomogr 1993;17:832–838.
14. Cline HE, Lorensen WE, Souza SP, et al. 3-D surface rendered MR images of the brain and its vasculature. J Comput Assisted Tomogr 1991;15:344–351.
15. Magnusson M, Lenz R, Danielsson PE. Evaluation of methods for shaded surface display of CT volumes. Comput Med Imaging Graph 1991;15:247–256.
16. Rubin GD, Dake MD, Napel S, et al. Spiral CT of renal artery stenosis: comparison of three-dimensional rendering techniques. Radiology 1994;190:181–189.
17. Drebin RA, Carpenter L, Hanrahan P. Volume rendering. Comput Graphics 1988;22:65–74.
18. Levoy M. Methods for improving the efficiency and versatility of volume rendering. Prog Clin Biol Res 1991; 363:473–488.
19. Rusinek H, Mourino MR, Firooznia H, et al. Volumetric rendering of MR images. Radiology 1989;171:269–272.
20. Fishman EK, Drebin B, Magid D, et al. Volumetric rendering techniques: applications for three-dimensional imaging of the hip. Radiology 1987;163:737–738.
21. Rubin GD, Beaulieu CF, Argiro V, et al. Perspective volume rendering of CT and MR images: applications for endoscopic imaging. Radiology 1996;199:321–330.
22. Johnson PT, Heath DG, Bliss DF, et al. Three-dimensional CT: real-time interactive volume rendering. AJR Am J Roentgenol 1996;167:581–583.
23. Kuszyk BS, Heath DG, Bliss DF, et al. Skeletal 3-D CT: advantages of volume rendering over surface rendering. Skeletal Radiol 1996;25:207–214.
24. Hara AK, Johnson CD, Reed JE, et al. Colorectal polyp detection with CT colonography: two- versus three-dimensional techniques. Work in progress [see Comments]. Radiology 1996;200:49–54.
25. Hara AK, Johnson CD, Reed JE, et al. Detection of colorectal polyps by computed tomographic colonography: feasibility of a novel technique. Gastroenterology 1996;110:284–290.
26. Ferretti GR, Vining DJ, Knoplioch J, et al. Tracheobronchial tree: three-dimensional spiral CT with bronchoscopic perspective. J Comput Assisted Tomogr 1996;20:777–781.
27. Vining DJ, Liu K, Choplin RH, et al. Virtual bronchoscopy. Relationships of virtual reality endobronchial simulations to actual bronchoscopic findings. Chest 1996;109:549–553.
28. Naidich DP, Grudrn JF, McGuinness G, et al. Volumetric (helical/spiral) CT (VCT) of the airways. J Thorac Imaging 1997;12:11–28.
29. Kimura F, Shen Y, Date S, et al. Thoracic aortic aneurysm and aortic dissection: new endoscopic mode for three-dimensional CT display of aorta. Radiology 1996;198:573–578.
30. Vining DJ, Zagoria RJ, Liu K, et al. CT cystoscopy: an innovation in bladder imaging. AJR Am J Roentgenol 1996;166:409–410.
31. Sommer FG, Olcott EW, Ch'en IY, et al. Volume rendering of CT data: applications to the genitourinary tract. AJR Am J Roentgenol 1997;168:1223–1226.
32. Paik DS, Beaulieu CF, Jeffrey RB, et al. Automated flight path planning for virtual endoscopy. Med Phys 1998; 25:629–637.
33. Beaulieu CF, Jeffrey RB Jr, Karadi C, et al. Display modes for CT colonography, part II: blinded comparison of axial CT and virtual endoscopic and panoramic endoscopic volume-rendered studies. Radiology 1999;212:203–212.

Protocol 1:
TRACHEOBRONCHIAL TREE (Fig. 1)

INDICATION: *Intrabronchial masses, extrinsic compression of bronchi, bronchial strictures*

SCANNER SETTINGS: kV(p): 120–140
mA: 200–300

ORAL CONTRAST: None

PHASE OF RESPIRATION: Suspended inspiration

ROTATION TIME: Minimum

ACQUISITION SLICE THICKNESS: 1.00–1.25 mm

PITCH: 1.5–2.0

RECONSTRUCTION SLICE THICKNESS/INTERVAL FOR FILMING: *Thickness:* 1.25 mm
Reconstruction: 0.5–0.8 mm
Film: Every fourth image

ANATOMIC COVERAGE:
   SUPERIOR EXTENT: Base of tongue
   INFERIOR EXTENT: Lung bases

IV CONTRAST: None

COMMENTS:
1. Caudal to cranial scanning minimizes breathing artifacts near the diaphragm.
2. Reconstruction FOV 18–20 cm, standard kernel.
3. Review for respiratory motion artifacts and rescan if necessary.

SEGMENTATION: None

VISUALIZATION:

CPRs (can be augmented with oblique
  orthogonal reformations)
External surface displays (central airways
  only)
  Upper threshold: −700 to −350 HU
Internal surface displays or volume
  rendering
  Lower threshold/transition zone: −700 to
  −900 HU

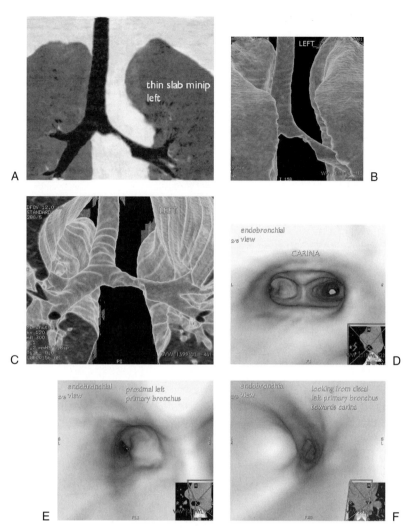

FIG. 1. A: Thin-slab minimum intensity projection of the proximal airways demonstrates a mass on the inferior aspect of the horizontal portion of the left main stem bronchus. Thin-slab minimum intensity projections are less operator-dependent than are curved planar reformations, which can provide a similar visualization; however, air within the bronchus surrounding an endobronchial lesion may result in underestimation of the size of the endobronchial lesion on a minimum intensity projection. **B, C:** Volume renderings obtained with an opacity transfer function that has a narrow spike to 100% opacity at −500 HU and has 0% opacity elsewhere provides an appearance similar to a traditional air-contrast examination. The walls of the airways are shown in relief and subtle details in mural irregularity are illustrated. Note the irregularity associated with the mass in the left mainstem bronchus including a small region of ulceration. **D, E, F:** Perspective shaded surface displays rendered from within the airways are created by applying a threshold at −500 HU. **(D)** is from the upper thoracic trachea viewed inferiorly and allows visualization of the carina with the mass in the left mainstem bronchus. **(E)** demonstrates the mass from the origin of the left mainstem bronchus from a perspective that is very similar to that which would be viewed during fiber-optic bronchoscopy. **(F)** is obtained from within the left lower lobe bronchus looking proximally and demonstrates the inferior relationships of the endobronchial mass, which is a perspective that cannot be acquired with a fiber-optic bronchoscope.

Protocol 2:
COLON (Fig. 2)

INDICATION: *Colonic polyps/masses*

SCANNER SETTINGS: kV(p): 120–140
                                        mA: 40–60

ORAL CONTRAST: None

RECTAL CONTRAST: Air insufflation via 12–16 Fr rubber tube

PHASE OF RESPIRATION: Suspended inspiration

ROTATION TIME: Minimum

ACQUISITION SLICE   2.5 mm
   THICKNESS:

PITCH: 0.75 (HQ = 3:1)

RECONSTRUCTION SLICE   *Thickness:* 2.5 mm
   THICKNESS/INTERVAL   *Reconstruction:* 0.5–0.8 mm
   FOR FILMING: *Film:* Every fourth image

ANATOMIC COVERAGE:
   SUPERIOR EXTENT: 1 cm above upper extent of colon on scout
   INFERIOR EXTENT: Anus

IV CONTRAST: None

COMMENTS: 1. Consider additional prone scan if
                                           substantial retained fluid on initial scan.
                                        2. Consider IV glucagon on additional
                                           prone scan if incomplete distention on
                                           initial scan.
                                        3. Reconstruction FOV to include colon,
                                           standard kernel.

SEGMENTATION: None

VISUALIZATION:

CPRs (can be augmented with oblique orthogonal reformations).

External surface displays
Upper threshold: −700 to −350 HU

Internal surface displays or VR
Lower threshold/transition zone: −850 to 900 HU

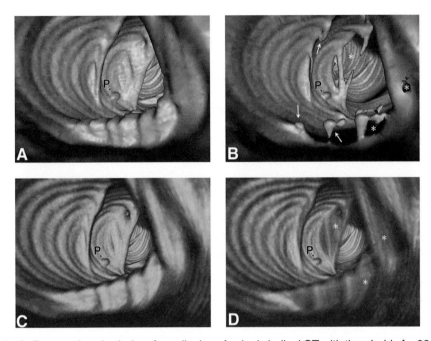

FIG. 2. A: Perspective shaded surface display of colonic helical CT with threshold of −980 HU, which is optimal for displaying the interior of the colon, and **(B)** threshold of −930 HU, which is too high. Portions of the colonic wall are not rendered and present as holes (*) or intraluminal juxtamural structures (*arrows*) that could be misinterpreted as polyps. A 5-mm polyp is visible in all views (P). **C:** Perspective volume rendering with an opacity curve that renders all voxels above −980 as 80% to 100% opaque is free from both artifactual wall discontinuities and juxtamural structures. **D:** Perspective volume rendering with a different opacity curve that renders the lower densities more transparently–creates a whispy appearance to the thinner structures (*). Frank discontinuities as seen with surface displays are not created. The presence of semi-transparent cues on volume rendered images **(C, D)** results in easier detection of errors than on surface displays **(A, B)**. Once detected, the opacity curve can be adjusted and the image rendered in 10 to 20 seconds. (Reprinted from Rubin, GD, Beaulieu CF, Argiro V et al. Perspective Volume Rendering of CT in MR Images: Applications for Endoscopic Imaging. Radiology:1996;199:321–330, with permission.)

Protocol 3:
INTRACRANIAL CT ANGIOGRAPHY (Fig. 3)

INDICATION:

Aneurysms or arterial occlusive disease from atherosclerosis, atheroembolization, or dissection

SCANNER SETTINGS:

kV(p): 120–140
mA: 250–300

ORAL CONTRAST:

None

PHASE OF RESPIRATION:

Quiet ventilation

ROTATION TIME:

Minimum

ACQUISITION SLICE THICKNESS:

0.5–1.25 mm

PITCH:

1.5–2.0

RECONSTRUCTION SLICE THICKNESS/INTERVAL FOR FILMING:

Thickness: 0.6–1.25 mm
Reconstruction: 50% of effective
   section thickness (0.3–0.6 mm)

ANATOMIC COVERAGE:
  SUPERIOR EXTENT:
  INFERIOR EXTENT:

Cranial vertex
Base of sella turcica

IV CONTRAST:

Concentration:	LOCM 300–320 mg iodine/mL
Rate:	4 mL/sec
Scan Delay:	Timed in internal carotid arteries
Total Volume:	100–120 mL

COMMENTS:

1. Scan caudal to cranial to avoid cavernous carotid obscuration from filling of the cavernous sinus.
2. Angle gantry (10–20 degrees) to avoid superimposition of artifacts from dental fillings onto pertinent vasculature.
3. Reconstruction FOV 10–15 cm, standard kernel.

SEGMENTATION:

Usually not necessary for STS-MIP, superior to inferior orthographic SSD/VR, and all perspective renderings.

ROI or region growing can be used to remove anterior, posterior, and lateral margins of the skull.

If base of skull subtraction is necessary, then region growing can identify and subtract skull; however, this can be difficult and may require additional localized ROI editing to disconnect skull base from blood vessels in some regions.

VISUALIZATION:

STS-MIP—transverse, coronal

Orthographic and external perspective surface displays or VRs (external perspective rendering eliminates necessity of segmentation)
Upper threshold: 150–300 HU

Internal surface display or VR
Lower threshold: 150–250 HU

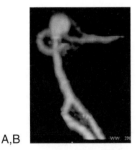
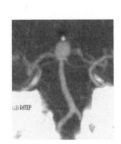
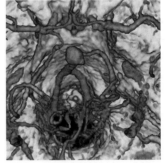

A,B

C

FIG. 3. A: Maximum intensity projection of the distal vertebral arteries, basilar artery and posterior cerebral arteries are demonstrating a basilar tip aneurysm. This required manual removal of all bones and other high attenuation structures in order to visualize the anatomy and the main associated arterial branches. The process of manual segmentation can be labor intensive. **B:** This thin slab maximum intensity projection, which was created by orienting an oblique plane parallel to the basilar artery and widening it to create a 1-cm thick slab through which a maximum intensity projection was created, allows visualization of the same anatomy in **(A)** yet without the need for manual editing. **C:** Volume rendering of the skull base not only allows appreciation of the basilar tip aneurysm, adjacent arterial branches, and the remainder of the circle of Willis, but also allows appreciation of 3D relationships that may be useful for the treating physician to better understand the specific location of branch origins relative to the aneurysm.

Protocol 4:
CAROTID, VERTEBRAL, AND INTRACRANIAL ARTERIES (Fig. 4)

INDICATION:	*Atherosclerotic occlusive disease or dissection*
SCANNER SETTINGS:	kV(p): 120–140 mA: 220–300
ORAL CONTRAST:	None
PHASE OF RESPIRATION:	Suspended inspiration after hyperventilation
ROTATION TIME:	Minimum
ACQUISITION SLICE THICKNESS:	1.00–1.25 mm
PITCH:	1.5–2.0
RECONSTRUCTION SLICE THICKNESS/INTERVAL FOR FILMING:	*Thickness:* 1.25 mm *Reconstruction:* 50% of effective section thickness (0.5–0.6 mm)

ANATOMIC COVERAGE:
  SUPERIOR EXTENT:
  INFERIOR EXTENT:
	
	Cranial vertex
	Mid aortic arch

IV CONTRAST:

Concentration:	LOCM 300–320 mg iodine/mL
Rate:	4 mL/sec
Scan Delay:	Timed in internal carotid arteries
Total Volume:	100–120 mL

COMMENTS:	1. Reconstruction FOV 15 cm, standard kernel. 2. Caudal to cranial scan direction
SEGMENTATION	None for CPR or STS-MIP. (carotid portion only; for intracranial CTA, see Protocol 3):

Bone removal by region-growing or ROI
editing. For removal of opacified jugular
vein (orthographic surface display and
VRs), additional detailed ROI editing to
disconnect carotid arteries from jugular
veins before removal by region growing.

VISUALIZATION   CPR, STS-MIP (oblique)
(carotid portion only;
for intracranial CTA,
see Protocol 3):
External surface displays (limited utility,
especially when calcium is present).
Upper threshold: 100–200 HU

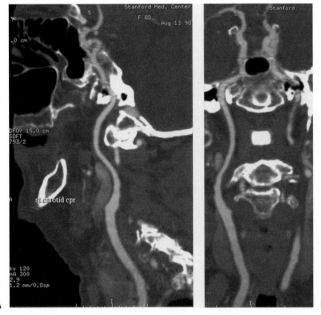

A   B

FIG. 4. A, B: Curved sagittal and coronal reformations through the right common and internal
carotid arteries readily demonstrate a normal vessel lumen along its entire course.

Figure continues

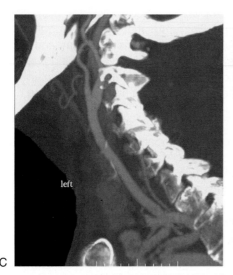

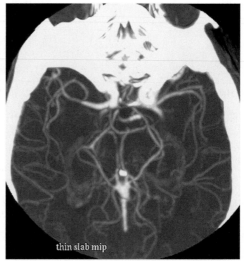

C   D

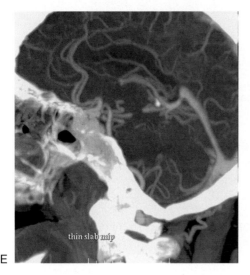

E

FIG. 4. *Continued.* **C:** Thin-slab maximum intensity projections allow simultaneous visualization of the proximal external as well as the internal carotid and common carotid arteries. The advantage of the slab MIP is that the course of these vessels can be visualized free of the distortions that are inherent in the curved planar reformations. A limitation of the slab MIP however is the fact that a portion of the body of C2 is obscuring the internal carotid artery just distal to the carotid bulb. **D, E:** Thin-slab MIP views from the same CT scan as in **A** through **C** demonstrate transverse and sagittal visualization of intracranial arteries and veins. At a workstation, these planes can be viewed in a stacked mode and the user may page through the contents of the cranium along any arbitrary plane allowing interactive visualization of all arterial and venous branches without selection of complex rendering parameters or the need to perform preliminary segmentation.

Protocol 5:
THORACIC AORTA (Fig. 5)

INDICATION:	*Aneurysm, dissection, intramural hematoma/ulceration, trauma, coarctation, anomalies*
SCANNER SETTINGS:	kV(p): 120–140 mA: 250–300
ORAL CONTRAST:	None
PHASE OF RESPIRATION:	Suspended inspiration after hyperventilation
ROTATION TIME:	Minimum
ACQUISITION SLICE THICKNESS:	2.5–3.0 mm
PITCH:	1.5
RECONSTRUCTION SLICE THICKNESS/INTERVAL FOR FILMING:	*Thickness:* 1.25–3.0 mm *Reconstruction:* 50% of effective section thickness (1.3–1.5 mm)
ANATOMIC COVERAGE: **SUPERIOR EXTENT:** **INFERIOR EXTENT:**	 Base of neck Celiac origin

IV CONTRAST:

Concentration:	LOCM 300–320 mg iodine/mL
Rate:	5 mL/sec
Scan Delay:	Timed in aortic arch (time both true and false lumen in presence of dissection and select intermediate delay time)
Total Volume:	75–100 mL

COMMENTS:
1. Venous access via right upper extremity.
2. Reconstruction FOV 24–30 cm, standard kernel.

SEGMENTATION: None for CPR.
                                        Bone removal by ROI editing for SSD.

VISUALIZATION: CPRs.
                                        External surface display or VRs (MIP rarely
                                            useful for the thoracic aorta).
                                            Upper threshold: 150–300 HU

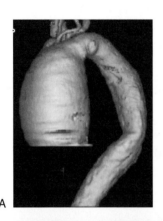
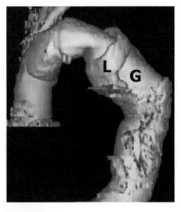

FIG. 5. Shaded surface displays or volume renderings tend to be the preferred means for assessing the thoracic aorta, which is a large structure that frequently is associated with complex
surface features and branch relationships. **A:** Shaded surface display of a patient with a large
ascending aortic aneurysm demonstrates the relationship of the aneurysm to the brachio-
cephalic branches. An ulceration within the proximal descending thoracic aorta is viewed *en
fosse*. This surface feature would not be displayed if a maximum intensity projection were used
to visualize this anatomy. **B:** Shaded surface display of a different patient following placement
of an elephant trunk graft (G) within the proximal aspect of the descending thoracic aorta. Contrast flow within the native descending thoracic aortic lumen (L) can be visualized to encase the
graft. **C:** In the setting of intraluminal abnormalities such as aortic dissection, curved planar reformations, demonstrated in a different patient, are preferred which allow visualization of the
true (T) and false (F) lumina as well as of the intimal flap *arrow*.

Protocol 6:
ABDOMINAL AORTA AND ILIAC ARTERIES
(Fig. 6)

INDICATION:	*Aneurysm, atherosclerotic occlusive disease, dissection*
SCANNER SETTINGS:	kV(p): 120–140 mA: 200–300
ORAL CONTRAST:	None
PHASE OF RESPIRATION:	Suspended inspiration
ROTATION TIME:	Minimum
ACQUISITION SLICE THICKNESS:	1.0–2.5 mm
PITCH:	1.5
RECONSTRUCTION SLICE THICKNESS/INTERVAL FOR FILMING:	*Thickness:* 1.25–3.0 mm *Reconstruction:* 50% of effective section thickness (0.6–1.5 mm)

ANATOMIC COVERAGE:
  SUPERIOR EXTENT:
  INFERIOR EXTENT:
	
	Aortic hiatus of diaphragm
	Lesser trochanter of femurs

IV CONTRAST:

Concentration:	LOCM 300–320 mg iodine/mL
Rate:	4 mL/sec
Scan Delay:	Timed in supraceliac aorta
Total Volume:	100–120 mL

COMMENTS:	Reconstruction FOV: 28–32 cm
SEGMENTATION:	None for CPR. *Bone removal:* 1. Highest threshold to isolate blood vessels and bones without losing important aortic branches.

2. ROI editing to disconnect arteries and bones (typically superior gluteal arteries exiting pelvis and regions of lumbar osteophytes).
3. Region-growing removal of blood vessels.
4. Dilation 3–5 pixels
5. Subtraction (Boolean operation) of resultant data set from original data.

Note: If technique described is unavailable, then more time-consuming ROI editing is necessary.

Additional limited ROI or region-growing removal of venous structures and celiac/mesenteric arterial branches may occasionally be necessary.

VISUALIZATION:

CPRs.

External surface renderings or VRs.
  Upper threshold: 150–300 HU

MIP (visualization of calcified plaque on external wall of aneurysm).

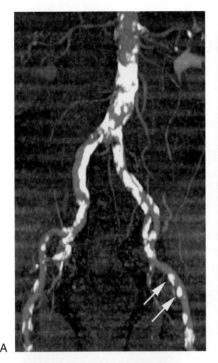

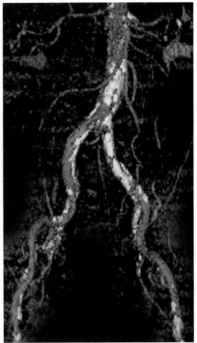

A

B

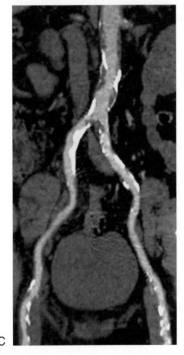

C

FIG. 6. A : Maximum intensity projection of the abdominal aorta and iliac arteries in a patient with extensive calcified atherosclerotic plaque. The plaque obscures the majority of the lumen making it impossible to determine the residual luminal caliber within these vessels. Two arrows indicate regions of calcification within the left external iliac artery that are not seen in a volume rendering **(B)**. These calcifications lie on the posterior wall of the external iliac artery and therefore cannot be visualized on the frontal volume rendering. Note that less calcium is seen on the volume rendering; however, the lumen, particularly in the distal abdominal aorta and within the left common iliac arteries, is obscured by circumferential calcification. **C:** Composite of two curved planar reformations including both the right and left iliac arteries demonstrates the importance of curved planar reformations in assessing the residual lumen when there is substantial mural calcium present. Note that no hemodynamically significant stenoses are evident within the distal aorta or the left common iliac artery. Moreover, the curved planar reformation allows visualization of both calcified as well as non-calcified atheromatous plaque. A limitation of the curved planar reformation is that branches of the aorta or iliac arteries may not be visualized such as the internal iliac arteries, which can be seen in both **A** and **B**.

Protocol 7:
COMBINED THORACIC AND ABDOMINAL AORTA (Fig. 7)

INDICATION:	*Aneurysm or dissection*
SCANNER SETTINGS:	kV(p): 120–140 mA: 200–300
ORAL CONTRAST:	None
PHASE OF RESPIRATION:	Suspended inspiration
ROTATION TIME:	Minimum
ACQUISITION SLICE THICKNESS:	1.0–2.5 mm
PITCH:	1.5
RECONSTRUCTION SLICE THICKNESS/INTERVAL FOR FILMING:	*Thickness:* 1.25–3.0 mm *Reconstruction:* 50% of effective section thickness (0.7–1.5 mm)

ANATOMIC COVERAGE:
  SUPERIOR EXTENT:
  INFERIOR EXTENT:
	
	Base of neck
	Lesser trochanter of femurs

IV CONTRAST:

Concentration:	LOCM 300–320 mg iodine/mL
Rate:	4 mL/sec
Scan Delay:	Timed in supraceliac aorta
Total Volume:	120–150 mL

COMMENTS:	None
SEGMENTATION:	*Chest:* Same as for thoracic aorta. *Abdomen:* Same as for abdominal aorta.
VISUALIZATION:	*Chest:* Same as for thoracic aorta. *Abdomen:* Same as for abdominal aorta.

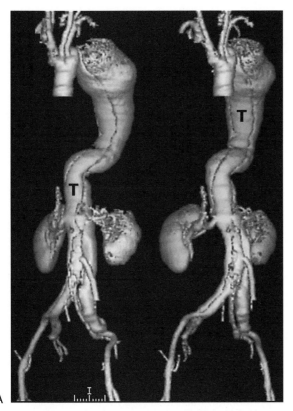
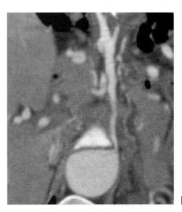

FIG. 7. Shaded surface displays obtained with two different obliquities illustrate imaging of the entire aortoiliac system in a patient with an extensive type B aortic dissection. The surface display allows visualization of the true lumen (T) along its entire course and its relationship to aortic branches. Both shaded surface displays and volume renderings are particularly useful when the relationship of aortic branches to the aorta is important to assess in 3D. Curved planar reformations can be of great value as well, particularly for defining the origins of branches in the setting of aortic dissection **(B)**. This curved planar reformation through the superior mesenteric artery demonstrates its narrowed ostium originating from the false (posterior) lumen. A curved planar reformation of the thoracic aorta in this patient is in Figure 5C.

Protocol 8:
RENAL ARTERIES (Fig. 8)

INDICATION: *Atherosclerotic occlusive disease, assessment of potential living renal donors*

SCANNER SETTINGS: kV(p): 120–140
mA: 300

ORAL CONTRAST: None

PHASE OF RESPIRATION: Suspended inspiration after hyperventilation

ROTATION TIME: Minimum

ACQUISITION SLICE THICKNESS: 1.00–1.25 mm

PITCH: 1.5

RECONSTRUCTION SLICE THICKNESS/INTERVAL FOR FILMING: *Thickness:* 1.25 mm
Reconstruction: 50% of effective section thickness (0.6 mm)

ANATOMIC COVERAGE:
SUPERIOR EXTENT: Superior aspect of kidneys or superior mesenteric artery, whichever is more cephalad
INFERIOR EXTENT: Inferior aspect of kidneys or to common iliac bifurcation, whichever is more caudal

IV CONTRAST:

Concentration:	LOCM 300–320 mg iodine/mL
Rate:	5 mL/sec
Scan Delay:	Timed in abdominal aorta
Total Volume:	100–140 mL

COMMENTS:
1. Reconstruction FOV 18–24 cm, standard kernel.
2. Delayed scout with 80 kV obtained 5 min after injection in potential renal donors. Repeat once if ureteral opacification is inadequate.

SEGMENTATION: None for CPR and STS-MIP.
Bone removal by ROI editing for SR/VR and MIP.

VISUALIZATION: CPRs (best for stenosis associated with calcification; must have curved coronal and curved transverse reformations to assess eccentric plaque).
STS-MIP.
SR/VR (renal donors only):
Upper threshold: 150–300 HU
MIP (as needed).

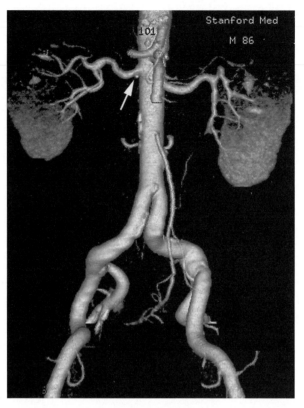

A

FIG. 8. A: Volume rendering of the renal arteries demonstrates a small calcification on the in-ferior surface of the proximal right renal artery (*arrow*). The benefit of the volume rendering is that the numerous hilar branches are demonstrated and their spatial relationships can be ap-preciated. Note that the proximal celiac axis and superior mesenteric artery can be visualized as well, although the proximal SMA obscures the proximal left renal artery. A small accessory renal artery to the upper pole of the left kidney is not well visualized due to the lower limit of the opacity transfer function falling above the attenuation value of this accessory renal artery. This opacity transfer function selection was likely based upon the desire to minimize visualization of stray voxels due to non-vascular tissues thus limiting the visualization of the accessory renal artery. **B:** Three centimeter thick maximum intensity projection oriented coronally and axially **(C)** demonstrates the same calcification as was observed in **(A)**(*arrows*). Note that the renal artery appears to be minimally narrowed at its origin on the coronal view; however, it has a greater than 50% narrowing on the transverse section. Perpendicular views should always be acquired to assess stenosis as atherosclerosis typically involves vessels eccentrically. Note also that the accessory renal artery to the left upper pole is visualized over its entire length as well as a substantial intrarenal portion on the coronal MIP **(B)**, which does not suffer from the limitations of applying an opacity transfer function for volume rendering. **D, E:** Curved planar reformations oriented coronally and axially demonstrates similar anatomy to as seen on the thin-slab MIPs **(B, C)** . Note however that fewer renal hilar branches can be visualized and that the accessory renal artery to the left kidney is not visualized either as these curves include the main renal course only. The right renal artery origin stenosis, seen on the transverse view **(E)**, does not demonstrate the calcification. The calcification is present only on the inferior aspect of the vessel and was included on the transverse MIP **(C)** because it "projected through" from the inferior aspect of the vessel. Curved planar reformations are probably the most reliable means of assessing vascular stenosis and although two perpendicular CPR's are minimally re-quired, optimal assessment of a vessel should involve multiple CPR's at a variety of angular orientations about the median centerline of the vessel.

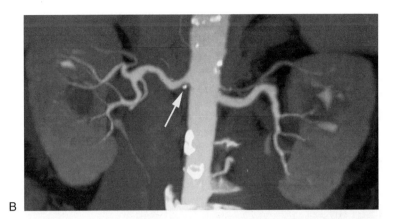

B

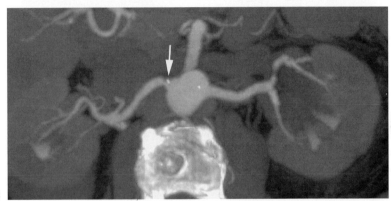

C

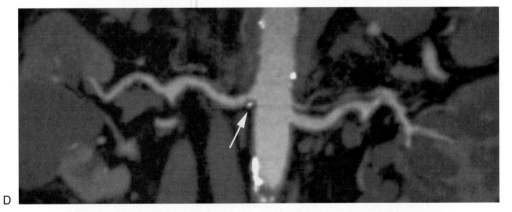

D

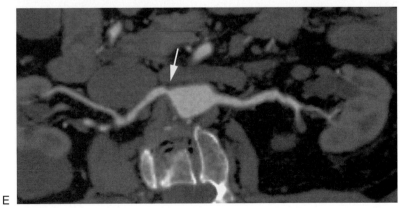

E

Protocol 9:
AORTOGRAM AND LOWER EXTREMITY RUN-OFF (Fig. 9)

INDICATION:	*Lower extremity claudication, rest pain, or limb-threatening ischemia, aneurysm*
SCANNER SETTINGS:	kV(p): 120–140 mA: 200–300
ORAL CONTRAST:	None
PHASE OF RESPIRATION:	Suspended inspiration through abdomen and pelvis, quiet breathing through legs
ROTATION TIME:	Minimum
ACQUISITION SLICE THICKNESS:	1.0–2.5 mm
PITCH:	1.5
RECONSTRUCTION SLICE THICKNESS/INTERVAL FOR FILMING:	*Thickness:* 1.25–3.0 mm *Reconstruction:* 50% of effective section thickness (0.6–1.5 mm)

ANATOMIC COVERAGE:
  SUPERIOR EXTENT:
  INFERIOR EXTENT:
	
	Celiac origin
	Through feet

IV CONTRAST:	**Concentration:**	LOCM 300–320 mg iodine/mL
	Rate:	3.8–4.0 mL/sec
	Scan Delay:	Timed in supraceliac aorta
	Total Volume:	150–180 mL

COMMENTS:	1. Tape knees and ankles together. 2. No pillow under knees. 3. Avoid patients who are diabetic due to difficult analysis of infrapopliteal arteries in the presence of extensive calcification.

SEGMENTATION: None for CPR and STS-MIP.
Bone removal:
Same as for abdominal aorta and iliac arteries for vessels above the lower calves.
ROI editing in lower calves and feet.
Isolate each side to render separately for MIP rotations.

VISUALIZATION: CPRs (best for stenosis associated with calcification; must have curved coronal and curved sagittal reformations to assess eccentric plaque).
MIP: break volume into four to five levels. Create 180 degree rotations every 15 degrees for each leg at each level.
Optional: SR/VR (with bones):
Upper threshold: 150–300 HU

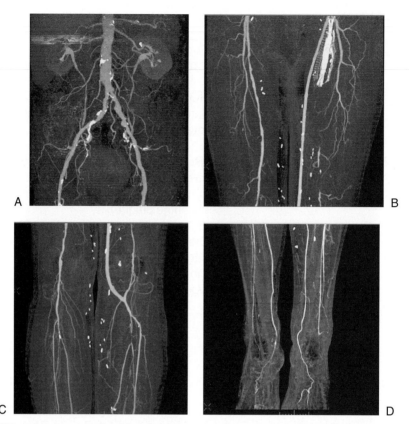

FIG. 9. CT aortogram run-off study is broken up into four maximum intensity frontal projections that include the aorta and iliac arteries **(A)** the superficial femoral arteries **(B)**, the popliteal and proximal calf arteries **(C)** and the distal cath and pedal vessels **(D)**. Maximum intensity projections allow visualization of the entirety of the arterial tree however they can be very time consuming to create due to the necessity of removing all the bones. If the bones were included in the rendering, then the arteries would be obscured. Although volume rendering would allow the arteries to be visualized relative to the bone, the fact that the arteries of the lower extremities coarse both anterior as well as posterior to the bone makes it impossible to visualize all vessels on a single view. Rendering of the lower extremity arteries in association with the bone should be reserved for applications where simultaneous bone visualization is important (Figure 10). This patient demonstrates extensive atherosclerotic plaque within the distal aorta, common iliac arteries, right superficial femoral artery, and in the infrapopliteal arteries. The left superficial femoral artery is occluded and patency of a bypass graft can be visualized with retrograde filling of the distal native superficial femoral artery. Two high attenuation structures lateral to the bypass graft in the left thigh proximally correspond to preciously placed grafts that have thrombosed. High attenuation vascular clips can be seen on the medial aspect of both legs and are indications of saphenous vein procurement for coronary artery bypass grafting.

Protocol 10:
LOWER EXTREMITY (Fig. 10)

INDICATION:	*Mapping distal run-off after insufficient MRI or conventional angiographic assessment, assessment of infrapopliteal arterial anatomy before fibular graft donation*
SCANNER SETTINGS:	kV(p): 120–140 mA: 300
ORAL CONTRAST:	None
PHASE OF RESPIRATION:	Breathing
ROTATION TIME:	Minimum
ACQUISITION SLICE THICKNESS:	1.0–1.25 mm
PITCH:	1.5
RECONSTRUCTION SLICE THICKNESS/INTERVAL FOR FILMING:	*Thickness:* 1.25 mm *Reconstruction:* 50% of effective section thickness (0.6 mm)
ANATOMIC COVERAGE: **SUPERIOR EXTENT:** **INFERIOR EXTENT:**	Femoral condyles Through feet

IV CONTRAST:

Concentration:	LOCM 300–320 mg iodine/mL
Rate:	3.8–4 mL/second
Scan Delay:	Timed in supraceliac aorta
Total Volume:	150–180 mL

COMMENTS:

Assessment of both legs/feet:
1. Tape knees and ankles together.
2. No pillow under knees.
3. Avoid patients who are diabetic due to difficult analysis of infrapopliteal arteries in the presence of extensive calcification.

Assessment of one leg/foot:
1. Flex leg that will not be imaged so that plantar surface of foot is on the CT table and positioned adjacent to the knee of the leg to be imaged.
2. Position the leg to be imaged in the scanner isocenter.

SEGMENTATION:

None for CPR.
Bone removal:
Same as for abdominal aorta and iliac arteries for vessels above the lower calves.
ROI editing in lower calves and feet
When both legs are imaged, isolate each side to render separately for MIP rotations.

VISUALIZATION:

CPRs (as needed).
MIP: Break volume into four to five levels. Create 180 degree rotations every 15 degrees for each leg at each level.
SR/VR (with bones):
Upper threshold: 150–300 HU

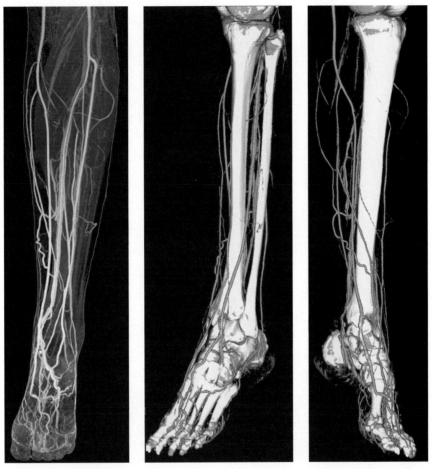

A,B   C

FIG. 10. A: Frontal maximum intensity projection of the left lower leg in a patient with an arteriovenous malformation involving the dorsum of the left foot with a nidus at the base of the second digit. Simultaneous visualization of numerous arteries and veins are demonstrated. The maximum intensity projection which was created after manual removal of the bones allows visualization of all patent arterial and venous branches however their superimposition makes appreciation of their relative 3D relationships very difficult. **B through E:** Volume renderings obtained at varying obliquities prior to removal of the bones allow for a substantially improved appreciation of the spatial relationships of these abnormal arteries and veins. The location of the AVM nidus and extensive venous collaterals on the dorsum of the foot are appreciated more readily than are seen on the MIP **(A)**. Three dimensional views such as these volume renderings can be valuable when bony landmarks are important for localizing specific branches for percutaneous access.

Figure continues

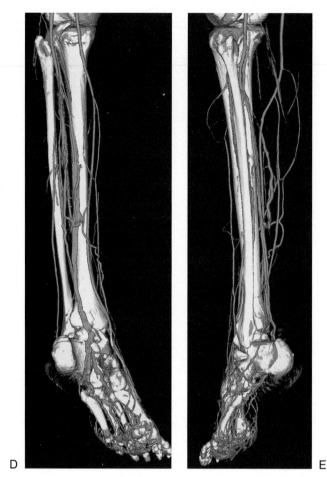

FIG. 10. *Continued.*

Subject Index

Subject Index

Note: Page numbers followed by f indicate figures; page numbers followed by t indicate tables.